FRONTIERS IN NEURODEGENERATIVE DISORDERS AND AGING: FUNDAMENTAL ASPECTS, CLINICAL PERSPECTIVES AND NEW INSIGHTS

NATO Science Series

A series presenting the results of scientific meetings supported under the NATO Science Programme.

The series is published by IOS Press and Kluwer Academic Publishers in conjunction with the NATO Scientific Affairs Division.

Sub-Series

I.	Life and Behavioural Sciences	IOS Press
II.	Mathematics, Physics and Chemistry	Kluwer Academic Publishers
III.	Computer and Systems Sciences	IOS Press
IV.	Earth and Environmental Sciences	Kluwer Academic Publishers
V.	Science and Technology Policy	IOS Press

The NATO Science Series continues the series of books published formerly as the NATO ASI Series.

The NATO Science Programme offers support for collaboration in civil science between scientists of countries of the Euro-Atlantic Partnership Council. The types of scientific meeting generally supported are "Advanced Study Institutes" and "Advanced Research Workshops", although other types of meeting are supported from time to time. The NATO Science Series collects together the results of these meetings. The meetings are co-organized by scientists from NATO countries and scientists from NATO's Partner countries – countries of the CIS and Central and Eastern Europe.

Advanced Study Institutes are high-level tutorial courses offering in-depth study of latest advances in a field.
Advanced Research Workshops are expert meetings aimed at critical assessment of a field, and identification of directions for future action.

As a consequence of the restructuring of the NATO Science Programme in 1999, the NATO Science Series has been re-organized and there are currently five sub-series as noted above. Please consult the following web sites for information on previous volumes published in the series, as well as details of earlier sub-series:

http://www.nato.int/science
http://www.wkap.nl
http://www.iospress.nl
http://www.wtv-books.de/nato_pco.htm

Series I: Life and Behavioural Sciences - Vol. 358 ISSN: 1566-7693

Frontiers in Neurodegenerative Disorders and Aging: Fundamental Aspects, Clinical Perspectives and New Insights

Edited by

Tomris Özben

Akdeniz University, Medical Faculty, Department of Biochemistry, Antalya, Turkey

and

Mordechai Chevion

The Dr. W. Ganz Chair of Heart Studies, The Hebrew University-Hadassah Medical School, Jerusalem, Israel

IOS Press

Amsterdam • Berlin • Oxford • Tokyo • Washington, DC

Published in cooperation with NATO Scientific Affairs Division

Proceedings of the NATO Advanced Research Workshop on
Frontiers in Neurodegenerative Disorders and Aging: Fundamental Aspects, Clinical Perspectives and New Insights
27 May 2003 – 1 June 2003
Antalya, Turkey

ISBN 1 58603 428 6
Library of Congress Control Number: 2004105156

Publisher
IOS Press
Nieuwe Hemweg 6B
1013 BG Amsterdam
Netherlands
fax: +31 20 620 3419
e-mail: order@iospress.nl

Distributor in the UK and Ireland
IOS Press/Lavis Marketing
73 Lime Walk
Headington
Oxford OX3 7AD
England
fax: +44 1865 75 0079

Distributor in the USA and Canada
IOS Press, Inc.
5795-G Burke Centre Parkway
Burke, VA 22015
USA
fax: +1 703 323 3668
e-mail: iosbooks@iospress.com

PRINTED IN THE NETHERLANDS

Foreword

This book brings together some of the foremost researchers in the field of aging and neurodegenerative diseases and presents up-to-date information concerning new developments in this exciting area of research in quite separate fields of biomedical science. It includes a wide range of issues such as basic and applied concepts, methods, and techniques used in this area. The chapters examine and evaluate our understanding of the pathogenetic mechanisms involved in these fields such as increased protein oxidation and macromolecular modifications associated with aging, a novel strategy for the visualization of ROS-induced protein oxidation and protection by antioxidants in living cells using fluorescent probes, thermochemiluminescence (TCL) methodology for determination of the oxidative status of biological systems in experimental and clinical setups, protein degradation, proteasome inactivation observed in the aging process or caused by oxidative stress. Other topics addressed are the oxidative stress theory of aging, oxidation and removal of protein aggregates in neurodegeneration, causes and consequences of oxidative stress in Alzheimer disease, assessment of antioxidants as a therapeutic for neurodegenerative diseases, rafts and prions, the many forms of the prion protein and its subcellular pathways, signaling pathways in protection of neural tissues by ischemic and drug-induced preconditioning, folding of proteins associated with neurodegenerative disorders and aging, neuroprotection in immuno-mediated neurodegeneration from infection to autoimmunity.

For the past two decades, research directed toward the basic understanding of biological aging mechanisms and possible aging interventions have given us new insights into the molecular bases and the biological events that contribute to age-related deterioration. Aging can be considered as the product of an interaction between genetic, environmental, and lifestyle factors, which in turn influences longevity that varies between and within species. Aging is not a disease, rather it contributes to the susceptibility to disease. The distinction between the biological aging process and age-related disease processes may be the first step towards understanding the basic mechanisms involved in biological aging. To date, the consensus among researchers broadly views the concept of biological aging as an organism's failure to maintain homeostasis. The causal factors that underlie the time-dependent, deleterious processes of aging have not yet been well defined, and no single adequate molecular explanation for aging is currently available. To develop a scientific base, a spectrum of new and innovative strategies and approaches are being applied to modulate the aging process at the level of cells, tissues, organs and organisms.

As life expectancy continues to increase, the burden of neurodegenerative diseases is growing. Neurodegenerative disorders are a group of diseases in which there is a loss of a defined population of neurons within the central nervous system, leading to progressive neurological diseases. The loss of neurons leads to the development of a range of clinical features, some of which respond to symptomatic drug treatment but none of which are amenable to cure, because the treatments simply try to replace missing or disordered transmitters rather than to arrest or replace the lost neurons. Developing effective means of preventing these disorders and of treating them when they do occur is a paramount challenge.

This book contains the proceedings of the NATO Advanced Research Workshop (ARW) on "Frontiers in Neurodegenerative Disorders and Aging. Fundamental Aspects, Clinical Perspectives and New Insights" which was held in Antalya, Turkey from 27 May-1 June, 2003. It presents the contents of the lectures and a selection of invited contributions from the experts in the field. The proceedings offer a comprehensive account of the most important topics discussed at the Workshop. This book is a comprehensive and reference work, which reflects the knowledge of leading experts in the field. The chapters are of considerable interest to scientists and clinicians working in this fertile area of research. The book contains 21 chapters, it is supported by over 2500 references, and contains a vast amount of schemes, figures and tables, and is intended to make the proceedings accessible to a large audience.

Tomris Özben
Mordechai Chevion
Editors

Contents

Frontiers in Neurodegenerative Disorders and Aging:
Fundamental Aspects, Clinical Perspectives and New Insights
T. Özben and M. Chevion (Eds.)
IOS Press, 2004

Age-Related Changes in the Degradation of Oxidized Proteins

Katrin Merker and Tilman Grune
Neuroscience Research Center, Medical Faculty (Charité), Humboldt University Berlin, Schumannstr. 20/21, 10117 Berlin, Germany
(tilman.grune@charite.de)

Abstract: One of the common features of cells derived from senescent tissues are the accumulated high molecular weight fluorophores (lipofuscin). It is generally accepted that the common origin of this fluorescent material are oxidized, non-degraded proteins. Several proteolytic pathways are responsible for degradation and elimination of unfolded, wrong folded, oxidized or other abnormal proteins. Therefore, malfunctions in these degradation systems seems to be responsible for the non-efficient degradation and consequently the accumulation of these abnormal proteins. Accumulated unfolded and modified proteins undergo further transformation via an array of chemical rcactions leading to the final formation of high molecular weight fluorescent material. In this review we try to concentrate on the different mechanisms involved in the degradation of non-functional proteins and their changes during the aging process.

1. Introduction

The protein pool in cells is in a constant state of turnover. This turnover is controlled and regulated by two processes: protein synthesis and protein degradation. Due to the up and down regulation of individual proteins the cells are able to maintain their functionality and to respond to environmental needs. However, age related changes in cellular metabolism are also visible in the protein turnover. So it is known that the overall protein turnover is declining. Furthermore some changes in the proteolytic capacity of intracellular proteases are abundant during aging. We try here to summarize the today's knowledge about the age related changes in the proteolytic systems and to present the results of the malfunction of these systems on the oxidation status of the protein pool and the accumulation of oxidized proteins.

2. Protein oxidation and protein aggregate formation

During their life-time cells are exposed to a changing level of oxidants. These oxidants are either scavenged or detoxified by numerous defense systems or interact with cellular macromolecules, e.g. proteins. The degree of protein oxidation caused by a given oxidant is dependent on many factors, including the nature, relative location and flux rate of the oxidant and the antioxidants available. In dependency of these conditions protein changes via oxidants are able to induce structural changes of the protein or oxidize amino acid side chains. Numerous amino acids are known to be susceptible to oxidation. Amino acids with aromatic side chains are primary targets of free radical action. The oxidation of leucine results in the formation of various hydoxyleucines, histidine oxidation to form aspartate or asparagine, and the methionine oxidation to methionine sulfoxide. The structural changes induced by oxidants include the unfolding of proteins, the fractionation or the formation of proteins prone to aggregation [1-6]. Oxidative polypeptide chain fragmentation results not in peptides, like those formed during proteolytic degradation of polypeptides, but in fragments with derivatized terminal amino acids. Protein aggregates are formed in a multi-step reaction beginning with the unfolding of proteins due to oxidation. This unfolding is accompanied by the exposure of hydrophobic protein moieties to the protein surface and the formation of free electrical charges. The following hydrophobic or electrochemical interaction leads to the formation of primary protein aggregates and which later on cross-link and form insoluble protein aggregates, accumulating in cells [1-4]. One of the most thoroughly investigated cross-links is the formation of a 2,2′-biphenyl cross-link by two tyrosyl radicals [6]. The formation of -S-S-bonds due to free radical action also seems to be fairly common. These aggregates of oxidized proteins are chemically not inert, but are able to react with other cellular components including lipids, carbohydrates and nucleic acids aggregates [1-9]. This aggregated material might be autophogozytosed resulting in a major accumulation of this material in lysosomes. The presence of catalytically active iron in lysosomes facilitate further oxidation processes [10, 11]. It was supposed, that the final step of the process of cross-linking of proteins is the formation of an insoluble, fluorescent material accumulating within aged cells. This material is called lipofuscin, ceroid or AGE-pigment-like fluorophores by various authors [12, 13]. It is believed that all these pigments have the same principal origin, although there might be tissue-specific or disease-connected differences [13-17].

One of the highlights of the aging process is the accumulation of these cross-linked aggregates. This was shown preferentially for the aging of postmitotic cells [10, 18-20]. It is, therefore, generally accepted that oxidation of proteins is one of the primary steps in the formation of lipofuscin-like material. Therefore, we summarize in the following chapter the knowledge about the degradation of oxidized proteins.

3. Degradation of oxidized proteins and the changes during the aging process

Mammalian cells contain major proteolytic systems, as the lysosomal cathepsins, the cytoskeletal calpains and the proteasomal system, which is located within the cytosol and the nuclei of cells. Whereas the proteasomal system is able to degrade the bulk of intracellular proteins, the lysosomal cathepsins are able to degrade proteins within phagosomes and autophagosomes. On the other hand calpains are involved in the degradation of cytoskeletal proteins. The proteasomal system is responsible for the degradation of the intracellular oxidized proteins, whereas it is now known that cathepsins are able to degrade oxidatively–modified extracellular proteins. The relationship between protein oxidation and proteolysis is today well established [1-9, 21-44]. These findings have been obtained with purified proteins and proteases in *in vitro* experiments as well as with diverse mammalian cell types. In purified systems the usage of various proteasome preparations have clearly indicated, that this protease is able to selectively recognize and degrade oxidized proteins [45]. From the results of these studies it has been concluded that proteins are inherently susceptible to oxidative modifications or damage followed by enhanced proteolytic susceptibility. However, our own studies have consistently demonstrated an increase in protein degradation following moderate oxidative damage, whereas extensive oxidative damage causes decreased proteolysis due to cross-linking, aggregation or decreased solubility of the substrates [32-35, 38-40, 43, 44]. The malfunction of proteolytic systems in the early degradation of moderately oxidized proteins and the inability to degrade extensively oxidized proteins may contribute to certain disease states and the aging process [46-48].

4. The Proteasomal System and its age related changes

The proteasome is a large multicatalytic protease, that exists in all eucaryotic cells, and is responsible for a major part of intracellular proteolysis [9, 48-53]. The proteasome core complex is a 700 kDa barrel like structure, which is also referred to as the 20S proteasome, containing 2 sets of seven α- and seven β-subunits. The subunits are arranged in four rings [54]. This 20S proteasomal particle is the central part of highly regulated proteolytic system. Today several regulatory mechanisms for the core proteasome are known, including the 19S 'ball' regulator, the 11S regulator, phosphorylation processes, subunit exchanges and HSP-binding. The binding of the regulatory 19S complex to both ends of the 20S core complex results in the formation of the 26S proteasome, which is able to degrade poly-ubiquitinated proteins in an ATP-dependent process. There is a several-fold excess of free 20S particles in comparison to the amount of the 19S regulator and 11S regulator together [55-57]. ATP usually stimulate intracellular proteolysis by the 26S proteasome [54]. The 19S regulator has two major functions: recognition of multi-Ub-conjugated proteins and their unfolding to allow entry into the proteasomal particle [53, 54, 57]. The poly-Ub-chain is responsible for the recognition of the substrate by the 26S proteasome [58, 59]. Ubiquitin is a small, highly conserved peptide that forms polymere chains binding to potential proteasome substrates, marking them for proteolytic degradation. The formation of poly-ubiquitin chains is an enzymatically controlled process, catalyzed by the ubiquitin-conjugation system, composed of a multitude of enzymes.

It is generally believed that the 20S proteasome core complex is sufficient for degradation of oxidized proteins [25, 28, 32-35, 38-42, 60, 61]. We have previously demonstrated a significant decline of 26S proteasome activity following oxidative stress [60, 61]. Others have shown a reversible reduction of the activity of Ub-system by rapid oxidative stress [31, 36, 37]. It appears to be clear that severe oxidative stress decreases the activity of the 26S proteasome-mediated pathways in a dose-dependent manner [41, 42 62-65]. Therefore, the 26S proteasome appears to be more sensitive to oxidative stress than the 20S form [60, 61, 65, 66]. All these results let us suggest a major participation of the 20S proteasome in the removal of oxidativly modified or damaged proteins.

The observed age-related accumulation of oxidized cross-linked material may be the result of both - increased protein oxidation followed by aggregation and/or declined protein breakdown and a malfunction of the proteasomal system. Several of the present studies measured the activity of the 20S proteasome using various model substrates. Carney et al. [67],

Stadtman et al. [68] and Starke-Reed and Oliver [69] demonstrated that the proteasomal activity is declining in the brain and liver during aging. Several authors reported no changes in the activity of the proteasomal system during aging of houseflies [70] or in the rat liver [71]. Since these experiments are performed under various conditions it is difficult to evaluate the results of these studies. The usage of fluorogenic peptide substrates was seriously doubted by Cao and Cutler [72]. Since these substrates allow only the investigation of certain function of the proteasomal complex. On the other hand the usage of a set of various fluorogenic peptide substrates gives more insight in the changes of different catalytic properties of the proteasome. In several studies it was reported, that only the peptidylglutamyl hydrolyzing activity of the proteasome was severely affected during aging [73-75]. Although the trypsin-like activity is also oxidation-dependent, it seems to be protected during aging due to the interaction of the proteasome with HSP90 [74]. It seems to be reasonable, that on the other hand the investigations of the proteolytic enzymes by using potentially natural substrates [71] - in this case oxidized proteins - seems to be much more reliable, than the exploration of artificial fluorogenic peptide substrates, which are very common in proteolysis research today.

Our own group was able to show that all three proteaomal activities (chymotrypsin-like, trypsin-like and peptidyl-glutamylhydrolysing activity) are declining in cellular senescence [19, 20, 76]. This is true as well for the proliferative senescence [19, 76] as for the aging of non-dividing cells [20]. Interestingly no concordant decline of the proteasomal amount could be detected, indicating a post-translational inactivating mechanism for the proteasome. However, mainly the cytosolic proteasome is affected by these changes, whereas the nuclear proteasome is more stable during the aging process and is less inactivated during senescence [77].

5. Proteolytic Pathways in Lysosomes after Oxidative Stress

Lysosomes take also part in the degradation of oxidatively modified proteins although their role is not well understood. The selective transport of certain cytosolic and organelle proteins into lysosomes for degradation appears to be important [78-80]. Whether here exists some preference for oxidized proteins remains unknown. On the other hand it is still believed that preferably exogenous proteins taken up by cells are degraded within lysosomes by a group of proteases called cathepsins. In the past years a lot of data relating oxidative stress and lysosomes were collected. Regarding the degradation of oxidized (mainly extracellular) proteins within lysosomes there are many conflicting results in the literature. A poor degradation and accumulation within lysosomes was described for oxidized apoB of oxidized LDL [81-83]. It has to be mentioned, that oxidation during preparation of oxidized LDL according to standard protocols might be strong due to the chain-reaction of lipid peroxidation. Therefore, a heavily cross-linked apoB can be the result of this particular oxidation procedure. More detailed analysis were performed by our group demonstrating a clear oxidation dependent uptake and degradation of extracellular oxidized proteins by macrophages and microglial cells [84]. Furthermore, we were able to show that also heavily oxidized and cross-linked proteins and even lipofuscin particles itself are taken up by cells [85].

Lysosomes and lysosomal cathepsins are also affected by age. There exist evidence, that the number and size of lysosososomes is increasing during aging. Secondly, an impairment of the degradation of long lived proteins (which are believed to be degraded within lysosomes) was measured in senescent fibroblasts [86, 87] and in the liver of old rats [88]. A clear decline in lysosomal cathepsin activity could also be observed in senescent fibroblasts [19, 20]. Furthermore, an accumulation of protein aggregates can be observed after inhibiting lysosomal cathepsins [50].

6. Metabolic effects of accumulated oxidized/cross-linked protein material

It was believed for some time that the accumulated lipofuscin-like material or oxidized/cross-linked proteins are pure waste disposals of the cells. Today it seems to be clear, that such material is influencing the cellular metabolism and several enzymatic pathways. With other words lipofuscin is not an metabolic and chemically inert material. Due to the various components of the lipofuscin on the surface of these particles are numerous active groups, like sulfhydryl, hydroxy, aldehydic, ketonic, amino groups and other. These are able to react with other components of the cell.

Lipofuscin is in particular influencing the proteolytic degradation machineries. So it was found by us that lipofuscin is able to bind the proteasome and inhibit it [85]. Interestingly, this is true also for other accumulated protein aggregates, like the paired helical filaments in Alzheimer's disease [90]. Furthermore, in several neurdegenerative diseases accumulated protein aggregates are ubiquitinated, indicating the reaction with the ubiquitination cascade.

We were able to show that fibroblasts fed with lipofuscin are loosing some of there proteasomal activity, indicating some movement of the lipofuscin from the vesicle compartment into the cytosol. The most likely possibility is a lysosomal disruption, which leads to a liberation of the lipofuscin into the cytosol. Additionally a high lipofuscin content is accompanied by some activation/induction of the lysosomal cathepsins perhaps via the formation of additional lysosomes.

In our opinion these metabolic effects of lipofuscin are only the beginning of the discovery of further metabolic effects of oxidized/cross-linked material.

7. Summary

The currently available data let us suggest that the overall protein turnover, the activity of the proteasome and the lysosomal cathepsins are decreasing during the aging of cells. This is paralleled by the accumulation of oxidized proteins and lipofuscin and a reduced response of the proteolytic machinery to oxidative stress. The proteasomal system seems to be responsible to degrade the vast amount of oxidatively damaged intracellular proteins. Due to the accumulating lipofuscin the cytosolic proteasome becomes more and more inactivated, whereas the nuclear proteasomal system seems to be stabilized. On the other hand mammalian cells are able to take up oxidized extracellular proteins and to degrade them.

Clearly one can expect in these processes cell type and tissue specific reactions, which are still largely unknown. Therefore, the investigation of the age-related cell type specific changes in the proteolytic systems is of major importance in the near future.

References

[1] Davies, K.J.A. (1987) Protein damage and degradation by oxygen radicals: I. general aspects. J. Biol. Chem. *262*, 9895-9901.
[2] Davies, K.J.A., Delsignore, M.E., and Lin, S.W. (1987) Protein damage and degradation by oxygen radicals: II. Modification of amino acids. J. Biol. Chem. *262*, 9902-9907
[3] Davies, K.J.A., and Delsignore, M.E. (1987) Protein damage and degradation by oxygen radicals: III. Modification of secondary and tertiary structure. J. Biol. Chem. *262*, 9908-9913.
[4] Davies, K.J.A., Lin, S.W., and Pacifici, R.E. (1987) Protein damage and degradation by oxygen radicals: IV. Degradation of denatured protein. J. Biol. Chem. *262*, 9914-9920
[5] Stadtman, E.R. (1993) Oxidation of free amino acids and amino acid residues in proteins by radiolysis and by metal-catalyzed reactions. Annu. Rev. Biochem. *62*, 797-821.
[6] Vogt W. (1995) Oxidation of methionyl residues in proteins: tools, targets, and reversal. Free Radic. Biol. Med. *18*, 93-105.
[7] Giulivi, C., and Davies, K.J.A. (1993) Dityrosine and tyrosine oxidation products are endogenous markers for the selective proteolysis of proteasome. J. Biol. Chem. *268*, 8752-8759
[8] Pacifici, R.E., Kono, Y., and Davies, K.J.A. (1993) Hydrophobicity as the signal for selective degradation of hydroxyl radical modified hemoglobin by the multicatalytic proteinase complex, proteasome. J. Biol. Chem. *268*, 15405-15411.
[9] Grune, T., Reinheckel, T., and Davies, K.J.A. (1997) Degradation of oxidized proteins in mammalian cells. FASEB J. *11*, 526-534
[10] Terman, A., and Brunk, U.T. (1998) Ceroid/lipofuscin formation in cultured human fibroblasts: the role of oxidative stress and lysosomal proteolysis. Mech. Ageing Dev. *104*, 277-291.
[11] Zs.-Nagy, I., Streiber, J., and Jeney F. Induction of age pigment accumulation in the brain cells of young male rats through iron-injection into the cerebrospinal fluid. In: Kitani K, Ivy GO, Shimasaki H (eds): Lipofuscin and ceroid pigments. Basel: S. Karger; 1995:145-156.
[12] Yin, D. Studies on age pigments evolving into a new theory of biological aging. In: Kitani K, Ivy GO, Shimasaki H (eds): Lipofuscin and ceroid pigments. Basel: S. Karger; 1995:159-170.
[13] Yin, D. (1996) Biochemical basis of lipofuscin, ceroid, and age pigment-like fluorophores. Free Radic. Biol. Med. *21*, 871-888.
[14] Jolly, R.D., Douglas, B.V., Davey, P.M., and Roiri JE. Lipofuscin in bovine muscle and brain: a model for studying age pigment. In: Kitani K, Ivy GO, Shimasaki H (eds): *Lipofuscin and ceroid pigments.* Basel:S. Karger; 1995: 283-293.
[15] Katz, M.L., Christianson, J.S., and Norbury, N.E. (1994) Lysine methylation of mitochondrial ATP synthase subunit c stored in tissues of dogs with hereditary ceroid lipofuscinosis. J. Biol. Chem. *269*, 9906-9911.
[16] Fearnley, I.M., Walker, J.E., and Martinus, R.D. (1990) The sequence of the major protein stored in ovine ceroid lipofuscinosis is identical with that of the dicyclohexylcarbodiimide-reactive proteolipid of mitochondrial ATP synthase. J. Biochem. *268*, 751-758.
[17] Hunt, J.V., Bottoms, M.A., and Clare, K. (1994) Glucose oxidation and low-density lipoprotein-induced macrophage ceroid accumulation: possible implications for diabetic atherosclerosis. J. Biochem. *300*, 243-249.
[18] Nakano, M., Oenzil, F., and Mizuno, T. Age-related changes in the lipofuscin accumulation of brain and heart. In: Kitani K, Ivy GO, Shimasaki H (eds): Lipofuscin and ceroid pigments. Basel: S. Karger; 1995:69-77.
[19] Sitte, N., Merker, K., von Zglinicki, T., Grune, T., and Davies, K.J.A. (2000) Protein oxidation and degradation during cellular senescence of human BJ-fibroblasts: Part I - Effects of proliferative senescence. FASEB J. *14*, 2495-2502.
[20] Sitte, N., Merker, K., von Zglinicki, T., Davies, K.J.A., and Grune, T. (2000) Protein oxidation and degradation during cellular senescence of human BJ-fibroblasts: Part II - Aging of non-dividing cells. FASEB J. *14*, 2503-2510.
[21] Rivett, A.J. (1985) Preferential degradation of the oxidatively modified form of glutamine synthetase by intracellular mammalian proteases. J. Biol. Chem. *260*, 300-305.
[22] Rivett, A.J. (1985) Purification of a liver alkine protease which degrades oxidatively modified glutamine synthetase: Characterization as a high molecular weight cysteine proteinase. J. Biol. Chem. *260*, 12600-12606.

[23] Davies, K.J.A., and Goldberg, A.L. (1987) Proteins damaged by oxygen radicals are rapidly degraded in extracts of red blood cells. J. Biol. Chem. *262*, 8227-8234

[24] Giulivi, C., and Davies, K.J.A. (1994) Dityrosine: a marker for oxidatively modified proteins and selevtive proteolysis. Meth. Enzymol. *233*, 363-371.

[25] Salo, D.C., Pacifici, R.E., and Davies, K.J.A. (1990) Superoxide dismutase undergoes proteolysis and fragmentation following oxidative modification and inactivation. J. Biol. Chem. *265*, 11919-11927.

[26] Stadtman, E.R. (1986) Oxidation of proteins by mixed-function oxidation systems: Implication in protein turnover, aging and neutrophil function. TIBS *11*, 11-12.

[27] Stadtman, E.R., and Oliver, C.N. (1991) Metal-catalyzed oxidation of proteins: Physiological consequences. J. Biol. Chem. *266*, 2005-2008.

[28] Pacifici, R.E., Salo, D.C., Lin, S.W., and Davies, K.J.A. (1989) Macroxyproteinase (M.O.P.): A 670 kDa proteinase comlex that degrades oxidatively denatured proteins in red blood cells. Free Radic. Biol. Med. *7*, 521-536.

[29] Pacifici, R.E., and Davies, K.J.A. (1990) Protein degradation as an index of oxidative stress. Meth. Enzymol. *186*, 485-502.

[30] Levine, R.L., Williams, J.A., and Stadtman, E.R. (1904) Carbonyl assays for determination of oxidatively modified proteins. Meth. Enzymol. *233*, 346-357.

[31] Shang, F., and Taylor, A. (1995) Oxidative stress and recovery from oxidative stress are associated with altered ubiquitin conjugating and proteolytic activities in bovine lens epithelial cells. Biochem. J. *307*, 297-303

[32] Grune, T., Reinheckel, T., Joshi, M., and Davies, K.J.A. (1995) Protein degradation in cultured liver epithelial cells during oxidative stress: role of the multicatalytic proteinase complex, proteasome. J. Biol. Chem. *270*, 2344-2351.

[33] Grune, T., Reinheckel, T., and Davies, K.J.A. (1996) Degradation of oxidized proteins in K562 human hematopoietic cells by proteasome. J. Biol. Chem. *271*, 15504-15509

[34] Grune, T., Blasig, I.E., Sitte, N., Roloff, B, Haseloff, R., and Davies, K.J.A. (1998) Peroxynitrite increases the degradation of aconitase and other cellular proteins by proteasome. J. Biol. Chem. *273*, 10857-10862.

[35] Grune, T., Klotz, L.O., Gieche, J., Rudeck, M., and Sies, H. (2001) Protein oxidation and proteolysis by the nonradical oxidants singlet oxygen or peroxynitrite. Free Radic. Biol. Med. *30*, 1243-1253.

[36] Jahngen-Hodge, J., Obin, M.S., Gong, X., Shang, F., Nowell, T.R. Jr, Gong, J., Abasi, H., Blumberg, J., and Taylor, A. (1997) Regulation of ubiquitin-conjugating enzymes by glutathione following oxidative stress. J. Biol. Chem. *272*, 28218-28226.

[37] Obin, M.S., Shang, F., Gong, X., Handelman, G., Blumberg, J., and Taylor, A. (1998) Redox regulation of ubiquitin-conjugating enzymes: mechanistic insights using the thiol-specific oxidant diamide. FASEB J. *12*, 561-569.

[38] Ullrich, O., Sitte, N., Sommerburg, O., Sandig, V., Davies, K.J.A., and Grune, T. (1999) Influence of DNA binding on the degradation of oxidized histones by the 20S proteasome. Arch. Biochem. Biophys. *362*, 211-216.

[39] Ullrich, O., Reinheckel, T., Sitte, N., Hass, R., Grune, T., and Davies K.J.A. (1999) Poly-ADP-ribose polymerase activates nuclear proteasome to degrade oxidatively damaged histones. Proc. Natl. Acad. Sci. USA *96*, 6223-6228.

[40] Ullrich, O., Diestel, A., Bechmann, I., Homberg, M., Grune, T., Hass, R., and Nitsch, R. (2001) Turnover of oxidatively damaged nuclear proteins in BV-2 microglial cells is linked to their activation state by poly-ADP-ribose polymerase. FASEB J. *15*, 1460-1462.

[41] Shringarpure, R., Grune, T., Sitte, N., and Davies, K.J.A. (2000) 4-Hydroxynonenal-modified amyloid-β peptide inhibits the proteasome: possible importance for Alzheimer`s disease. Cell. Mol. Life Sci. *57*, 1802-1809.

[42] Shringarpue, R., Grune, T., Mehlhase, J., and Davies, K.J.A. (2003) Ubiquitin conjugation is not required for the degradation of oxidized proteins by proteasome. J. Biol. Chem. *278*, 311-318.

[43] Mehlhase, J., Gieche, J., Ullrich, O., Sitte, N., and Grune, T. (2000) LPS-induced protein oxidation and proteolysis in BV-2 microglial cells. IUBMB life *50*, 331-335.

[44] Gieche, J., Mehlhase, J., Licht, A., Zacke, T., Sitte, N., and Grune, T. (2001) Protein oxidation and proteolysis in RAW264.7 macrophages: effects of PMA activation. Biochim. Biophys. Acta *1538*, 321-328

[45] Lasch, P., Petras, T., Ullrich, O., Backmann, J., Naumann, D., and Grune, T. (2001) Hydrogen peroxide-induced structural alterations of RnaseA. J. Biol. Chem. *276*, 9492-502.

[46] Butterfield, L.H., Merino, A., Golub, S.H., and Shau, H. (1999) From cytoprotection to tumor suppression: the multifactorial role of peroxiredoxins. Antioxid. Redox. Signal. *1*, 385-402
[47] Christen, Y. (2000) Oxidative stress and Alzheimer disease. Am. J. Clin. Nutr. *71*, 621s-629s.
[48] Merker, K., and Grune, T. (2000) Proteolysis of oxidized proteins and cellular senescence. Exp. Gerontol. *35*, 779-786.
[49] Rivett, A.J. (1993) Proteasomes: multicatalytic proteinase complexes. Biochem. J. *291*, 1-10
[50] Ciechanover, A. (1994) The ubiquitin-proteasome proteolytic pathway. Cell *79*, 13-21.
[51] Goldberg, A.L., Akopain, T.N., Kisselev, A.F., Lee, D.H., and Rohrwild, M. (1997) New insights into the mechanisms and importance of the proteasome in intracellular protein degradation. Biol. Chem. *378*, 131-140
[52] Tanaka, K. (1998) Proteasomes: structure and biology. J. Biochem. *123*, 195-204.
[53] Voges, D., Zwickl, P., and Baumeister, W. (1999) The 26S proteasome: a machine designed for controlled proteolysis. Annu. Rev. Biochem. *68*, 1015-1068.
[54] Coux, O., Tanaka, K., and Goldberg, A.L. (1996) Structure and functions of the 20S and 26S proteasomes. Annu. Rev. Biochem. *65*, 801-847.
[55] Yang, Y, Fruh, K., Ahn, K., and Peterson, P.A. (1995) In vivo assembly of the proteasomal complexes, implications for antigen processing. J. Biol. Chem. *270*, 27687-27694.
[56] Russel, S.J., Steger, K.A., Johnston, S.A. (1999) Subcellular localization, stoichiometry, and protein levels of 26S proteasome subunits in yeast. J. Biol. Chem. *274*, 21943-21952.
[57] Brooks, P., Fuertes, G., Murray, R.Z., Bose, S., Knecht, E., Rechsteiner, M.C., Hendil, K.B., Tanaka, K., Dyson, J., and Rivett, A.J. (2000) Subcellular localization of proteasome and their regulatory complexes in mammalian cells. Biochem. J. *346*, 155-161.
[58] Beal, R.E., Toscano-Cantaffa, D., Young, P., Rechsteiner, M., and Pickart, C.M. (1998) The hydrophobic effect contributes to polyubiquitin chain recognition. Biochemistry *37*, 2925-2934.
[59] Thrower, J.S., Hoffman, L., Rechsteiner, M., and Pickart, C.M. (2000) Recognition of the polyubiquitin proteolytic signal. EMBO J. *19*, 94-102.
[60] Reinheckel, T., Sitte, N., Ullrich, O., Kuckelkorn, U., Grune, T. (1998) Comparative resistance of 20S and 26S proteasome to oxidative stress. Biochem. J. *335*, 637-642.
[61] Reinheckel, T., Ullrich, O., Sitte, N., Grune, T. (2000) Differential impairment of 20S and 26S proteasome activities in human hematopoietic K562 cells during oxidative stress. Arch. Biochem. Biophys. *377*, 65-68.
[62] Okada, K., Wangpoengtrakul, C., Osawa, T., Toyokuni, S., Tanaka, K., and Uchida, K. (1999) 4-Hydroxy-2-nonenal-mediated impairment of intracellular proteolysis during oxidative stress. J. Biol. Chem. *274*, 23787-23793.
[63] Keller J.N., and Markesbery W.R. (2000) Proteasome inhibition results in increased poly-ADP--ribosylation: implications for neuron death. J. Neurosci. Res. *61*, 436-442
[64] Keller J.N., Hanni K.B., and Markesbery W.R. (2000) Impaired proteasome function in Alzheimer's disease. J. Neurochem. *75*, 436-439
[65] Shang, F., Nowell, T.R. Jr., and Taylor, A. (2001) Removal of oxidatively damaged proteins from lens cells by the ubiquitin-proteasome pathway. Exp. Eye Res. *73*, 229-238.
[66] Davies, K.J.A. (2001) Degradation of oxidized proteins by the 20S proteasome. Biochimie *83*, 301-310.
[67] Carney, J.M., Starke-Reed, P.E., and Oliver, C.N. (1991) Reversal of age-related increase in brain protein oxidation, decrease in enzyme activity, and loss in temporal and spatial memory by chronic administration of the spin-trapping compound *N-tert*-butyl-a -phenylnitone. Proc Natl Acad Sci USA. *88*, 3633-3636.
[68] Stadtman, E.R., Starke-Reed, P.E., and Oliver, C.N. Protein modification in aging. In: Emerit I and Chance B (eds.) Free Radicals and Aging. Basel, Birkhäuser Verlag; 1992: 64-72.
[69] Starke-Reed, P.E., and Oliver, C.N. (1989) Protein oxidation and proteolysis during aging and oxidative stress. Arch. Biochem. Biophys. *275*, 559-567.
[70] Agarwal, S., and Sohal, R.S. (1994) Aging and proteolysis of oxidized proteins. Arch. Biochem. Biophys. *309*, 24-28.
[71] Sahakian, J.A., Szwedam L.I., Friguet, B., Kitani, K., and Levine, R.L. (1995) Aging of the liver: proteolysis of oxidatively modified glutamine synthetase. Arch. Biochem. Biophys. *318*, 411-417.
[72] Cao, G., and Cutler, R.G. (1995) Protein oxidation and aging. Arch. Biochem. Biophys. *320*, 195-201.
[73] Conconi, M., Szweda, L.I,, and Levine, R.L. (1996) Age-related decline of rat liver multicatalytic proteinase activity and protection from oxidative inactivation by heat-shock protein 90. Arch. Biochem. Biophys. *331*, 232-240.
[74] Conconi, M., and Friguet, B. (1997) Proteasome inactivation upon aging and on oxidation-effect of HSP 90. Mol. Biol. Rep. *24*, 45-50.

[75] Anselmi, B., Conconi, M., Veyrat-Durebex, C., Turlin, E., Biville, F., Alliot, J., and Friguet, B. (1998) Dietary self-selection can compensate an age-related decrease of rat liver 20S proteasome activity observed with standard diet. J. Gerontol. *53*, B173-B179.
[76] Sitte, N., Merker, K., von Zglinicki, T., and Grune, T. (2000) Protein oxidation and degradation during proliferative senescence of human MRC-5 fibroblasts. Free Rad. Biol. Med. *28*, 701-708.
[77] Merker. K., Ullrich, O., Schmidt, H., Sitte, N., and Grune, T. (2003) Stability of the Nuclear Protein Turnover During Cellular Senescence of Human Fibroblasts (Submitted).
[78] Dean, R.T. (1975) Concerning a possible mechanism for selective capture of cytoplasmic proteins by lysosomes. Biochem. Biophys. Res. Commun. *67*, 604-609
[79] Dean, R.T. (1975) Direct evidence of importance of lysosomes in degradation of intracellular proteins. Nature (London). *257*, 414-416
[80] Cuervo, A.M., Knecht, E., Terlecky, S.R., and Dice, J.F. (1995) Activation of a selective pathway of lysosomal proteolysis in rat liver by prolonged starvation. Am. J. Physiol. *269*, C1200-C1208.
[81] Jessup, W., Mander, E.L., and Dean, R.T. (1992) The intracellular storage and turnover of apolipoprotein B of oxidized LDL in macrophages. Biochim. Biophys. Acta *1126*, 167-177.
[82] Grant, A.J., Jessup, W., and Dean, R.T. (1992) Accelerated endocytosis and incomplete catabolism of radical-damaged protein. Biochim. Biophys. Acta *1134*, 203-209
[83] Dhaliwal, B.S., and Steinbrecher, U.P. (2000) Cholesterol delivered to macrophages by oxidized low density lipoprotein is sequestered in lysosomes and fails to efflux normally. J. Lipid Res. *41*, 1658-1665
[84] Stolzing, A., Wengner, A., and Grune, T. (2002) Degradation of oxidized extracellular proteins by microglia. Arch. Biochem. Biophys. *400*, 171-179.
[85] Sitte, N., Huber, M., Grune, T., Ladhoff, A., Doecke, W.D., Zglinicki, T., and Davies, K.J.A. (2000) Proteasome inhibition by lipofuscin/ceroid during postmitotic ageing of fibroblasts. FASEB J. *14*, 1490-1498.
[86] Dice, J.F. (1993) Cellular and molecular mechanisms of aging. Physiol. Rev. *73*, 149-59
[87] Okada AA, Dice JF.Altered degradation of intracellular proteins in aging human fibroblasts. Mech Ageing Dev 1984 Aug;26(2-3):341-56
[88] Lavie, L., Reznick, A.Z., and Gershon, D. (1982) Decreased protein and puromycinyl-peptide degradation in livers of senescent mice. Biochem. J. *202*, 47-51
[89] Ivy, G.O., Schottler, F., Wenzel, J., Baudry, M., and Lynch, G. (1984) Inhibitors of lysosomal enzymes: accumulation of lipofuscin-like dense bodies in the brain. Science *226*, 985-7
[90] Keck, S., Nitsch, R., Grune, T., Ullrich, O. (2003) Proteasome inhibition by paired helical filament-tau in brains of patients with Alzheimer's disease. J. Neurochem. *85*, 115-122

The Proteasome and its Involvement in Aging

Anne–Laure Bulteau and Bertrand Friguet
Laboratoire de Biologie et Biochimie Cellulaire du Vieillissement, Université Paris 7 – Denis Diderot, 2 Place Jussieu, 75251 Paris Cedex 05, France

Abstract: Aging is characterised by the accumulation of potentially harmful altered proteins that could lead to gradual deterioration of cellular functions and eventually result in increased probability of death. Metabolic turnover of proteins thus plays an essential role in maintaining life of an organism. It is suspected that the proteasome is one of the key factors controlling the age-dependent turnover of intracellular proteins. This hypothesis is based on the observation that the proteasome is responsible for the degradation of oxidized, aggregated and misfolded proteins. Because of the role played by the protesome in the maintenance of cellular homeostasis, the observation of decline in proteasome activity with aging demonstrates that proteasome is involved in the aging process. Following an updated description of proteasome structure and function, this review will present recent findings that have evidenced age-related decline of proteasome activity and discuss the mechanisms underlying proteasome inhibition as well as the relation between impairment of proteasome function and deregulation of cellular homeostasis.

1. Introduction

The proteasomal pathway is responsible for a large percentage of cellular protein degradation including the control of processes essential for cell viability, such as cell regulation, signal transduction and the degradation of oxidized and misfolded proteins [1-3]. This proteolytic complex exists in different oligomeric assemblies, e.g the 20S and 26S. The 20S and 26S proteasome are functionally distinct in both their substrate preference and requirement for ATP. For example, it has been shown in vitro that the 20S proteasome degrades oxidized proteins in an ATP-independent manner and has been suggested as a primary mechanism for degrading damaged proteins following an oxidative insult [2]. In contrast, the 26S proteasome requires ATP for activation and is responsible for most cellular degradation of both ubiquitinated [4] and some non-ubiquitinated proteins [5]. With aging, a loss of proteasome function has been reported in many different tissues [6-9]. This loss is correlated with an increase in oxidized proteins. Since the proteasome is responsible for the degradation of oxidized proteins, this age-related decline in function suggests that aged tissue is at greater risk for the damage associated with oxidative stress [10-13]. Therefore, a crucial question is to define whether and how the proteasome is implicated in the age-related accumulation of damaged proteins. The focus of this review is to discuss what is presently known about the effects of aging on proteasome biology, discuss how such alterations may occur and describe how these alterations may play a role in age-related increases in protein oxidation.

2. Proteasome Biology

The proteasome was observed for the first time by Harris [14] in human erythrocytes and is ubiquitous among eukaryotic cells. The 20S proteasome, a 700 kDa multiproteolytic complex, represents up to 1 % of soluble cellular proteins [15]. In the mammalian cell, this complex constitutes the main non-lysosomal proteolytic machinery implicated in protein degradation. The proteasome plays a crucial role in the turnover of cytosolic proteins but is not only a "housekeeping" enzyme. In fact, beside eliminating abnormal proteins that are either misfolded or altered, it also participates to the activation of essential functions of the cell. Indeed, the proteasome is implicated in a broad range of cellular pathways [16,17] such as apoptosis [18,19], cell cycle [20], cell differentiation [21], DNA repair [22, 23] and degradation of many of important rate-limiting enzymes in metabolic pathways (Figure 1).

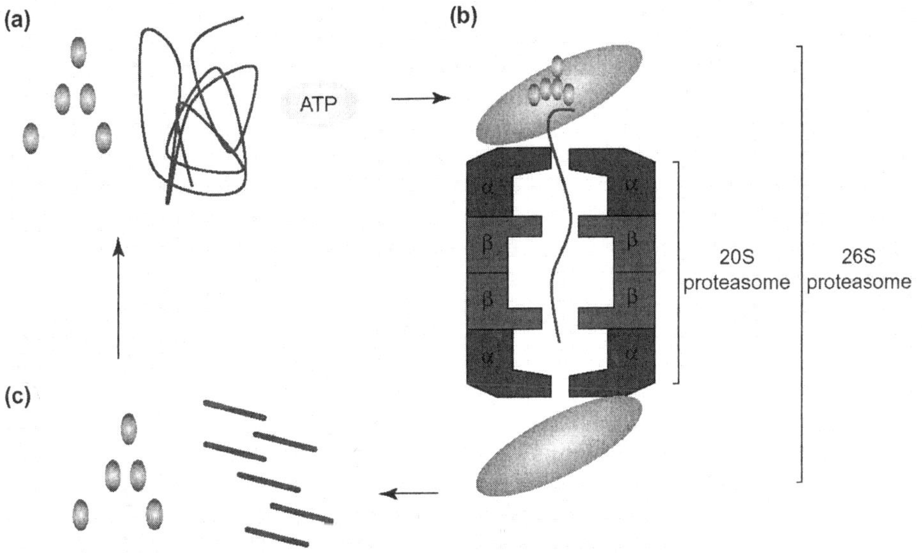

Figure 1. Degradation by the 26S proteasome requires multiple steps. Proteins must be ubiquitinated first (a), unfolded (b) in order to be degraded (c).

2.1 Structure and Organisation

The 20S proteasome is located in the cytosol, in the nucleus and is associated to the endoplasmic reticulum [24]. It can be easily visualised by electron microscopy and exhibits a cylinder shape of about 15 nm length and 11 nm diameter [25]. Its quaternary structure consists of four stacked rings containing each seven subunits of 21 to 35 kDa [26]. The X-ray diffraction analysis of the yeast proteasome clearly showed three cavities of about 5 nm diameter each [27]. The α subunits form the outer rings of the cylinder while the β subunits

inhibition [89]. Moreover, intracellular accumulation of lipofuscin upon loading of WI 38 fibroblasts with ceroid was found associated with a decline of proteasome activity, suggesting that lipofuscin may be implicated in proteasome inhibition in living cells [90].

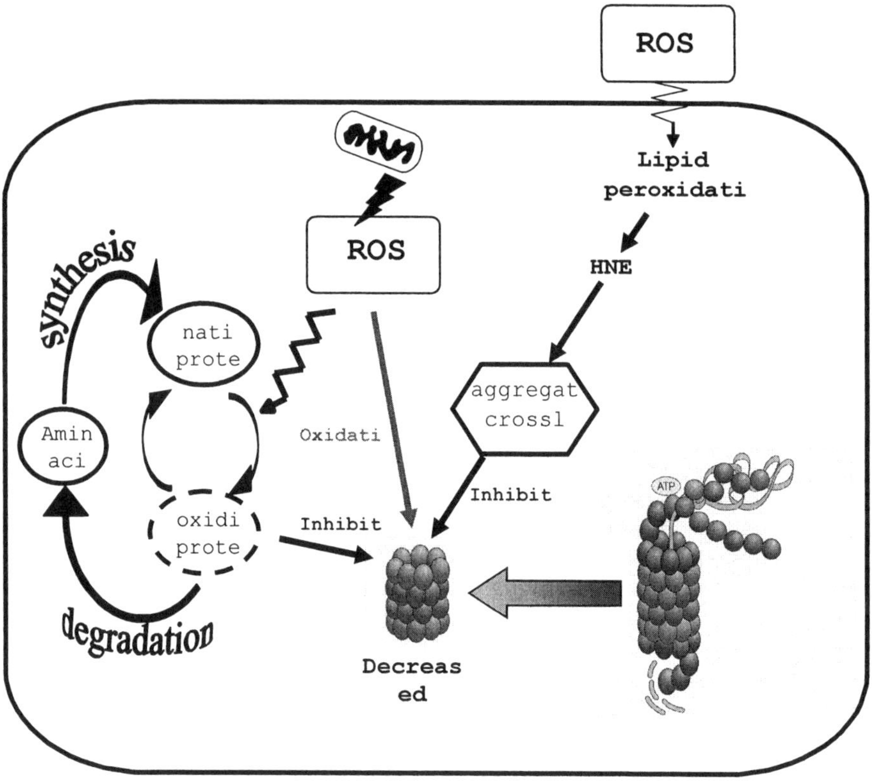

Figure 2. Impairment of proteasome structure and function in aging. The loss of proteasome activity with age can be explained by three different mechanisms: decreased proteasome expression, oxidative alterations of the proteasome or inhibition by cross-limked proteins.

4. Conclusions

It is becoming clear that damaged proteins accumulate while protein turnover declines with age. Evidence has also been provided that the activity of the proteasome which is a major cytosolic degradation system is impaired with age. Depending on the tissue or cellular system investigated the age- and disease-related loss of proteasome activity appears to be the results of combined effects (Figure 2): a decreased proteasome expression; structural modifications and inhibitory damaged proteins. Developing a better understanding of the changes in proteasome biology in aging is critical because it will aid in the development of potential therapeutic interventions designed to preserve necessary proteasome function.

References

[1] Coux, O., Tanaka, K. & Goldberg, A.L. (1996) Structure and functions of the 20S and 26S proteasomes. Annu Rev Biochem, 65, 801-847.
[2] Davies, K.J. (2001) Degradation of oxidized proteins by the 20S proteasome. Biochimie, 83, 301-10.
[3] Carrard, G., Bulteau, A.L., Petropoulos, I. & Friguet, B. (2002) Impairment of proteasome structure and function in aging. Int J Biochem Cell Biol, 34, 1461-74.
[4] Hochstrasser, M. (1996). Ubiquitination-dependent protein degradation. genetics. 30, 405-39
[5] Kisselev, A.F.,Akopian, T.N., Woo, K.M. and Goldberg, A.l. (1999). The size of peptides generated from protein by mamalian 26s and 20s proteasome. Implication for understanding the dgradative mechanism and antigen presentation.J. Biol.chem. 274, 3363-71.
[6] Carney, j.m., starke-reed, p.e., oliver,c.n., landum,r.w., cheng, m.s., wu, j.f., floyd, r.a. (1991). Reversal of age-related increase in brain protein oxidation, decrease in enzyme activity, and loss in temporal and spatial memory by chronic administration of the spin-trapping compound N-tert-butyl-alpha-phenylnitrone. Proc.Natl.acad.sci.Usa. 88, 3633-3636.
[7] Dunlop, R.A., Rodgers, K.J. & Dean, R.T. (2002) Recent developments in the intracellular degradation of oxidized proteins. Free Radic Biol Med, 33, 894-906.
[8] Shringarpure, R. & Davies, K.J. (2002) Protein turnover by the proteasome in aging and disease. Free Radic Biol Med, 32, 1084-.
[9] Szweda, P.A., Friguet, B. & Szweda, L.I. (2002) Proteolysis, free radicals, and aging. Free Radic Biol Med, 33, 29-36.
[10] Beckman, K.B. & Ames, B.N. (1998) The free radical theory of aging matures. Physiol Rev, 78, 547-81.
[11] Stadtman, E.R. (1992) Protein oxidation and aging. Science, 257, 1220-4.
[12] Davies, K.J. (1993) Protein modification by oxidants and the role of proteolytic enzymes. Biochem Soc Trans, 21, 346-53.
[13] Stadtman, E.R. (1990) Metal ion-catalyzed oxidation of proteins: biochemical mechanism and biological consequences. Free Radic Biol Med, 9, 315-25.
[14] Harris, J.R. (1968) Release of a macromolecular protein component from human erythrocyte ghosts. Biochim Biophys Acta, 150, 534-7.
[15] Tanaka, K., Ii, K., Ichihara, A., Waxman, L. & Goldberg, A.L. (1986) A high molecular weight protease in the cytosol of rat liver. I. Purification, enzymological properties, and tissue distribution. J Biol Chem, 261, 15197-203.
[16] Ciechanover, A., Orian, A. & Schwartz, A.L. (2000) The ubiquitin-mediated proteolytic pathway: mode of action and clinical implications. J Cell Biochem Suppl, 34, 40-51.
[17] Lecker, S.H., Solomon, V., Mitch, W.E. & Goldberg, A.L. (1999) Muscle protein breakdown and the critical role of the ubiquitin- proteasome pathway in normal and disease states. J Nutr, 129, 227S-237S.
[18] Chang, Y.C., Lee, Y.S., Tejima, T., Tanaka, K., Omura, S., Heintz, N.H., Mitsui, Y. & Magae, J. (1998) mdm2 and bax, downstream mediators of the p53 response, are degraded by the ubiquitin-proteasome pathway. Cell Growth Differ, 9, 79-84.
[19] Drexler, H.G. (1998) Review of alterations of the cyclin-dependent kinase inhibitor INK4 family genes p15, p16, p18 and p19 in human leukemia-lymphoma cells. Leukemia, 12, 845-59.
[20] King, R.W., Deshaies, R.J., Peters, J.M. & Kirschner, M.W. (1996) How proteolysis drives the cell cycle. Science, 274, 1652-9.
[21] Helin, K. (1998) Regulation of cell proliferation by the E2F transcription factors. Curr Opin Genet Dev, 8, 28-35.
[22] Gillette, T.G., Huang, W., Russell, S.J., Reed, S.H., Johnston, S.A. & Friedberg, E.C. (2001) The 19S complex of the proteasome regulates nucleotide excision repair in yeast. Genes Dev, 15, 1528-39.
[23] Pajonk, F. & McBride, W.H. (2001) The proteasome in cancer biology and treatment. Radiat Res, 156, 447-59.
[24] Kruger, E., Kloetzel, P.M. & Enenkel, C. (2001) 20S proteasome biogenesis. Biochimie, 83, 289-93.
[25] Voges, D., Zwickl, P. & Baumeister, W. (1999) The 26S proteasome: a molecular machine designed for controlled proteolysis. Annu Rev Biochem, 68, 1015-68.

[26] Lowe, J., Stock, D., Jap, B., Zwickl, P., Baumeister, W. & Huber, R. (1995) Crystal structure of the 20S proteasome from the archaeon T. acidophilum at 3.4 A resolution. Science, 268, 533-9.
[27] Groll, M., Ditzel, L., Lowe, J., Stock, D., Bochtler, M., Bartunik, H.D. & Huber, R. (1997) Structure of 20S proteasome from yeast at 2.4 A resolution [see comments]. Nature, 386, 463-71.
[28] Brannigan, J.A., Dodson, G., Duggleby, H.J., Moody, P.C., Smith, J.L., Tomchick, D.R. & Murzin, A.G. (1995) A protein catalytic framework with an N-terminal nucleophile is capable of self-activation. Nature, 378, 416-9.
[29] Seemuller, E., Lupas, A., Stock, D., Lowe, J., Huber, R. & Baumeister, W. (1995) Proteasome from Thermoplasma acidophilum: a threonine protease. Science, 268, 579-82.
[30] Brannigan, J.A. & Dodson, G.G. (1997) A short cut for the immune system. Nat Struct Biol, 4, 334-8.
[31] Chen, P. & Hochstrasser, M. (1996) Autocatalytic subunit processing couples active site formation in the 20S proteasome to completion of assembly. Cell, 86, 961-72.
[32] Kisselev, A.F., Akopian, T.N., Castillo, V. & Goldberg, A.L. (1999) Proteasome active sites allosterically regulate each other, suggesting a cyclical bite-chew mechanism for protein breakdown. Mol Cell, 4, 395-402.
[33] Orlowski, M., Cardozo, C. & Michaud, C. (1993) Evidence for the presence of five distinct proteolytic components in the pituitary multicatalytic proteinase complex. Properties of two components cleaving bonds on the carboxyl side of branched chain and small neutral amino acids. Biochemistry, 32, 1563-72.
[34] Meng, L., Mohan, R., Kwok, B.H., Elofsson, M., Sin, N. & Crews, C.M. (1999) Epoxomicin, a potent and selective proteasome inhibitor, exhibits in vivo antiinflammatory activity. Proc Natl Acad Sci U S A, 96, 10403-8.
[35] Dick, L.R., Cruikshank, A.A., Grenier, L., Melandri, F.D., Nunes, S.L. & Stein, R.L. (1996) Mechanistic studies on the inactivation of the proteasome by lactacystin: a central role for clasto-lactacystin beta-lactone. J Biol Chem, 271, 7273-6.
[36] Fenteany, G., Standaert, R.F., Lane, W.S., Choi, S., Corey, E.J. & Schreiber, S.L. (1995) Inhibition of proteasome activities and subunit-specific amino-terminal threonine modification by lactacystin. Science, 268, 726-31.
[37] Kroll, M., Arenzana-Seisdedos, F., Bachelerie, F., Thomas, D., Friguet, B. & Conconi, M. (1999) The secondary fungal metabolite gliotoxin targets proteolytic activities of the proteasome. Chem Biol, 6, 689-98.
[38] Rock, K.L., Gramm, C., Rothstein, L., Clark, K., Stein, R., Dick, L., Hwang, D. & Goldberg, A.L. (1994) Inhibitors of the proteasome block the degradation of most cell proteins and the generation of peptides presented on MHC class I molecules. Cell, 78, 761-71.
[39] Mellgren, R.L. (1997) Specificities of cell permeant peptidyl inhibitors for the proteinase activities of mu-calpain and the 20 S proteasome. J Biol Chem, 272, 29899-903.
[40] Kisselev, A.F. & Goldberg, A.L. (2001) Proteasome inhibitors: from research tools to drug candidates. Chem Biol, 8, 739-58.
[41] Ma, C.P., Slaughter, C.A. & DeMartino, G.N. (1992) Identification, purification, and characterization of a protein activator (PA28) of the 20 S proteasome (macropain). J Biol Chem, 267, 10515-23.
[42] Watanabe, N. & Yamada, S. (1996) Activation of 20S proteasomes from spinach leaves by fatty acids. Plant Cell Physiol, 37, 147-51.
[43] Groll, M., Bajorek, M., Kohler, A., Moroder, L., Rubin, D.M., Huber, R., Glickman, M.H. & Finley, D. (2000) A gated channel into the proteasome core particle. Nat Struct Biol, 7, 1062-7.
[44] Kohler, A., Cascio, P., Leggett, D.S., Woo, K.M., Goldberg, A.L. & Finley, D. (2001) The axial channel of the proteasome core particle is gated by the Rpt2 ATPase and controls both substrate entry and product release. Mol Cell, 7, 1143-52.
[45] Braun, B.C., Glickman, M., Kraft, R., Dahlmann, B., Kloetzel, P.M., Finley, D. & Schmidt, M. (1999) The base of the proteasome regulatory particle exhibits chaperone-like activity. Nat Cell Biol, 1, 221-6.
[46] Kloetzel, P.M. (2001) Antigen processing by the proteasome. Nat Rev Mol Cell Biol, 2, 179-87.
[47] Deveraux, Q., Ustrell, V., Pickart, C. & Rechsteiner, M. (1994) A 26 S protease subunit that binds ubiquitin conjugates. J Biol Chem, 269, 7059-61.
[48] van Nocker, S., Sadis, S., Rubin, D.M., Glickman, M., Fu, H., Coux, O., Wefes, I., Finley, D. & Vierstra, R.D. (1996) The multiubiquitin-chain-binding protein Mcb1 is a component of the 26S proteasome in Saccharomyces cerevisiae and plays a nonessential, substrate-specific role in protein turnover. Mol Cell Biol, 16, 6020-8.
[49] Dubiel, W., Pratt, G., Ferrell, K. & Rechsteiner, M. (1992) Purification of an 11 S regulator of the multicatalytic protease. J Biol Chem, 267, 22369-77.

[50] Rivett, A.J., Bose, S., Brooks, P. & Broadfoot, K.I. (2001) Regulation of proteasome complexes by gamma-interferon and phosphorylation. Biochimie, 83, 363-6.
[51] Tanahashi, N., Murakami, Y., Minami, Y., Shimbara, N., Hendil, K.B. & Tanaka, K. (2000) Hybrid proteasomes. Induction by interferon-gamma and contribution to ATP-dependent proteolysis. J Biol Chem, 275, 14336-45.
[52] Berlett, B.S. & Stadtman, E.R. (1997) Protein oxidation in aging, disease, and oxidative stress. J Biol Chem, 272, 2013-20316.
[53] Shringarpure, R., Grune, T., Mehlhase, J., davies, K.J. (2003) Ubiquitin conjugaison is not required for the degradation of oxidized proteins by proteasome. J Biol Chem, 278, 311-318.
[54] Grune, T., Reinheckel, T. & Davies, K.J. (1997) Degradation of oxidized proteins in mammalian cells. Faseb J, 11, 526-34.
[55] Shang, F., Nowell, T.R., Jr. & Taylor, A. (2001) Removal of oxidatively damaged proteins from lens cells by the ubiquitin-proteasome pathway. Exp Eye Res, 73, 229-38.
[56] Friguet, B., Bulteau, A.L., Chondrogianni, N., Conconi, M. & Petropoulos, I. (2000) Protein degradation by the proteasome and its implications in aging. Ann N Y Acad Sci, 908, 143-54.
[57] Gaczynska, M., Osmulski, P.A. & Ward, W.F. (2001) Caretaker or undertaker? The role of the proteasome in aging. Mech Ageing Dev, 122, 235-54.
[58] Goto, S., Takahashi, R., Kumiyama, A.A., Radak, Z., Hayashi, T., Takenouchi, M. & Abe, R. (2001) Implications of protein degradation in aging. Ann N Y Acad Sci, 928, 54-64.
[59] Grune, T. (2000) Oxidative stress, aging and the proteasomal system. Biogerontology, 1, 31-40.
[60] Keller, J.N., Gee, J. & Ding, Q. (2002) The proteasome in brain aging. Ageing Res Rev, 1, 279-93.
[61] Conconi, M., Szweda, L.I., Levine, R.L., Stadtman, E.R. & Friguet, B. (1996) Age-related decline of rat liver multicatalytic proteinase activity and protection from oxidative inactivation by heat-shock protein 90. Arch Biochem Biophys, 331, 232-40.
[62] Shibatani, T., Nazir, M. & Ward , W.F. (1996) Alterations of rat liver 20 S proteasome activities by age and food restriction. J Gerontol Biol Sci, 51, 316-322.
[63] Anselmi, B., Conconi, M., Veyrat-Durebex, C., Turlin, E., Biville, F., Alliot, J. & Friguet, B. (1998) Dietary self-selection can compensate an age-related decrease of rat liver 20 S proteasome activity observed with standard diet. J Gerontol A Biol Sci Med Sci, 53, B173-9.
[64] Hayashi, T. & Goto, S. (1998) Age-related changes in the 20S and 26S proteasome activities in the liver of male F344 rats. Mech Ageing Dev, 102, 55-66.
[65] Bulteau, A., Petropoulos, I. & Friguet, B. (2000) Age-related alterations of proteasome structure and function in aging epidermis. Exp Gerontol, 35, 767-77.
[66] Carrard, G., Dieu, M., Toussaint, O., Raes, M. & Friguet, B. (2003) Impact of ageing on proteasome structure and function in human lymphocytes. Int J Biol Cell Bioch, 35, 728-739.
[67] Chondrogianni, N., Petropoulos, I., Franceschi, C., Friguet, B. & Gonos, E.S. (2000) Fibroblast cultures from healthy centenarians have an active proteasome [In Process Citation]. Exp Gerontol, 35, 721-8.
[68] Keller, J.N., Hanni, K.B. & Markesbery, W.R. (2000) Possible involvement of proteasome inhibition in aging: implications for oxidative stress. Mech Ageing Dev, 113, 61-70.
[69] Merker, K., Sitte, N. & Grune, T. (2000) Hydrogen peroxide-mediated protein oxidation in young and old human MRC- 5 fibroblasts. Arch Biochem Biophys, 375, 50-4.
[70] Ponnappan, U., Zhong, M. & Trebilcock, G.U. (1999) Decreased proteasome-mediated degradation in T cells from the elderly: A role in immune senescence. Cell Immunol, 192, 167-74.
[71] Bulteau, A.L., Szweda, L.I. & Friguet, B. (2002) Age-dependent declines in proteasome activity in the heart. Arch Biochem Biophys, 397, 298-304.
[72] Petropoulos, I., Conconi, M., Wang, X., Hoenel, B., Bregegere, F., Milner, Y. & Friguet, B. (2000) Increase of oxidatively modified protein is associated with a decrease of proteasome activity and content in aging epidermal cells. J Gerontol A Biol Sci Med Sci, 55, B220-7.
[73] Lee, C.K., Klopp, R.G., Weindruch, R. & Prolla, T.A. (1999) Gene expression profile of aging and its retardation by caloric restriction. Science, 285, 1390-3.
[74] Ly, D.H., Lockhart, D.J., Lerner, R.A. & Schultz, P.G. (2000) Mitotic misregulation and human aging. Science, 287, 2486-92.
[75] Bardag-Gorce, F., Farout, L., Veyrat-Durebex, C., Briand, Y. & Briand, M. (1999) Changes in 20S proteasome activity during ageing of the LOU rat. Mol Biol Rep, 26, 89-93.
[76] Conconi, M., Petropoulos, I., Emod, I., Turlin, E., Biville, F. & Friguet, B. (1998) Protection from oxidative inactivation of the 20S proteasome by heat- shock protein 90. Biochem J, 333, 407-15.

[77] Conconi, M. & Friguet, B. (1997) Proteasome inactivation upon aging and on oxidation-effect of HSP 90. Mol Biol Rep, 24, 45-50.

[78] Glockzin, S., von Knethen, A., Scheffner, M. & Brune, B. (1999) Activation of the cell death program by nitric oxide involves inhibition of the proteasome. J Biol Chem, 274, 19581-6.

[79] Reinheckel, T., Sitte, N., Ullrich, O., Kuckelkorn, U., Davies, K.J. & Grune, T. (1998) Comparative resistance of the 20S and 26S proteasome to oxidative stress. Biochem J, 335, 637-42.

[80] Arrigo, A.P. (2001) Hsp27: novel regulator of intracellular redox state. IUBMB Life, 52, 303-7.

[81] Verbeke, P., Clark, B.F. & Rattan, S.I. (2001) Reduced levels of oxidized and glycoxidized proteins in human fibroblasts exposed to repeated mild heat shock during serial passaging in vitro. Free Radic Biol Med, 31, 1593-602.

[82] Gomes-Marcondes, M.C. & Tisdale, M.J. (2002) Induction of protein catabolism and the ubiquitin-proteasome pathway by mild oxidative stress. Cancer Lett, 180, 69-74.

[83] Sitte, N., Merker, K., Von Zglinicki, T., Grune, T. & Davies, K.J. (2000) Protein oxidation and degradation during cellular senescence of human BJ fibroblasts: part I--effects of proliferative senescence. Faseb J, 14, 2495-502.

[84] Keller, J.N., Huang, F.F., Zhu, H., Yu, J., Ho, Y.S. & Kindy, T.S. (2000) Oxidative stress-associated impairment of proteasome activity during ischemia-reperfusion injury. J Cereb Blood Flow Metab, 20, 1467-73.

[85] Okada, K., Wangpoengtrakul, C., Osawa, T., Toyokuni, S., Tanaka, K. & Uchida, K. (1999) 4-Hydroxy-2-nonenal-mediated impairment of intracellular proteolysis during oxidative stress. Identification of proteasomes as target molecules. J Biol Chem, 274, 23787-93.

[86] Bulteau, A.L., Lundberg, K.C., Humphries, K.M., Sadek, H.A., Szweda, P.A., Friguet, B. & Szweda, L.I. (2001) Oxidative modification and inactivation of the proteasome during coronary occlusion/reperfusion. J Biol Chem, 25, 25.

[87] Friguet, B., Stadtman, E.R. & Szweda, L.I. (1994) Modification of glucose-6-phosphate dehydrogenase by 4-hydroxy-2- nonenal. Formation of cross-linked protein that inhibits the multicatalytic protease. J Biol Chem, 269, 21639-43.

[88] Friguet, B. & Szweda, L.I. (1997) Inhibition of the multicatalytic proteinase (proteasome) by 4-hydroxy-2-nonenal cross-linked protein. FEBS Lett, 405, 21-5.

[89] Bulteau, A.L., Moreau, M., Nizard, C. & Friguet, B. (2002) Impairment of proteasome function upon UVA- and UVB-irradiation of human keratinocytes. Free Radic Biol Med, 32, 1157-70.

[90] Sitte, N., Huber, M., Grune, T., Ladhoff, A., Doecke, W.D., Von Zglinicki, T. & Davies, K.J. (2000) Proteasome inhibition by lipofuscin/ceroid during postmitotic aging of fibroblasts. Faseb J, 14, 1490-8.

Frontiers in Neurodegenerative Disorders and Aging:
Fundamental Aspects, Clinical Perspectives and New Insights
T. Özben and M. Chevion (Eds.)
IOS Press, 2004

Role and Physiological Implications of Methionine Oxidation within Proteins

Stéphanie Vougier and Bertrand Friguet
Laboratoire de Biologie et Biochimie Cellulaire du Vieillissement, Université Paris 7 – Denis Diderot, 2 Place Jussieu, 75251 Paris Cedex 05, France

Abstract. Methionine and cysteine in proteins are the first targets of reactive oxygen species (ROS). Protein oxidation is generally associated with a loss of protein function and oxidized protein accumulation can alter cell function. Methionine and cysteine oxidations are the only reversible amino acid modifications. In particular, methionine oxidation leads to methionine sulfoxide which can be reduced by the peptide methionine sulfoxide reductases (Msr) system. In addition to its repair role, this enzymatic system has been implicated in the fight against oxidative stress and in the redox regulation of protein function. The importance of the Msr system in aging and in age-related pathologies is also reported.

1. Introduction

During aerobic respiration in the mitochondria, oxygen can be incompletely reduced and generates reactive oxygen species (ROS) including hydrogen peroxide, superoxide and hydroxyl radicals. ROS can also result from environmental stresses [1, 2]. ROS attack depletes reduced glutathione (GSH) and leads to oxidative modifications of macromolecules such as DNA, lipids and proteins. Within proteins, the side chain of sulfur-containing amino acid residues (cysteine and methionine) are the most sensitive to ROS [3, 4]. The mild oxidation of cysteine and methionine generates intra- and inter-molecular disulfide bridges, sulfenic acid and methionine sulfoxide respectively. In addition, peroxynitrite $ONOO^-$, which is generated by the reaction of nitric oxide with superoxide anions, can nitrate tyrosine residues [5], oxidize cysteine [6] and methionine residues [7, 8]. The oxidative modification of other amino acid residues can lead to carbonyl derivatives.

In the cell, the redox status is tightly controlled and oxidized proteins are continuously eliminated. Upon oxidative stress in the cell, ROS formation is increased and the balance between the rate of formation of oxidized proteins and their elimination is disrupted. The production of ROS is a source of physiological dysfunction associated to several age-related changes and to degenerative pathologies, where oxidized proteins tend to accumulate. As observed in reperfusion injury, inflammatory processes, rheumathoid arthritis and pulmonary emphysema [9-14], an excess of ROS production results in an increased rate of oxidation that can alter the function of proteins.

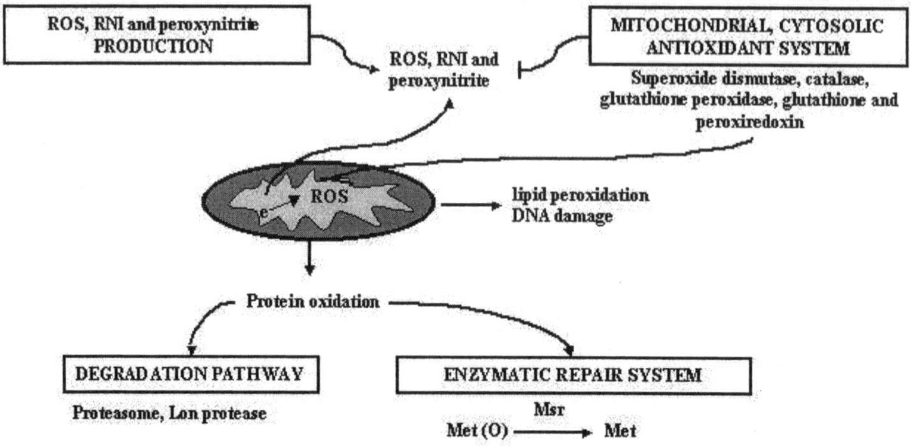

Figure 1. Maintenance mechanisms of cellular redox status and degradation / repair enzymatic pathways of oxidized proteins. Mitochondria are the major source of ROS. Some cytosolic and mitochondrial antioxidant systems can eliminate ROS, RNI (reactive nitrogen intermediate) and peroxynitrite. Indeed, these oxidant species can modify lipids, DNA and in particular proteins. To prevent oxidized protein accumulation, modified proteins can be dregraded or repaired by the Msr system.

2. Oxidation of sulfur-amino acids

2.1 Cysteine oxidation

The redox status of cysteine residues in the catalytic site of enzymes is important, since the sulfhydryl groups are described as nucleophilic agents in many redox reactions (glyceraldehyde 3-phosphate dehydrogenase, glutathione reductase, thioredoxin, glutaredoxin and glutathione S-transferase) and in peptidase activity [15]. The oxidation of cysteine leads to a variety of products including intra- and inter-molecular disulfide bridges, sulfenic acid, sulfinic acid and sulfonic acid [16]. The disulfide br idges and sulfenic acid are reversibly reduced *in vivo* and *in vitro* by dithiothreitol. Cysteine reversible oxidation has been proposed as an important cellular redox sensor for some proteins [16]. The cytoplasm is a reductive environment due to high concentrations of reduced glutathione GSH, but oxidative stress can shift the equilibrium from thiol to disulfide. During oxidative stress, protein function can be altered as observed for peroxiredoxin I which is inactivated after oxidation of its catalytic cysteine [17].

The protein disulfide can be directly reduced non enzymatically by glutathione but the reaction is slow and inefficient. To avoid the accumulation of protein disuldfides, the cell has developed two major repair enzymatic systems: thioredoxin / thioredoxin reductase; glutaredoxin / glutathione reductase [18]. The thioredoxin and thioredoxin reductase system is mainly used to reduce the disulfide bridges of proteins. The sulfinic and sulfonic acids are described as irreversible modifications but recently, it has been shown that the active-site cysteine of peroxiredoxin I oxidized to sulfinic acid is rapidly reduced to the active thiol form in mammalian cells [19]. This new type of oxidized cysteine repair mechanism could regulate the function of various proteins. Finally, many reactive cysteines located at the protein surface may also act as antioxidant and protect the cell against oxidative stress [20].

2.2 Methionine oxidation

In the cell, the oxidation of methionine to methionine sulfoxide is a common post-translational modification since methionine residues are very sensitive to the action of ROS and reactive nitrogen intermediates. In the presence of stronger oxidants, methionine sulfoxide is further oxidized to methionine sulfone. These modifications can alter the function of the protein. Methionine oxidation changes the physical properties of the methionine side chain which is long, flexible and hydrophobic. In contrast, the methionine sulfoxide becomes a hydrophilic residue, closest to lysine since oxidation leads to substitute methionine by a polar amino acid [21]. The variation in hydrophibicity has more or less pronounced effect on protein function since methionine residues can be located within or exposed at the surface of the protein near to or far from the catalytic site. Methionine sulfoxide, as oxidized cysteine, can be reduced back enzymatically to methionine by the peptide methionine sulfoxide reductases system. Therefore, methionine oxidation can play a role in protein regulation.

3. Peptide methionine sulfoxide reductases system

The oxidation of methionine leads to a racemic mixture of both S and R diastereoisomeres methionine sulfoxide (Met-S(O) and Met-R(O)) (Figure 2). In *Escherichia coli*, the peptide methionine sulfoxide reductase A and peptide methionine sulfoxide reductase B (MsrA and MsrB) reduce free and protein-bound Met-S(O) and Met-R(O) respectively, in the presence of thioredoxin and thioredoxin reductase [22-25]. Other enzymatic systems in this bacteria named fMsrA and fMsrB reduce only free Met-S(O) and Met-R(O) respectively [26]. Recently, a new membrane-associated peptide methionine sulfoxide reductase activity has been detected in *Escherichia coli* and requires NADPH to reduce both S and R methionine sulfoxide [27]. In addition, an other soluble peptide methionine sulfoxide reductase A activity has been detected in a *msra / msrb* double mutant, so there appears in *Escherichia coli* at least six members of the peptide methionine sulfoxide reductase family [27].

In humans, one MsrA protein was described although two proteins : CBS-1 and the selenoenzyme SelX, exhibiting MsrB activity are known [28-31]. SelX and MsrA proteins have a nearly identical phylogenetic profile suggesting that these proteins were functionally linked [30]. Indeed, in *Neisseria gonorrhoeae*, MsrA, SelX and thioredoxin-fold domains are fused to a single protei n [30, 32].

In plants, the *Arabidopsis thaliana* genome contains at least five *msra* genes that encode for two different MsrA enzymes characterized in the cytosol and in the plasts. These isoforms shared 70% of protein sequence homology and are divergent by their pH optima and tissue localization [33].

MsrA and SelX are present in the majority of the organisms, only very few bacterial and archaeal organisms lacked the *msra* and *selx* genes suggesting that the peptide methionine sulfoxide reductases system has an important repair physiological role for the cell (see below) [30]. Moreover, the enzymes SelX and MsrA have been described as members of the original minimal gene set encoding proteins essential for cellular life [33].

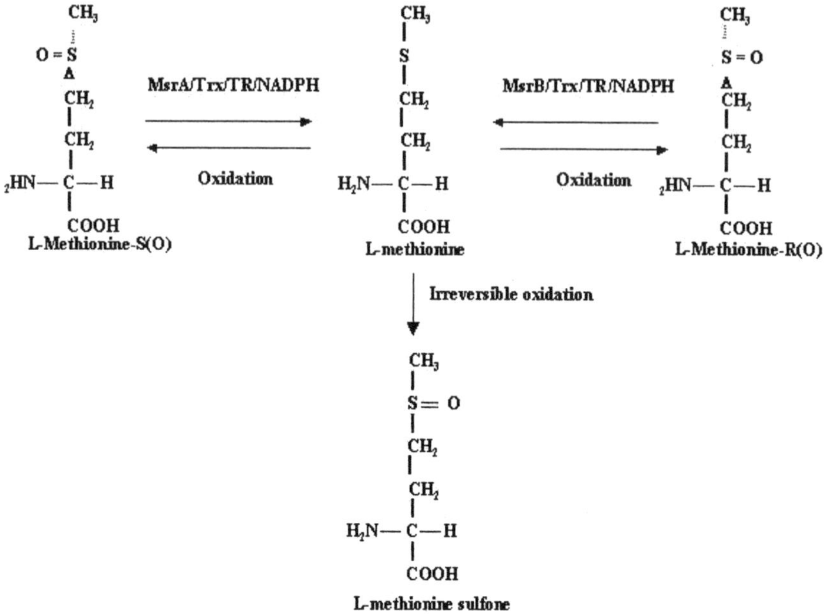

Figure 2. Shematic representation of the diastereoselective reduction of methionine sulfoxide by MsrA and MsrB. In the cell, the oxidation of methionine residues leads to a mixture of S and R diastereoisomeres of methionine sulfoxide. These diastereoisomeres are specifically reduced back to methionine by peptide methionine sulfoxide reductase A (MsrA) and peptide methionine sulfoxide reductase B (MsrB), respectively. These repair enzymes are regenerated by an electron donor system, thioredoxin (Trx), thioredoxin reductase (TR) and NADPH.

4. Mechanism and structure

MsrA is a well-characterized protein requiring a thioredoxin-regenerating system *in vivo*. Two crystal structures of bovine and *Escherichia coli* MsrA are available [34, 35]. This enzyme is folded in an α/β roll not found in other proteins with a large proportion of coil in the amino- and in the glycine rich carboxy-extremity. The catalytic mechanism involved three cysteine residues. First a cysteine attack, belonging to the consensus sequence GCFW leads to a sulfenic acid intermediate and release the reduced methionine. The sulfenic acid is reduced by way of thiol-disulfide exchanges between the catalytic cysteine and the two last cyteine residues, located in the carboxy-terminus coil, and by the thioredoxin-dependent recycling system [36, 37]. The crystal structure of the C-terminal MsrB domain of *Neisseria gonorrhoeae* PilB revealed no resemblance to the previously determined structure of MsrA [38] but the active sites of MsrA and MsrB domains show approximate mirror symmetry suggesting a similar catalytic mechanism.

In PilB of *Neisseria meningiditis*, the Cys-494 participates to the catalysis to form a sulfenic acid intermediate and this cysteine is regenerated by forming a disulfide bridge with Cys-439 and is then reduced by the thioredoxin system [39]. Mammalian SelX is a zinc-containing enzyme with a selenocysteine essential for maintaining high reducing MsrB activity [40]. The catalytic mechanism of the selenoenzyme SelX of *Drosophila melanogaster* implies a sulfenic acid intermediates on Cys-129 (or Selenocys-129). The major difference with MsrA is the regeneration of the thiolate which occurs either directly by thioredoxin or by a disulfide bond between Cys-129 and Cys-69 reduced by the thioredoxin system [41]. In the human CBS-1, Cys-169 corresponds to Selenocys-129 of human SelX and to Cys-494 of the PilB-MsrB domain and its substitution leads to an inactive enzyme, suggesting that this cysteine may be located in the active site [31].

5. Localisation in tissues

MsrA is an ubiquitous enzyme detected in all tissues investigated, but is expressed differentially indicating a specific physiological function. In rat, MsrA was detected by immunocytochemistry in liver, kidney, heart and brain [42] and a high expression of MsrA is observed in the same tissues in humans [28].

The hCBS-1 protein is expressed also in all tissues investigated : heart, skeletal muscle, liver kidney, and with a weaker signal in brain [31]. The high expression level of MsrA and hCBS-1 in liver and kidney suggests that both peptide methionine sulfoxide reductases may have an important anti-oxidant role in these detoxifying organs. The different expression patterns of MsrA and hCBS-1 in some tissues could also be due to the presence of other peptide methionine sulfoxide reductases as it is described in *Escherichia coli* [43].

6. Subcellular localisation

In rat liver cells, MsrA has been identified both in the cytosol and in the matrix of the mitochondria, a major site of ROS production [44]. A single msra gene encodes two proteins: one which is longer, bearing a cleavable mitochondrial signal peptide located in the amino-terminus extremity, and the other one which is a shorter cytosolic protein [44, 45]. This MsrA dual localisation reinforced its role in oxidative stress protection. We have also shown that cytosolic MsrA is oxidatively modified at its cysteine residues in sulfinic or sulfonic acid while mitochondrial MsrA was hardly affected. This enzyme could be regulated via the oxidation of its cysteine residues since three of them are implicated in the catalytic mechanism. Moreover, it has been shown in *Arabidopsis thaliana*, that multiple genes exist that encode at least two different MsrA distributed in the cytosol and in the plastids [33, 46].

7. Implications in pathologies

The accumulation of oxidized proteins has been associated to cellular dysfunction and pathologies. The processes that result in an excess of ROS production leading to oxidized proteins are ischemia / reperfusion, inflammation, rheumatoid arthritis and pulmonary emphysema [9-14]. In the two last pathologies, α_1-antiproteinase, the inhibitor of elastase, is inactivated when methionines are oxidized. An incubation with MsrA enzyme restores the activity of the inhibitor [47]. Methionine oxidation has been observed in aging and in several neurodegenerative diseases such as Alzheimer disease, cataract formation and pulmonary emphysema. Indeed, in all brains of Alzheimer disease patients, the MsrA activity decreased with a significant parallel elevation of oxidized proteins [48]. Whereas methionine sulfoxide residues are detected in more abundant amount in old cataract lenses, no decrease of MsrA activity was detected [49, 50].

The mRNA and protein levels as well as the activity of MsrA decreased with aging in rat liver and kidney [51]. This down-regulation of MsrA could explain, at least in part, the accumulation of oxidized proteins with aging. In all these processes, it will be interesting to determine if there is always a correlation between the progression of aging, or of the disease and alterations of the peptide methionine sulfoxide reductases system.

Moreover, MsrA is not expressed in tumour cell lines such as lymphoma cell lines whereas normal peripheral blood leukocytes express MsrA [28]. It will remain to be known if a relationship exists between the lack of MsrA and carcinogenesis. MsrA has been implicated in bacterial adherence since a MsrA mutant of *Streptococcus pneumoniae* binds more hardly to lung and vein epithelial cells [52] and MsrA has been described as a virulence factor for the plant pathogen *Erwinia chrysanthemi* [53].

8. Protection against oxidative stress

Enzymatic systems are able to fight against the accumulation of ROS. These systems include superoxide dismutase and catalase which remove superoxide ($O_2^{\cdot -}$) and hydrogen peroxide (H_2O_2) from the cytoplasm, respectively [20]. In addition, glutathione peroxidase reduce H_2O_2 to H_2O [20] with glutathione and the peroxidredoxin enzymes exert their protective antioxidant role in cells in reducing H_2O_2, peroxynitrite and a wide range of organic hydroperoxides ($ROOH + 2e^- \rightarrow ROH + H_2O$) [6, 54-56].

In addition to its repair activity, MsrA can act as an antioxidant enzyme and help the other enzymatic systems to remove ROS in the cell. Indeed, the exposed surface methionine residues could be oxidized with little effect on enzyme activity and protect the buried residues within the core of the protein. Within proteins such as glutamine synthetase, eight exposed surface methionine residues act as scavengers of ROS, which are reduced back to the methionine by the peptide methionine sulfoxide reductases system [3, 4]. MsrA and seleno-MsrB (SelX) are important in the maintenance of the cell redox status, since null-*msra* mutants in *Escherichia coli*, in *Saccharomyces cerevisiae,* in mice and null-*msrb* mutants in *Saccharomyces cerevisiae* and in *Arabidopsis thaliana* showed an increased sensitivity to oxidative stress [30, 32, 57-59]. Moreover, when *Drosophila melanogaster* and *Saccharomyces cerevisiae* overexpress MsrA protein, they better cope with oxidative stress and have an increased lifespan [59-61]. Human T lymphocytes transfected stably with bovine msra gene are more resistant to hydrogen peroxide than non-transfected cells [61]. Using a cDNA microarrays approach, the expression level of SelX and MsrA proteins is elevated in response to agents causing oxidative stress in *Escherichia coli* and *Saccharomyces cerevisiae*, which underscores the antioxidant role of MsrA and SelX [30]. In addition, it has been recently shown that null-*msra* mutant in mice fed a selenium-free diet exhibit an increased oxidative stress with a higher content of protein carbonyls and oxidized methionines which is correlated with a decrease of the seleno-MsrB mRNA, protein and activity levels in certain tissues [62].

9. Regulation of protein function

The oxidation of specific methionine residues in proteins resulting in a loss of function without pathological consequences strongly suggests a regulatory role for the peptide methionine sulfoxide reductases system. Indeed, oxidized calmodulin was identified *in vivo*, [63] and it has been shown that oxidation of methionine residues at position 144 and 145 in the calmodulin prevents the calcium fixation and the activation of the plasma membrane Ca-ATPase [64]. Incubation of calmodulin in the presence of MsrA restores its ability to activate the plasma membrane Ca-ATPase [65]. The inactivation of the voltage-dependent potassium channel is also modulated via methionine oxidation and reduction by MsrA. Indeed, when the methionine at position 3 is oxidized, the inactivation is prevented and is restored by co-expression with MsrA [66]. Moreover, oxidation of methionine at position 440 accelerates the inactivation of the voltage-dependent potassium channel so methionine oxidation may play a role in mediating the cellular responses in hypoxia / hyperoxia [67]. In addition, HIV-2 protease is inactivated by *in vitro* oxidation of Met-95 at the dimer interface and its enzymatic activity is partly restored by MsrA. The retroviral protease is inactivated after a minor modification, indicating that a putative protease inhibitor targeting the dimer interface could be developed [68].

The oxidation and reduction of methionine residues by the peptide methionine sulfoxide reductases may participate to a regulatory pathway implicated in signal transduction. The action of this enzymatic repair system could be regulated since a homologue of elongation factor1γ named EF1γ has been discovered recently to regulate *msra* gene expression in *Saccharomyces cerevisiae* [69].

10. Conclusions

All these data highlight the importance of methionine oxidation as a marker of oxidative stress and the implication of the peptide methionine sulfoxide reductases system in protein repair and in the fight against the accumulation of methionine sulfoxide in the cell.

During the aging process and in several neurodegenerative diseases as observed in Alzheimer disease, accumulation of oxidized methionines is correlated with a decrease of the MsrA activity. Nevertheless, it remains to be determined what is the real implication of MsrA and MsrB function disturbance, when it occurs, in the progression of neurodegenerative diseases and aging.

The function of several proteins can be regulated via methionine oxidation and reduction by MsrA and MsrB which can be compared to the phosphorylation / dephosphorylation process mediated by various kinases and phosphatases although no methionine oxidase has been identified yet. It will be interesting to determine if the regulation, via methionine oxidation/reduction, as observed with cysteine oxidation, is implicated in particular regulation pathways of signal transduction.

References

[1] Berlett, BS and Stadtman, ER (1997) Protein oxidation in aging, disease, and oxidative stress. J Biol Chem 272, 20313-20316

[2] Beckman, KB and Ames, BN (1998) The free radical theory of aging matures. Physiol Rev 78, 547-581

Frontiers in Neurodegenerative Disorders and Aging: Fundamental Aspects, Clinical Perspectives and New Insights
T. Özben and M. Chevion (Eds)
IOS Press, 2004

Activation of Human Neutrophils Leads to the Cross-linking of Tyrosyl Radicals to Endogenous Anti-inflammatory and Anti-bacterial proteins. Application of a Tyrosylating fluorophore.

Diana Avram[1], Edwin P. Romijn[2], Albert J.R. Heck[2] and Karel W.A. Wirtz[1]
[1] *Department of Biochemistry of Lipids, Center for Biomembranes and Lipid Enzymology, Institute of Biomembranes, Utrecht University, Padualaan 8, 3584 CH Utrecht and*
[2] *Department of Biomolecular Mass Spectrometry, Bijvoet Center and Utrecht Institute for Pharmaceutical Sciences, Utrecht University, Sorbonnelaan 16, 3584 CA Utrecht, The Netherlands*

Abstract: As part of the host defense against invading microorganisms polymorphonuclear neutrophils (PMNs) generate an oxidative burst as a result of which myeloperoxidase (MPO) utilizes hydrogen peroxide (H_2O_2) to convert L-tyrosine into tyrosyl radicals. These radicals can cross-link with free or protein-bound tyrosine residues to form dityrosine considered to be a marker of oxidative stress. Here we show that endogenous proteins of activated human PMNs are targets of tyrosyl radicals generated extracellularly. Up to recently the identification of tyrosylated proteins in an intact cell system remained elusive. We have developed a new strategy to identify these oxidatively modified proteins by using a membrane-impermeable tyrosylating fluorophore, i.e. fluorescein coupled to tyramine, in combination with proteomics techniques. By using this approach, proteins with anti-inflammatory and anti-bacterial properties were found to be tyrosylated. It remains to be established whether this post-translational modification affects the phagocytic function of PMNs

1. Introduction

Proinflammatory mediators are essential to life because of the immune responses evoked to ward off infection and to prevent malignant cell development. Key effectors in the host defense are polymorphonuclear neutrophils (PMNs) that represent the first cells in the peripheral blood attracted to the site of inflammation (1). Activation of PMNs triggers microbicidal mechanisms such as the release of proteolytic enzymes and antimicrobial peptides as well as the rapid production of reactive oxygen species (ROS), a phenomenon known as the oxidative burst.

In addition to their role in phagocytosis, PMNs potentiate inflammatory responses by releasing proinflammatory cytokines such as IL-1β, IL-8, and TNF-α, which can either prime

This work was supported with a grant of the Council for Chemical Sciences of the Netherlands Organization for Scientific Research (NWO-CW)

or activate the ROS production. Excessive or chronic release of ROS and other toxic products at the inflammatory locus can result in severe vascular or tissue injury. By accelerating their cell death program these proinflammatory agonists could also affect neutrophil functions. Therefore, PMNs responses as regulated by cytokines, serum factors and other immunomodulators (2) must be tightly controlled in order to maintain optimal antibacterial and tumoricidal activity.

The neutrophil oxidative burst is a process that is associated with extensive oxygen consumption upon NADPH oxidase complex assembly resulting in the generation of superoxide anion ($O_2^{\bullet -}$) (3). The relatively harmless $O_2^{\bullet -}$ dismutates spontaneously into hydrogen peroxide (H_2O_2) and forms other toxic agents such as hypochlorous acid (HOCl) by the action of the azurophilic granules-derived myeloperoxidase (MPO) in the presence of chloride. In a resting neutrophil, about 95% of the inactive NADPH oxidase (i.e., cytochrome b_{558}, which contains heme and flavins gp91phox, p21phox) is found in the membranes of subcellular granules and vesicles, and the rest resides in the plasma membrane (4),(5). The oxidase is a multicomponent transport chain that transfers electrons from NADPH to molecular oxygen. The phagocyte-specific heterodimeric transmembrane protein, cytochrome b_{558}, appears to be the terminal component of the oxidase responsible for the one-electron reduction of molecular oxygen (6).

- $$NADPH + O_2 \rightarrow NADP^+ + O_2^{\bullet -} \rightarrow H_2O_2$$

Activation of NADPH requires participation of the cytosolic components p67phox, p47phox, and p40phox, which together with the small GTP-binding protein p21rac are translocated to the cytochrome b membrane constituent (7). Some studies have provided evidence that a functional enzyme complex can also be formed directly in the granule membranes. This suggests that activated PMNs may be able to either release ROS extracellularly or retain the species within phagosomes or granules, depending on what receptors or signaling pathways are activated. The release of granulocytic enzymes with peroxidase and bactericidal activity such as MPO, elastase and lysozyme either to the outside of the cell or into the phagocytic vacuole (8) in tandem with ROS is absolutely required for optimal pathogen clearance. However, the cytotoxic action of these reactive agents is not limited exclusively towards foreign intruders or modified cells but also often damages normal cells or tissue surrounding an inflamed area. Oxidative damage involves the modification of nucleic acids, lipids and proteins. Here we will focus on the oxidation of tyrosine residues in proteins of activated neutrophils.

2. Oxidative modification of proteins via dityrosine formation

The recent finding that MPO-H_2O_2 oxidative system secreted by activated PMNs uses free L-tyrosine to generate a tyrosyl radical indicates that the enzyme converts the amino acid to a freely diffusible intermediate, which may undergo a dimerization reaction to yield the stable compound *o,o'*-dityrosine (9). Tyrosyl radicals can also cross-link to tyrosine residues yielding protein-bound dityrosine (tyrosylated proteins) (10). In addition, protein tyrosyl radicals can form intermolecular cross links as shown with calmodulin (11) and EGF receptor (12) which dimerize as a result of dityrosine bond formation. Intramolecular transfer of electrons between a tyrosyl radical and another amino acid may also occur as shown in *E. coli* ribonucleotide reductase (13). *In vitro* studies demonstrate that in addition to *o,o'*-dityrosine, hydroxyl radicals can also induce the formation of the unnatural amino acids *o*-tyrosine and *m*-tyrosine

(14,15). These tyrosine analogs could serve as markers of protein oxidation during aerobic metabolism, glycooxidation, and metal-catalyzed oxidation reactions.

Activated mice neutrophils produce *o,o'*-dityrosine cross-links in tissue proteins, which are subsequently excreted in urine as breakdown products (16). This strongly suggests that *in vivo* the oxidatively modified proteins are targets for proteolytic degradations and that the modified tyrosine residues cannot be converted into other compounds. Patients with septic shock markedly increased their output of *o,o'*-dityrosine into urine suggesting that systemic inflammation may be a potent source of oxidative stress in humans. The pathway promoting the generation of these abnormal amino acids involves the activation of phagocyte NADPH oxidase since mice deficient in gp91phox, one of the components of NADPH complex, failed to produce protein-bound *o,o'*-dityrosine.

3. Nitric oxide and nitrotyrosine

A considerable body of evidence has identified nitric oxide (NO) as a free radical signaling molecule involved in the immune defense both as a putative key mediator of tissue damage and as a regulatory molecule to inhibit the pathways leading to apoptosis. The dual role of NO is regulated by its reactivity state, the microenvironment and cell type. The cytotoxic potential of NO is clearly manifest in tandem with reactive oxygen intermediates released at the sites of activated neutrophils and macrophages. It has also been shown that during oxidative burst phagocytic cells can use $O_2^{\bullet-}$ to directly oxidize N(G)-hydroxy–L-arginine to NO, independent of NO-synthase. Decreased ROS production is often attributed to the reaction between NO and superoxide anion ($O_2^{\bullet-}$), which yields the powerful oxidant peroxynitrite ($ONOO^-$) (17). Although peroxynitrite is a potent nitrating agent of protein-associated tyrosine residues yielding 3-nitrotyrosine, some recent studies indicate that this nitration reaction occurs at unphysiological concentrations of peroxynitrite (18). Since dityrosine formation almost completely outcompetes tyrosine nitration at low steady-state concentrations of peroxynitrite it was suggested that another pathway involving nitric dioxide ($^{\bullet}NO_2$)-induced tyrosyl radical formation. According to this pathway (see Fig. 1), $^{\bullet}NO_2$ formed during homolytic cleavage of peroxynitrous acid (ONOOH) reacts with tyrosine (Tyr) to generate a tyrosyl radical (reaction a). This radical could react either with $^{\bullet}NO_2$ to yield 3-nitrotyrosine (reaction b) or dimerizes to form dityrosine (reaction c).

A major competing reaction is $^{\bullet}NO_2$ dimerization yielding N_2O_4. Recent studies suggest that about 30% of ONOOH is converted into $^{\bullet}NO_2$ and $^{\bullet}OH$, whereas the residual 70% undergoes rearrangement to nitric acid without free radical formation (19). Dityrosine formation may also involve hydroxyl radicals ($^{\bullet}OH$) since $^{\bullet}OH$ scavengers enhance peroxynitrite-mediated tyrosine nitration (20). It was hypothesized that $^{\bullet}OH$ can also react with tyrosyl radicals resulting in the formation of 3-hydroxytyrosine (dopa) (21). Based on these studies one may conclude that dityrosine formation represents the predominant end product of tyrosine oxidation at relatively low $NO/O_2^{\bullet-}$ fluxes that are likely to occur in most *in vivo* conditions. It has been suggested that dityrosine formation together with increased NO synthase expression may be a useful marker for peroxynitrite formation in tissues.

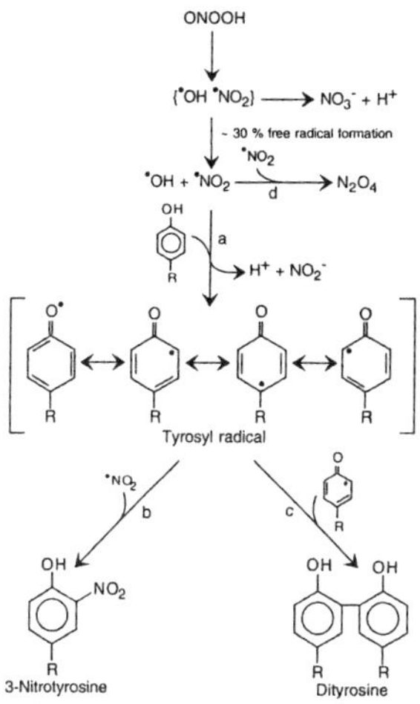

Figure 1. Hypothetical mechanism of nitrotyrosine and dityrosine formation by peroxinitrite according to ref. 13.

4. Dityrosine formation as a biomarker of aging and neurodegenerative diseases

High levels of oxidatively modified protein tyrosine residues, in particular protein-bound dityrosine products, have been detected in human atherosclerotic plaques, in the brain of elderly humans (22) and in age-related nuclear cataract (23). In the latter study additional tyrosine-specific oxidation products, such as dopa, *o*-tyrosine and *m*-tyrosine have been found to accumulate in long-lived proteins of human cataractous lenses. In aged non-cataractous lenses an increase of up to 30% has been observed for dityrosine whilst *o*-tyrosine was barely detectable. Five- to eight-fold elevated levels of dityrosine and nitrotyrosine have been detected in the ventricular cerebrospinal fluid and in the hippocampus and neocortical regions of the Alzheimer's disease brain as compared to normal subjects. This may indicate that the disease progression is associated with neutrophil infiltration into the brain inducing oxidative modifications of proteins. Thus dityrosine and nitrotyrosine could serve as stable biomarkers of neurologic oxidative degeneration.

5. Protein tyrosylation in neutrophils

Due to massive accumulation of phagocytes-derived toxic products in tissue or biologic fluids, proteins may become oxidatively modified at tyrosine residues providing markers for pathological conditions. Although the formation of *o,o'*-dityrosine cross-links in model proteins or lipoproteins was extensively characterized, the identity of proteins susceptible to tyrosyl radical attack in an intact cellular system is hampered by the lack of a specific antibody detecting the protein-bound dityrosine (tyrosylated proteins). Here we present a new strategy consisting of a tyrosylating agent – i.e. the tyrosine analogue, tyramine, coupled to fluorescein (TyrFluo)- able to cross-link to oxidized protein tyrosine residues (Fig. 2) in combination with proteomic analyses of tyrosylated proteins. We show that as a result of the oxidative burst endogenous proteins of activated neutrophils could be targets of tyrosyl radicals produced extracellularly.

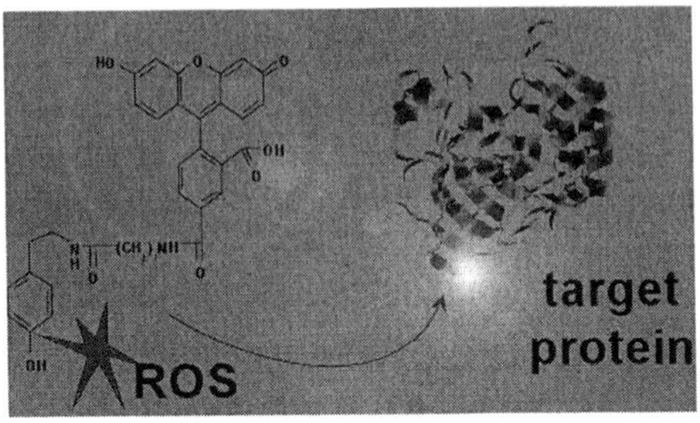

Figure 2. Chemical structure of the fluorescein-labeled tyramine (TyrFluo) and ROS-induced covalent coupling of this conjugate to oxidized tyrosine residues in a target protein

Upon protein kinase C activation neutrophils secrete MPO, which utilizes H_2O_2 to abstract a hydrogen atom from L-tyrosine residues present. In case the TyrFluo probe is present in the medium, fluorescent tyrosyl radicals generated can crosslink to protein tyrosyl radicals. By this mechanism the probe will covalently couple to oxidized proteins (Fig. 2). We observed by confocal microscopy that the activation of human neutrophils by PMA in the presence of rat-1 fibroblasts restricts the coupling of TyrFluo primarily to the neutrophil indicating that the tyrosyl radicals are formed in the immediate vicinity of the plasma membrane (Fig 3B). Compared to PMA-activated fibroblasts alone (Fig 3A) one can see that the fibroblasts become more intensely fluorescent when PMA is added in the presence of neutrophils. This indicates that the MPO-H_2O_2 oxidative system has the capacity to oxidize proteins of neighboring cells. Previously we showed that neutrophil activation results in the tyrosylation of extracellular matrix proteins of human endothelial cells(24). To assess the distribution of fluorescently labeled proteins in neutrophils

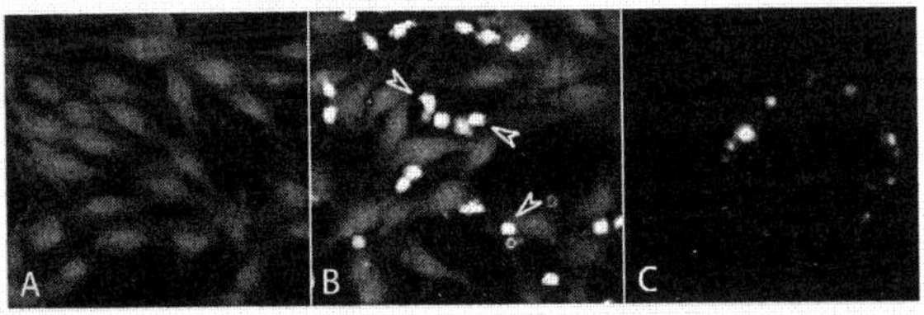

Figure 3. PMA-activation in the presence of TyrFluo induces an extensive fluorescent labeling of neutrophils as shown by confocal laser scanning fluorescent microscopy. A. PMA-activated rat-1 fibroblasts; B. PMA-activated neutrophils (see arrows) co-incubated with rat-1 fibroblasts; C. optical section of TyrFluo-labeled neutrophil upon PMA activation.

Optical sections of fixed cells were taken after 15 min of PMA-activation (Fig 3C). It appears that the bulk of fluorescence is present in relatively large intracellular compartments near the plasma membrane most likely reflecting the internalization of tyrosylated membrane proteins. Apparently after the initial labeling of proteins at the cell surface, oxidatively modified (tyrosylated) proteins were internalized, which most likely are to become degraded.

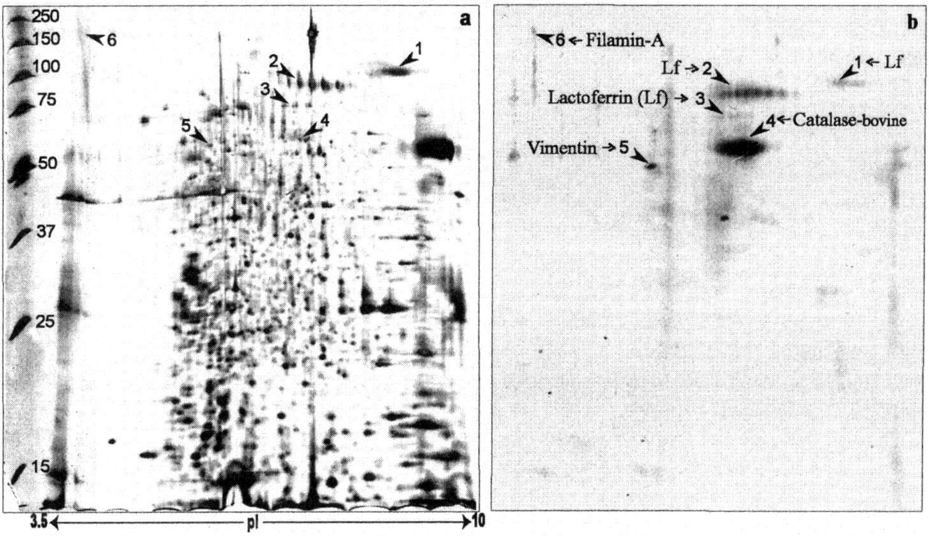

Figure 4. Two-dimensional maps of membrane-associated proteins from PMA-activated PMNs and the corresponding Western blot of tyrosylated proteins. A. silver-stained master map; B tyrosylation pattern of membrane-associated proteins

In order to identify the tyrosylated proteins after labeling with TyrFluo the neutrophils were lysed and the total membrane fraction isolated. The membrane-associated proteins were analyzed by two-dimensional electrophoresis (2D-PAGE) followed by Western blotting using anti-fluorescein antibody. The neutrophil membrane-associated proteome is presented in Fig 4a. The numbers indicate the proteins identified by mass spectrometry analysis and correspond with the proteins found to be tyrosylated after PMA-activation. As shown in Fig 4b, one of the major tyrosylated proteins identified was a neutral isoform of lactoferrin (number 2). This glycoprotein isoform (Mr 80 kDa) comprised a chain of seven spots, which may reflect different degrees of glycosylation. In addition, two other neutral isoforms (Mr 75 kDa and 85 kDa) were identified of which the 75 kDa form was slightly tyrosylated (number 3). The well-known basic isoform of lactoferrin (number 1, Mr 85 kDa), which we found to be exclusively present in the soluble fraction of the resting neutrophils (data not shown), is also tyrosylated. Another heavily tyrosylated protein was identified as bovine catalase (number 4), which was added to activated neutrophils to abolish further tyrosyl radical formation. Catalase in the process of decomposing H_2O_2 forms endogenous tyrosyl radicals(25). It could be that these radicals are involved in cross-linking TyrFluo tyrosyl radicals to the catalase itself which is then internalized similar to what has been observed for other heme proteins(26) (27). Two structural proteins, i.e. vimentin (number 5) and filamin A (number 6) were also found to be tyrosylated. The susceptibility of these two cytoskeletal proteins to tyrosyl radical attack may be explained by their binding to β-integrin receptors (8,28) mediating microfilament cytoskeleton rearrangements.

6. Concluding remarks

Knowledge about the identity of cellular proteins undergoing tyrosylation reactions could be helpful in understanding the importance of tyrosyl radicals generated by neutrophils under physiological and pathological conditions. In our study we show that the oxidative burst generated by activated neutrophils, results in the tyrosylation of lactoferrin, vimentin and filamin A. These proteins are known for their anti-inflammatory and anti-bacterial properties. So it has been established that by interacting with lipopolysaccharide (LPS) lactoferrin inhibits the binding of LPS to the CD14 receptors and, hence, the down-regulation of the proinflammatory cytokine cascade (29,30). Recently vimentin was found to be secreted by activated macrophages acting as a potent anti-bacterial protein (31). Although several studies assumed that the oxidative modification of tyrosine residues is detrimental, we consider the possibility that free or protein-bound tyrosyl radicals could also enhance the phagocytic functions of neutrophils. If true, it is likely that some of the oxidatively modified endogenous proteins express an enhanced anti-microbial activity. Therefore, it is of great interest to further investigate the neutrophil protein efficacy during the phagocytosis of bacteria under conditions of tyrosine oxidation.

References

[1] Babior, B. M. (1984) Oxidants from phagocytes: agents of defense and destruction Blood 64, 959-966

[2] Djaldetti, M., Salman, H., Bergman, M., Djaldetti, R., and Bessler, H. (2002) Phagocytosis--the mighty weapon of the silent warriors Microsc Res Tech 57, 421-431

[3] De Leo, F. R., Ulman, K. V., Davis, A. R., Jutila, K. L., and Quinn, M. T. (1996) Assembly of the human neutrophil NADPH oxidase involves binding of p67phox and flavocytochrome b to a common functional domain in p47phox J Biol Chem 271, 17013-17020

[4] Jesaitis, A. J., Buescher, E. S., Harrison, D., Quinn, M. T., Parkos, C. A., Livesey, S., and Linner, J. (1990) Ultrastructural localization of cytochrome b in the membranes of resting and phagocytosing human granulocytes J Clin Invest 85, 821-835

[5] Bjerrum, O. W., and Borregaard, N. (1989) Dual granule localization of the dormant NADPH oxidase and cytochrome b559 in human neutrophils Eur J Haematol 43, 67-77

[6] Ellis, J. A., Cross, A. R., and Jones, O. T. (1989) Studies on the electron-transfer mechanism of the human neutrophil NADPH oxidase Biochem J 262, 575-579

[7] Shatwell, K. P., and Segal, A. W. (1996) NADPH oxidase Int J Biochem Cell Biol 28, 1191-1195

[8] Borregaard, N., and Cowland, J. B. (1997) Granules of the human neutrophilic polymorphonuclear leukocyte Blood 89, 3503-3521

[9] Heinecke, J. W., Li, W., Daehnke, H. L., 3rd, and Goldstein, J. A. (1993) Dityrosine, a specific marker of oxidation, is synthesized by the myeloperoxidase-hydrogen peroxide system of human neutrophils and macrophages J Biol Chem 268, 4069-4077

[10] Heinecke, J. W., Li, W., Francis, G. A., and Goldstein, J. A. (1993) Tyrosyl radical generated by myeloperoxidase catalyzes the oxidative cross-linking of proteins J Clin Invest 91, 2866-2872

[11] Malencik, D. A., and Anderson, S. R. (1996) Dityrosine formation in calmodulin: cross-linking and polymerization catalyzed by Arthromyces peroxidase Biochemistry 35, 4375-4386

[12] van der Vliet, A., Hristova, M., Cross, C. E., Eiserich, J. P., and Goldkorn, T. (1998) Peroxynitrite induces covalent dimerization of epidermal growth factor receptors in A431 epidermoid carcinoma cells J Biol Chem 273, 31860-31866

[13] Katterle, B., Sahlin, M., Schmidt, P. P., Potsch, S., Logan, D. T., Graslund, A., and Sjoberg, B. M. (1997) Kinetics of transient radicals in Escherichia coli ribonucleotide reductase. Formation of a new tyrosyl radical in mutant protein R2 J Biol Chem 272, 10414-10421

[14] Leeuwenburgh, C., Rasmussen, J. E., Hsu, F. F., Mueller, D. M., Pennathur, S., and Heinecke, J. W. (1997) Mass spectrometric quantification of markers for protein oxidation by tyrosyl radical, copper, and hydroxyl radical in low density lipoprotein isolated from human atherosclerotic plaques J Biol Chem 272, 3520-3526

[15] Leeuwenburgh, C., Wagner, P., Holloszy, J. O., Sohal, R. S., and Heinecke, J. W. (1997) Caloric restriction attenuates dityrosine cross-linking of cardiac and skeletal muscle proteins in aging mice Arch Biochem Biophys 346, 74-80

[16] Bhattacharjee, S., Pennathur, S., Byun, J., Crowley, J., Mueller, D., Gischler, J., Hotchkiss, R. S., and Heinecke, J. W. (2001) NADPH oxidase of neutrophils elevates o,o'-dityrosine cross-links in proteins and urine during inflammation Arch Biochem Biophys 395, 69-77

[17] Modolell, M., Eichmann, K., and Soler, G. (1997) Oxidation of N(G)-hydroxyl-L-arginine to nitric oxide mediated by respiratory burst: an alternative pathway to NO synthesis FEBS Lett 401, 123-126

[18] Pfeiffer, S., Schmidt, K., and Mayer, B. (2000) Dityrosine formation outcompetes tyrosine nitration at low steady-state concentrations of peroxynitrite. Implications for tyrosine modification by nitric oxide/superoxide in vivo J Biol Chem 275, 6346-6352

[19] Merenyi, G., Lind, J., Goldstein, S., and Czapski, G. (1998) Peroxynitrous acid homolyzes into *OH and *NO2 radicals Chem Res Toxicol 11, 712-713

[20] van der Vliet, A., Eiserich, J. P., O'Neill, C. A., Halliwell, B., and Cross, C. E. (1995) Tyrosine modification by reactive nitrogen species: a closer look Arch Biochem Biophys 319, 341-349

[21] van der Vliet, A., O'Neill, C. A., Halliwell, B., Cross, C. E., and Kaur, H. (1994) Aromatic hydroxylation and nitration of phenylalanine and tyrosine by peroxynitrite. Evidence for hydroxyl radical production from peroxynitrite FEBS Lett 339, 89-92

[22] Kato, Y., Maruyama, W., Naoi, M., Hashizume, Y., and Osawa, T. (1998) Immunohistochemical detection of dityrosine in lipofuscin pigments in the aged human brain FEBS Lett 439, 231-234

[23] Fu, S., Dean, R., Southan, M., and Truscott, R. (1998) The hydroxyl radical in lens nuclear cataractogenesis J Biol Chem 273, 28603-28609

[24] Czapski, G. A., Avram, D., Sakharov, D. V., Wirtz, K. W., Strosznajder, J. B., and Pap, E. H. (2002) Activated neutrophils oxidize extracellular proteins of endothelial cells in culture: effect of nitric oxide donors Biochem J 365, 897-902

[25] Putnam, C. D., Arvai, A. S., Bourne, Y., and Tainer, J. A. (2000) Active and inhibited human catalase structures: ligand and NADPH binding and catalytic mechanism J Mol Biol 296, 295-309

[26] Cassidy, R. A., Burleson, D. G., Delgado, A. V., Kohler, D. J., Salin, M. L., and Pruitt, B. A., Jr. (2000) Effects of heme proteins on nitric oxide levels and cell viability in isolated PMNs: a mechanism of toxicity J Leukoc Biol 67, 357-368

[27] Baldus, S., Eiserich, J. P., Mani, A., Castro, L., Figueroa, M., Chumley, P., Ma, W., Tousson, A., White, C. R., Bullard, D. C., Brennan, M. L., Lusis, A. J., Moore, K. P., and Freeman, B. A. (2001) Endothelial transcytosis of myeloperoxidase confers specificity to vascular ECM proteins as targets of tyrosine nitration J Clin Invest 108, 1759-1770

[28] Stossel, T. P., Condeelis, J., Cooley, L., Hartwig, J. H., Noegel, A., Schleicher, M., and Shapiro, S. S. (2001) Filamins as integrators of cell mechanics and signalling Nat Rev Mol Cell Biol 2, 138-145

[29] Elass-Rochard, E., Legrand, D., Salmon, V., Roseanu, A., Trif, M., Tobias, P. S., Mazurier, J., and Spik, G. (1998) Lactoferrin inhibits the endotoxin interaction with CD14 by competition with the lipopolysaccharide-binding protein Infect Immun 66, 486-491

[30] Baveye, S., Elass, E., Fernig, D. G., Blanquart, C., Mazurier, J., and Legrand, D. (2000) Human lactoferrin interacts with soluble CD14 and inhibits expression of endothelial adhesion molecules, E-selectin and ICAM-1, induced by the CD14-lipopolysaccharide complex Infect Immun 68, 6519-6525

[31] Mor-Vaknin, N., Punturieri, A., Sitwala, K., and Markovitz, D. M. (2003) Vimentin is secreted by activated macrophages Nat Cell Biol 5, 59-63

The TCL Analyzer consists of two blocks: a sample preparation block and an analysis block. Tested fluid samples of 50 μl are distributed over the surface of a cylindrical aluminum tray (dimensions: diameter – 19mm, height - 3mm, thickness - 0.12mm), which is positioned inside the sample preparation block, tightly sealed and then vacuum – dried. The sample is then transferred to the analysis block, where the dish is mounted on a preheated oven with a constant temperature heater of 80° +/- 0.2 °C. Sequential photon counting, in counts per second (CPS) is performed by an electronic cathode tube (R6095P photomultiplier, Hamamatsu Photonics, Japan) with spectral response in the range of 300 – 650 nm wavelength, during 300 seconds. Total test time lasts less than 12 minutes. TCL curve is a computerized trend line of individual points, each of which represents the mean photon count during one second. (Fig. 2).

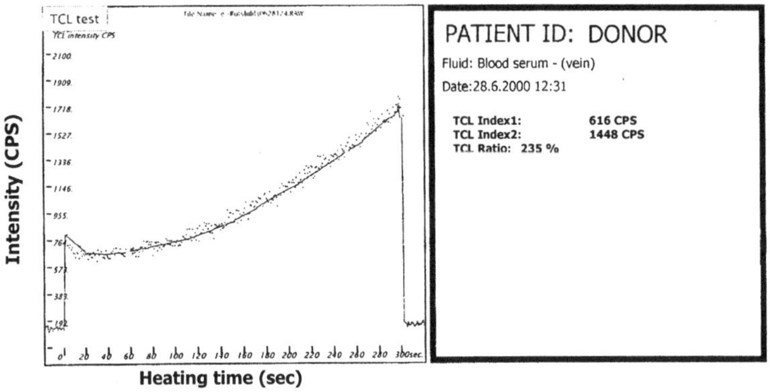

Figure 2. TCL kinetic curve of blood serum

Once reaching 50 seconds, photon readings were marked by low variation. In serum, the period between 50 and 280 seconds produced the most significant changes in photon reading and were highly reproducible. Beyond 280 seconds, photon reading did not produce any additional meaningful information.

2.2 TCL assay parameters

The parameters of the TCL kinetic curve that reflect Electronically Excited Species (EES) formation rate due to heat induced oxidative modification are: 1. TCL amplitude at 50 sec or TCL index 1, which reflects the baseline of heat induced EES formation rate. 2. TCL amplitude at 280 sec or TCL index 2, which reflects the end level of heat induced EES formation rate in TCL test time. 3. TCL ratio (TCL R) parameter (in %) reflects the heat-induced susceptibility to oxidative modification of the tested sample.

TCL R (%) = (TCL index 2 / TCL index 1) X 100

2.3. Reproducibility of the TCL test for blood serum.

The reproducibility of the TCL assay parameters for blood serum is +/- 8.6 %. TCL parameters in blood serum remain stable in room temperature (20 - 24 °C) for at least two hours after sample collection. The stable state of the parameters is evaluated with respect to daily kit.

3. Detection of Oxidative stress in vitro by TCL assay

3.1 TCL curve pattern of blood serum in acute hydrogen peroxide (HP) induced oxidative stress (OS)

Addition of HP to normal blood serum led to a dramatic increase of the intensity in the initial part of the TCL curve (Fig. 3), described by TCL–index 1, that indicates the elevation of the oxidative modification rate. The decrease TCL R reflects the decrease of susceptibility to oxidation of the sample during test due to prior oxidation in vitro by HP. Thus lower TCL R expresses more oxidized sample (Table 1).

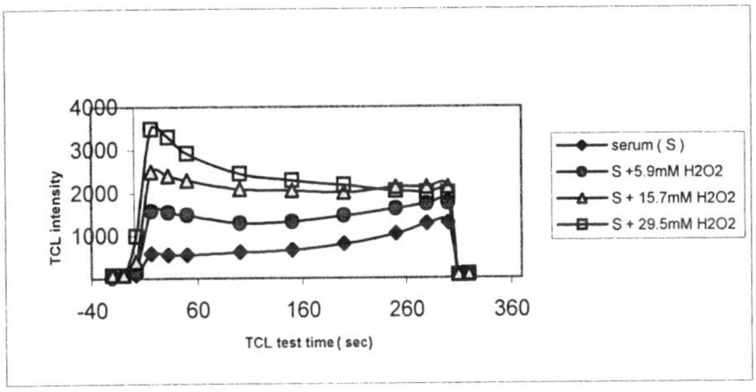

Figure 3. TCL kinetic curve of blood serum after addition of H_2O_2

Table 1. TCL curve parameters before and after adding H_2O_2

sample	TCL index 1(cps) test time 50 sec	TCL index 2 (cps) test time 280 sec	TCL - ratio (%)
Serum (S)	555	1287	232%
S + 5.9 mM H_2O_2	1490	1739	114%
S + 15.7 mM H_2O_2	2294	2134	93%
S + 29.5 mMH_2O_2	2928	2006	69%

3.2 TCL monitoring of the H_2O_2 Induced oxidative stress in serum

Six blood serum samples were examined by TCL method before addition of 2.95 mM H_2O_2 and 0.5 h, 1h, and 3 h after it. We found a time dependent increase in TCL- index-I and a decrease in the slope of the curve, by TCL ratio parameter (Fig.4).

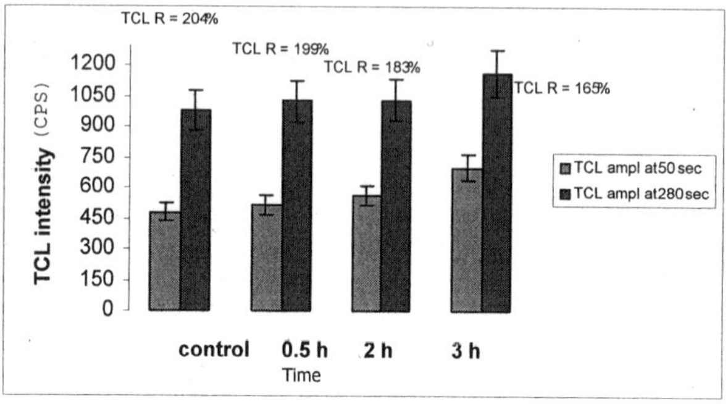

Figure 4. TCL ratio (TCL R) parameter in blood serum after addition of 2.95 mM H_2O_2 at various times of incubation.

4. TCL kinetic curve pattern and its parameters in detecting oxidized lipids and proteins

Bovine Serum Albumin (BSA) and linolenic acid were tested by TCL method before and after oxidation, as a model for detection of oxidized proteins and lipids by TCL assay. BSA, 10mg/ml, (Sigma, Ltd, U.S.A.) was oxidized by Fe^{3+} and ascorbic acid (19) and measured by TCL and protein carbonyl (20) before and after oxidation. In the protein carbonyl assay, BSA was added to 5ml of 2.5mM dinitrophenylhydrazine (DNPH), dissolved in 2 M HCL and incubated for 1 hour. After the DNPH reaction, proteins were precipitated with an equal volume of 20% (W/V) trichloroacetic acid, and the pellets were washed, once with 4 ml of 10% (W/V) trichloroacetic acid and three times with 4 ml of an ethanol: ethyl acetate mixture (1:1). Washings were achieved by mechanical disruption of the pellets in the washing solution using a small spatula, and repelleting by centrifugation at 6000g for 5 min. Finally, the precipitates were dissolved in 6 M guanidine-HCL solution, and the absorbance peak at 365nm was determined by spectral scanning at the range of 320 to 400 nm. Protein contents were determined on the HCL blank pellets using a bovine serum albumin standard curve in guanidine-HCL and reading the absorbance at 280 nm. Linolenic acid, (0.5 mM) was oxidized using an oxidation assay described by Kanner and Lapidot (21) and measured by TCL and by conjugated dienes (spectrophotometric technique) before and after oxidation (22).

Results: Basal TCL curve pattern of BSA showed a gradual increase in TCL amplitude starting at 50 sec (baseline of heat-induced EES formation rate - TCL Index I - first Parameter) following heating until 280 sec (Fig. 5A-1). After oxidation, TCL amplitude at 50 sec - TCL index (TCL – I) increased compared to the pre-oxidation level, and then gradually decreased until 280 sec. (Fig 5B-1). Basal TCL curve pattern of LA showed relatively stable TCL amplitude in the range of 50–280 sec. (Fig 5A-2). Following oxidation, TCL curve pattern changed in a similar manner to that of BSA (Fig 5B- 2). Concomitantly, the levels of protein carbonyls and conjugate dienes increased significantly (P<0.001 and P<0.001, respectively) after oxidation (Table 2).

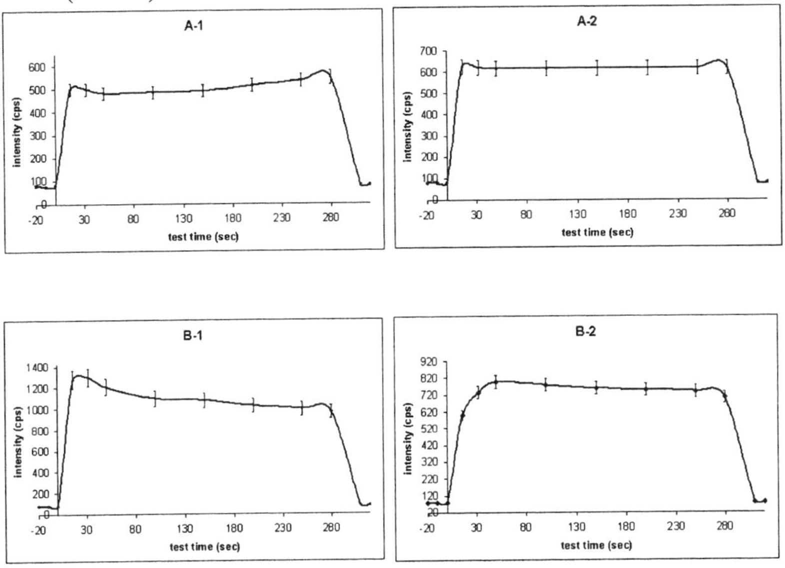

Figure 5. TCL kinetic curves of BSA (A-1 before oxidation, B-1 after oxidation), and Linolenic acid (A-2 before oxidation, B- 2 after oxidation)

Table 2. TCL and oxidative markers parameters of BSA and Linolenic acid before and after oxidation

Sample n = 6	TCL index 1 (CPS)	TCL index 2 (CPS)	TCL –R (%)	Protein Carbonyls (nmol/ml) n = 6	Conjugated dienes (nmol/ml) n = 6
BSA 10mg/ml	482±26	544±34	113 +/- 6.4	1.31+/-0.07	
Ox-BSA	1211±57	1040±43	86 +/- 4.3	1.75+/-0.09	
% of change Significance	+151% P<0.001	+91% P<0.001	-27 %	+33.5% P<0.001	
Linolenic acid 0.5mM	616±36	614±32	100		21±1.3
Ox-Linolenic acid	798±23	705±18	88 +/- 3.8		29±1.8
% of change Significance	29.5% P < 0.001	15 % P < 0.001	-12 %		38 % P < 0.001

Therefore, TCL reading during analysis indicates formation of unstable carbonyl fragments in the tested sample, which expresses its susceptibility to oxidation.

5. Correlation between TCL and a conventional oxidizability method.

5.1 AAPH induced oxidation and TCL method

We tested susceptibility to oxidation in 30 samples of blood serum from Chronic Heart Failure (CHF) patients using two methods: TCL assay and AAPH (100 mM) induced oxidation with measuring MDA by Thiobarbituric acid-reactive substances (TBARS) before and after adding AAPH. In this case we are using TBARS ratio parameter.

TBARS ratio = TBARS value after addition of AAPH / Initial TBARS value.

We found a significant correlation between AAPH induced oxidation and heat induced oxidation by TBARS ratio and by TCL ratio index ($r = 0.75$, $p < 0.01$) (Fig. 6). This correlation indicates that TCL ratio parameter reflects susceptibility to oxidation.

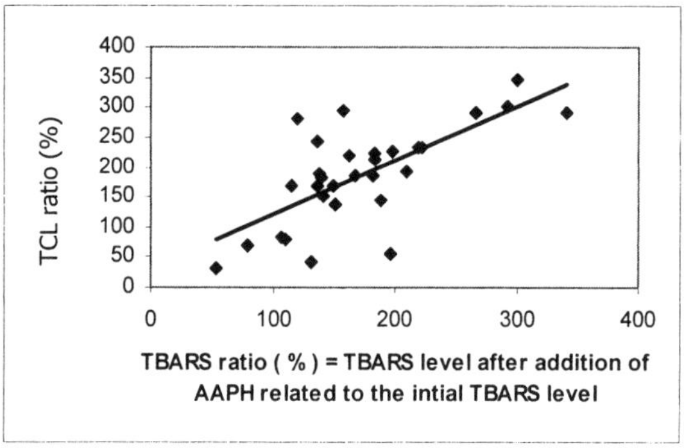

Figure 6. Correlation between TCL ratio parameters and ratio of TBARS in AAPH (100 mM) induced oxidation in CHF patients' sera ($n = 30$, $r = 0.75$, $p < 0.01$)

6. Clinical studies using TCL assay in blood serum and saliva

6.1 Enhanced oxidative stress and decreases susceptibility to oxidation of serum derived from septic patients

In the present study we investigated the extent of oxidative stress by measuring both protein and lipid oxidative products and oxidizability in serum derived from two groups of septic patients: surgery and non-surgery origin (23). For each patient, the oxidative state was assayed over a period of 7-21 days after clinical identification of sepsis. On the day of admission, the levels of lipid peroxides (LP) and of TBARS were significantly increased in serum obtained from all patients. Protein carbonyl concentrations, which were used as a marker of oxidized proteins, were also significantly increased in the patients (surgery and non-surgery origin) by 46% and 53% respectively compared to control group. There was no significant difference in the extent of oxidation between the two groups. The oxidizability was tested by AAPH – induced serum lipid peroxidation and TCL assay. The susceptibility to oxidation of the septic patients' serum was studied on the day of admission and was found to be reduced compared to the control group. AAPH-induced serum lipid peroxidation was decreased by 25-45% in all patients, in comparison to normal subjects.

Using TCL assay, we found a similar pattern of decreased susceptibility to oxidation of blood serum, a decrease of 28 % in the TCL ratio parameter, which indicates high-level prior (in vivo) oxidation. (Fig. 7).

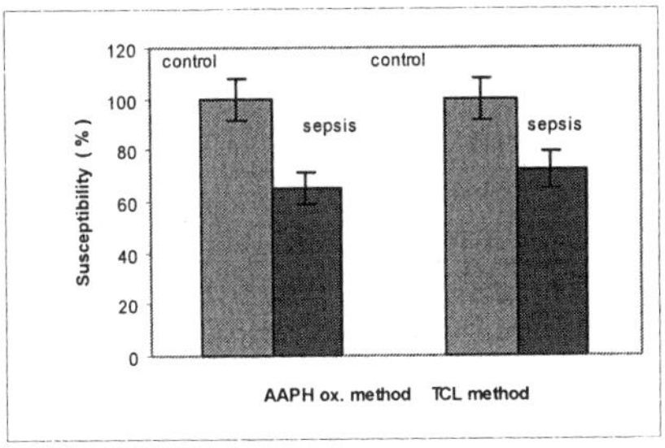

Figure 7. Decrease of susceptibility to lipid peroxidation by AAPH induced oxidation method and TCL method in septic patients' sera.

The results obtained in the present study demonstrate an enhanced oxidative stress and a decreased susceptibility to oxidation in septic patients.

6.2 Detection of smoking induced Oxidative Stress in blood serum by the TCL method. Relationship between TCL parameters in blood serum of smokers and biochemical indices of risk factors for cardiovascular disease (CVD).

Investigation of gas-phase cigarette smoke radicals by spin-trapping technique indicates high content of peroxy radicals (ROO•) and Nitric oxide (NO•), which led to oxidative stress. We tested blood serum samples of 534 non-smokers and 170 smoking persons. Results: We have found significant increase of TCL index 1 in the smokers group (574 +/- 125) compared to the non-smokers group (471 +/- 77) ($p < 0.001$) and significant decrease of TCL ratio in the smokers group (154 +/- 19) compared to the non-smokers group (172 +/- 17) ($p < 0.001$) (Table 3).

Table 3. TCL parameters in blood serum of non-smokers and smokers group.

Group N	TCL index 1	TCL index 2	TCL R parameter (%)
Non smokers N = 534	471 +/- 77	810 +/- 87	172 +/- 17
Smokers N = 170	574 +/- 125	883 +/- 92	154 +/- 19
% of change Significance	22 % P < 0.001	N.S.	-10.5 % P < 0.001

This result is consistent with changes of TCL pattern, which was found in cases of BSA and linolenic acid oxidation, and during serum oxidation by H_2O_2 in vitro. Correlation between TCL – index 1, and the age of the tested persons was found only for the smokers group ($r = 0.435$, $p = 0.005$). Moreover, we observed significant correlation between the average number of cigarettes smoked per day and TCL index ($r = 0.55$, $p < 0.001$) and also with the TCL Ratio parameter ($r = 0.41$, $P < 0.001$). The ratio parameter also correlates significantly with the level of blood serum glucose ($r = 0.22$, $p < 0.0028$) and CRP level (negative correlation $p < 0.05$). We obtained high significant correlation between TCL index 1 and LDL level ($r = 0.25$, $p = 0.0009$). TCL index 1 correlates with cholesterol (Chol), HDL (negative correlation) and CRP levels ($p < 0.01$). High significant correlation between the levels of maximum oxidative modification rate (TCL index 2) and CVD risk factors: blood serum glucose ($r = 0.307$), Chol. ($r = 0.361$), LDL ($r = 0.333$), Triglycerides ($r = 0.278$), was found ($p < 0.001$ for all of them), which indicates the role of these substances on TCL curve pattern formation i.e. oxidizability pattern formation. Our results demonstrate that the smokers' blood serum TCL parameters reflect the smoking induced oxidative stress and the possible relationship between TCL parameters and CVD risk factors development.

6.3 Smoking induced oxidative stress in saliva as detected by TCL

In Table 4, the TCL parameters of Index 1, Index 2, and TCLR were determined in saliva of non smokers and smokers. Overall, the results obtained in saliva were similar to the ones obtained in serum. Also in saliva Index 1 was higher in smokers compared to non smokers by almost 40% while Index 2 was higher about 30% and the difference in the two indices between non smokers and smokers were statistically significant respectively ($p<0.01$, $p< 0.02$). TCL ratio (TCLR), as was expected, decreased by 8% indicating that indeed saliva of smokers is more oxidized than that of non-smokers.

Table 4. TCL parameters in saliva for non smokers and smokers

Groups, n	TCL index 1 (cps)	TCL index 2 (cps)	TCL ratio (%)
non smokers n = 15	558 +/-151*	621 +/-164**	111%
smokers n = 15	779 +/- 244*	807 +/- 202**	103%
% change smokers vs. Non-smokers * p < 0.01 ** p< 0.02	39.6%	29.9%	-8%

7. Laboratory studies

7.1 Studies on cell culture lines

7.1.1 Detection of oxidative stress in models of neuronal cell lines (neuroblastoma and PC12) resulting from dopamine treatment, using TCL assay. (T. Mamou, M.Sc. student, G. Zozulya, PhD student. Instructor: Prof. A. Hochman).

Dopamine (DA) is an endogenous neurotransmitter that exerts cellular toxic effects through its oxidative metabolites. These products were shown to cause death of PC12 and mesencephalic melanoma, neuroblastoma, dorsal root ganglion neuronal cell cultures, as well as nigral cells death in the substantia nigra of Parkinson's disease patients (24,25). In previous studies we (26,27), and others have shown that dopamine caused apoptotic death of PC12 cells, and that cells could be rescued by incubation with antioxidants. In the present study we wanted to check if treatment of neuroblastome cells (SK-NMC) with dopamine caused oxidative damage. In addition we also tested the cells with ethanol, which may also cause cell death by a ROS-dependent mechanism.

Cells and cultures. Neuroblastoma SK-NMC cells were grown on RPMI medium with 20% fetal calf serum, and PC12 cells in DMEM medium with 8% fetal calf serum and 8% horse serum, in 24-well culture plates with a 13 mm cover glass at the bottom. Ethanol and dopamine were added after 24 hours, and counting and TCL analysis were performed after additional 24 hours. For TCL analysis the cover slides were transferred to the TCL Analyzer. Results: Treatment of SKNMC cells grown with serum with dopamine (DA) caused a dose-dependent death (Fig. 8). With 0.1 mM DA there was 70% survival and with 0.6 mM DA, 50% survival. Ethanol caused only 12% cell death. DA and ethanol treatment caused oxidative stress as was estimated by the TCL method. Cell death was proportional to oxidative damage: in the ethanol treated cells it was 11% relative to control, while in the DA-treated cells it was 184% and 266% with 0.1 mM and 0.6mM DA, respectively. Cells grown without serum were more sensitive to the toxic effect of DA but not to ethanol. Fig. 9 shows that 0.05 mM and 0.3 mM DA caused 11% and 65 % cell death, and ethanol treatment resulted in only 4% death. As in the serum-grown culture, Cell death was proportional to oxidative damage - in the ethanol treated cells TCL was 11% higher relative to control, while in the DA-treated cells it was 184% and 266%, with 0.1 mM and 0.6mM DA, respectively.

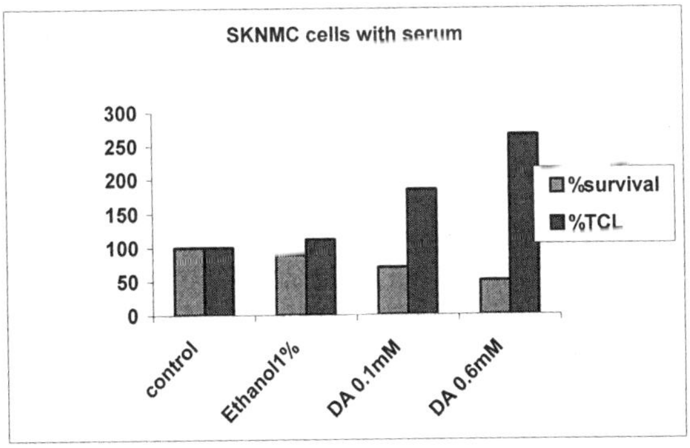

Figure 8. Effect of DA and ethanol treatment on survival and oxidative stress in SKNMC neuroblastoma cells grown with serum.

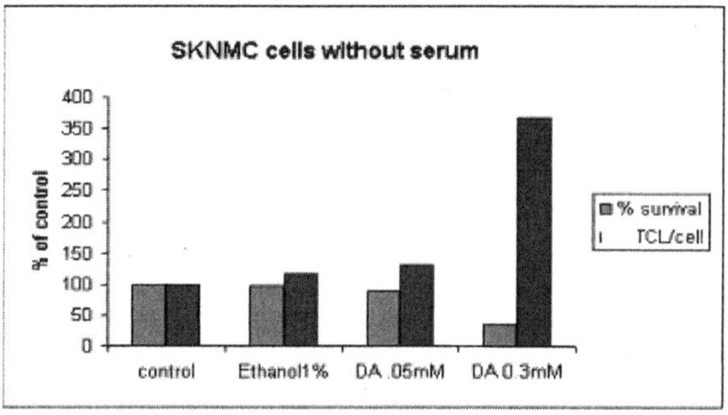

Figure 9. Effect of DA and ethanol treatment on survival and oxidative stress in SKNMC neuroblastoma cells grown without serum.

Interestingly, TCL parameter (% TCL/ 1 x 10 ^{5}cells) was linear with % of surviving cells, even if both experiments are combined (Fig. 10).

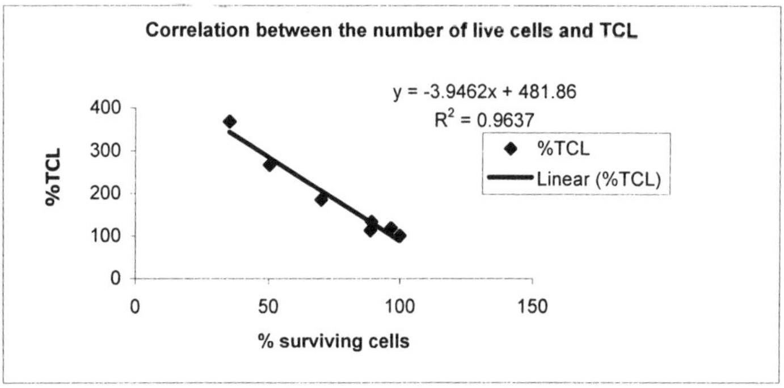

Figure 10. Correlation between the % of surviving cells and % of TCL/cell.

Addition of 0.3 mM dopamine to PC12 caused 35-50% cell death. TCL analysis of treated and untreated cultures revealed oxidative stress in the dopamine treated cells. Fig. 11 shows that there is a positive correlation between the cell numbers and the TCL ratio. Fig. 12 shows that treatment with dopamine resulted in a decrease in this ratio, but it was again linear with the number of cells. TCL ratio/1x10^5 cells, was lower in the treated culture (0.387) relative to the control (0.534), suggesting prevalence of oxidative stress in the former.

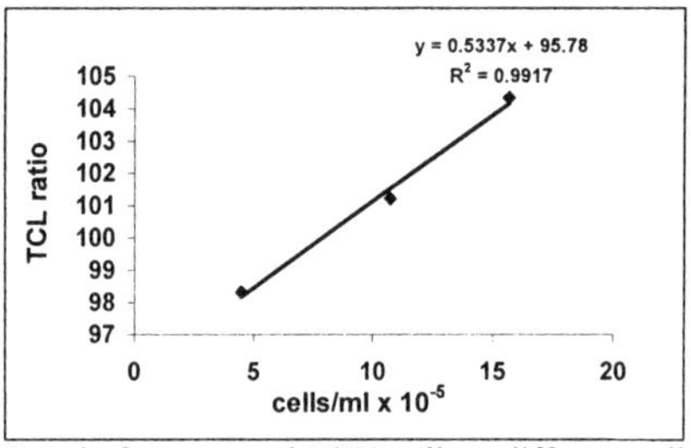

Figure 11. TCL ratio for untreated PC12 cells at different cell concentration

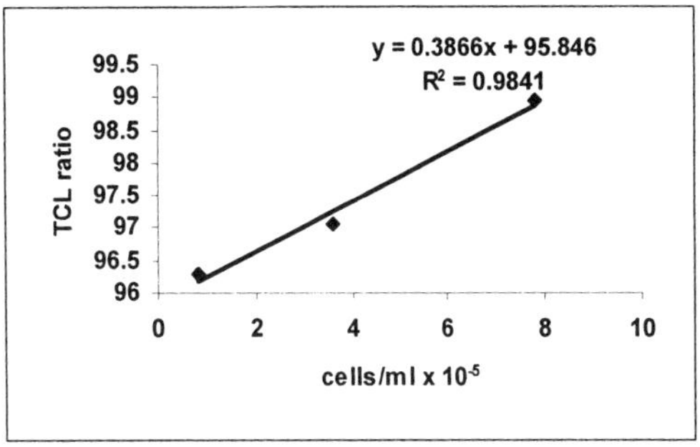

Figure 12. TCL ratio for untreated PC12 cells at different cell concentration

The data presented here confirm previous findings that dopamine caused a dose-dependent death of neuroblastoma cells and that this death was the result of oxidative stress. Oxidative stress was assessed by the TCL method. The TCL data showed positive correlation with the level of the stress, as it increased with increasing concentrations of DA. Furthermore TCL parameter (% TCL/1x105cells) showed negative correlation (R2=0.963) with % surviving cells, even if both experiments are combined. The decrease of TCL ratio found in PC12 cells treated with dopamine shows that the treatment caused oxidative stress to the cells. These findings suggest the TCL method may provide a reliable and easy-to-perform analytical approach for analyzing oxidative stress in whole cells.

7.1.2 Detection of oxidative stress in supernatant of cardiomyocytes during anoxia-reoxygenation

Numerous reports have demonstrated that oxygen free radicals are generated during the anoxia and reoxygenation. The superoxide anion radical is the major reactive oxygen species, generated in the mitochondria and is involved in the production of several potentially damaging species, i.e., hydrogen peroxide, hydroxyl radical and peroxynitrite, that leads to oxidative stress (28,29,30).

The aim of this study was to examine the use and practicality of the new Thermochemiluminescence (TCL) oxidizability assay for detection of oxidative stress in supernatant of cardiomyocytes during anoxia and followed by reoxygenation. Cell cultures of cardiomyocytes of three to four-day-old newborn Wistar rat were prepared as described elsewhere. Briefly, the hearts were removed from the newborns under sterile conditions, minced with scissors in Phosphate Buffered Saline (PBS, calcium and magnesium free) and incubated at room temperature with a dilution of 1:200 of RDB, a proteolytic digestive enzyme (a product of Ness Ziona biological institute, Israel) for 25 min. Then, the supernatant was collected, centrifuged and the cellular sediment was suspended in DMEM medium. The remaining tissues underwent about four more such treatments with RDB until very few cells could be found in the supernatant. All sediments of cells were pooled together and seeded in 35 mm Corning tissue culture dishes in DMEM medium plus 10% horse serum. Prior to the seeding, the dishes had been covered with 0.1% sterile gelatin for at least two hours. About 0.9 million cells were seeded in each plate. On the next day the medium was discarded and fresh one was introduced into the cultures. All the reagents in this study were purchased from Beit – Haemek biological industries, Israel.

Induction of anoxia and reoxygenation (AR), Collection of supernatant: The cultures samples were then subjected to anoxic incubation of another 120 minutes at 370 in a sealed chamber in which N2 (95%) and CO2 (5%) were gassed for 2 hours. Then the cultures were returned to the incubator for 1 hr reoxygenation. When the AR had been completed, the supernatants of the cultures were collected, centrifuged and were prepared for the TCL determinations.

Results: We found significant increase in the baseline of EES formation in supernatant by TCL index 1 (436+/ 13 cps) compared to the control group (394 +/-11 cps) (n = 6, p < 0.01) after AR treatment of cardiomyocytes. The positive TCL curve pattern of supernatant in control, after AR treatment of cardiomyocytes takes negative form (Fig. 13).

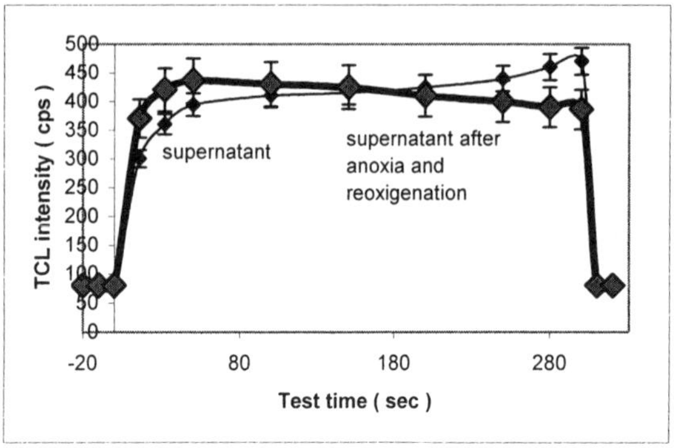

Figure 13. TCL kinetic curves of supernatant before and after AR treatment

TCL ratio after AR treatment was 96 +/- 11 % compared to the control group 113 +/- 9 % ($p < 0.05$). Therefore, the two TCL parameters indicate the active process of oxidative modification of proteins and lipids of a supernatant due to AR treatment of the cardiomyocytes.

7.2 Exposure of saliva ex vivo to cigarette smoke (CS) (in vitro model smoke induced oxidative stress as detected by TCL).

The major ROS and RNS in CS are lipid peroxyl radicals ($ROO^{\bullet}$) and Nitric oxide ($NO^{\bullet}$). Changes of TCL intensity and carbonyl formation in saliva were monitored during exposure to cigarette smoke. In Scheme 1 we show the possible mechanism generation of photon emission due to nitric oxide and peroxyl radical induced oxidative modification of lipids and proteins

The protein carbonyls assay is the best marker of oxidative damage of saliva proteins (32). Protein carbonyls determination in saliva was performed according to the procedure of Reznick and Packer (20). Vacuum-derived smoking apparatus was used for saliva protein damage model as previously described (33).

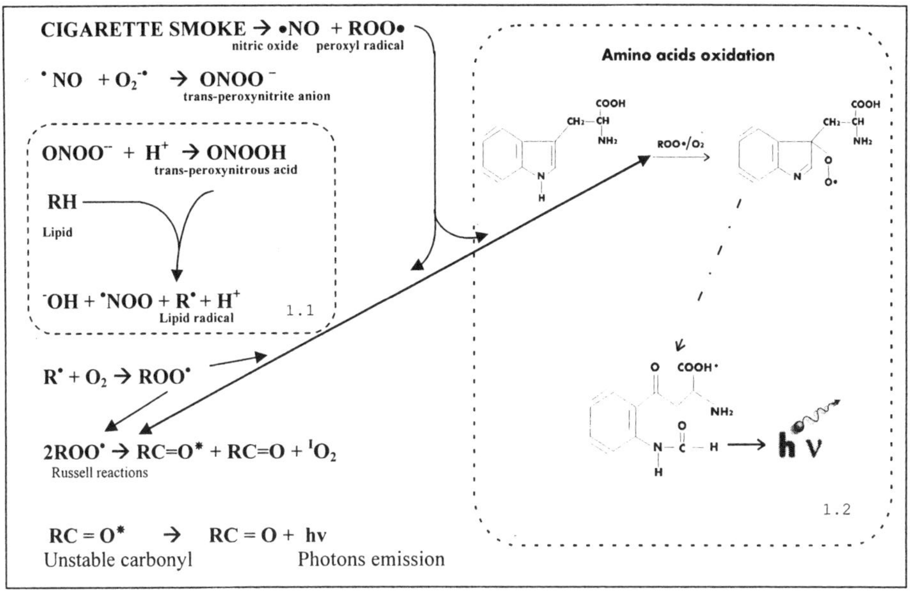

Scheme 1. Nitric oxide and peroxyl radical induced Electronically Excited Species and photon emission formation. [1.1 from (31), 1.2 from (17)]

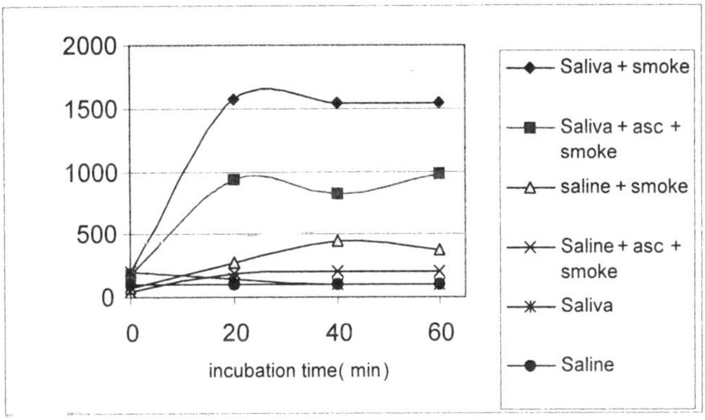

Figure 14. TCL intensity of saliva exposed to CS in the presence and absence of ascorbic acid.

Fig 14 shows the intensity of TCL in saliva exposed to CS and in the presence of ascorbic acid. Saliva was exposed to three puffs of CS at 0, 20 and 40 mins and samples were taken for measurements at 20, 40, and 60 mins. Saliva level of TCL intensity (Index 1) of control saliva was in the range of 200-300 cps. Exposure of saliva to CS for 60 mins increased the level to 1500 cps. However, incubation of saliva in the presence of 1 mM ascorbic acid and exposure to CS, reduced the effect of CS to 800-900 cps. In Fig 15 TCL studies were conducted on saliva exposed to CS and to CS plus alcohol. It can be seen that smoking for 60 mins increased the TCL intensity to1800 cps and upon addition of Ethanol (42%) to the exposed saliva, the increase was augmented to 2200 cps at 40 mins .

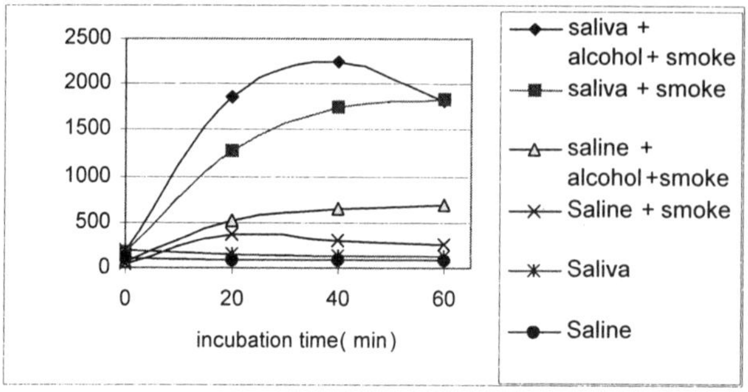

Figure 15. TCL intensity of saliva exposed to CS in the presence and absence of alcohol (42%).

8. Summary

The work described in this monograph presents a new approach to detection of oxidized lipids and proteins using TCL. This methodology is relatively simple to execute and uses the detection of photons emanating from excited carbonyls in biomolecules. The application of this assay has been used for both clinical and laboratory studies and showed that this technology can be applied very efficiently to detect oxidations in biological systems as well as in pathological conditions.

References

[1] Kontush A. and Beisigel U. Measurement of oxidizability of blood plasma. Method in Enzymol, 1999; 299; 35 – 49

[2] Karmansky I., Shnaider H., Palant A., Gruener N. Plasma lipid and susceptibility to of low-density lipoproteins to oxidation in male patients with stable coronary artery disease. Clinical Biochemistry, 1996; 29; 573 – 79.

[3] Haffener SM, Agil A., Mykkanen L., Stern MP., Jialal I. Plasma oxidizability in subjects with normal glucosetolerance, ompaired glucose tolerance, and NIDDM. Diabetes Care, 1995; 18: 646-53.

[4] Salonen GT., Nyyssonen K., Salonen R., Porkkala-Sarataho E., Tuomainen TP., Diczfalusy U., Bjorkhem I. Lipoprotein Oxidation and progression of carotid atherosclerosis. Circulation, 1997; 95:840-45.

[5] Toikka JO.,Niemi P., Ahotura M., Noniikoski H., Ronnemmaa T., Viikari JS., Hartiala JJ., Raitakari OT.Decreased large artery distensibility in borderline hypertension is related to increased in vivo low-density lipoprotein oxidation. Scand J Clin Lab Invest, 2002; 62: 301 – 6.

[6] Schnitzer, E., Pinchuk I., Bor A., Fainaru M., Samuni A. M., Lichtenberg D. Lipid oxidation in unfractionated serum and plasma. Chemistry and Physics of Lipids, 1998; 92:151-17.

[7] Schnitzer E., Pinchuk I., Fainaru M., Schafere Z., Lichtenberg, D. Copper – induced oxidation in unfractionated plasma- the lag preceding oxidation as a measured of oxidation resistance. Biochemical and Biophysical Research Communications, 1995; 216:854-861.

[8] Pinchuk I. and Lichtenberg D. The mechanism of action of Antioxidants against lipoprotein peroxidation, evaluation based on kinetic experiments. Prog. Lipid Res, 2002; 41: 279-319.

[9] Shnizer S., Kagan T., Lanir A., Maor I., Reznick AZ. Modification and oxidation of lipids and proteins in human serum detected by thermochemiluminescence. Luminescence, 2003; 18: 90 –96.

[10] Russell GA. Deuterium-isotope effects in the autoxidation of aryl alkyl hydrocarbons. Mechanism of the interaction of peroxy radicals. J Am. Chem. Soc., 1957; 79 :3871-3877.

[11] Adam W, Beinhauer A, Hauer H. Activation parameters and excitation yields of 1,2- dioxetane chemiluminescence. Handbook of organic photochemistry, 1989; 2: 271-327.

[12] Kopecky KR., Mumford C. Luminescence in the thermal decomposition of 3,3,4-trimethyl- 1,2-dioxetane. Can.J.Chem., 1969 ;47: 709-711.

[13] Schulte-Herbruggen T, Sies H. The peroxidase/oxidase activity of soybean lipoxygenase—II.Triplet carbonyls and red photoemission during polyunsaturated fatty acid and glutatione oxidation. Photochem. Photobiol, 1989; 49 :705-710.

[14] Boverus A, Cadenas E, Chance B. Low-level Chemiluminescence of the lipoxygenase reaction. Photobiochem. Photobiophys, 1980; 1;175-172.

[15] Cadenas E, Sies H. Low-level chemiluminescence of liver microsomal fractions initial by tert–butyl hydroperoxide. Eur. J. Biochem, 1982; 124: 349-356.

[16] Timmins GS, Santos RE, Whitwood AC, Catalani LH, Di Mascio P, Gilbert BC, Bechara EJ. Lipid peroxidation–dependent chemiluminescence from the cyclization of alkylperoxyl radicals to dioxetane radical intermediates. Chem. Res. Toxicol, 1997; 10:1090-1096.

[17] Aspee A, Lissi E.A. Kinetics and mechanism of the chemiluminescence associated with the free radical-mediated oxidation of amino acids. Luminescence, 2000; 15:273-282.

[18] Sudhakar K, Phillips CM, Williams SA, Vanderkooi JM Excited state of tryptophan in code parvalbumin. Identification of a short-lived emitted triplet state at room temperature. Biophysic J., 1993; 64:1503-1511.

[19] Levine RL, Rivett AJ. Oxidative modification of glutamine synthatase: covalent and conformational changes which control susceptibility to proteolysis. Basic Life Sci., 1988; 49: 541-544.

[20] Reznick AZ, Packer L. Oxidative damage to proteins: Spectrophotometric methods for carbonyl assay. Methods Enzymol., 1994; 233: 357–63.

[21] Kanner J and Lapidot T. The stomach as a bioreactor: Dietary lipid peroxidation in the gastric fluid and the effects of plant-derived antioxidants. Free Rad Biol Med., 2001; 31: 1388-95.

[22] Aviram M and Vaya J. Markers for low-density lipoprotein oxidation. Method Enzymol., 2001; 333:244-256.

[23] Maor I., Dor Y., Shnizer S., Kagan T., Lanir A. Enhanced Oxidative stress and decreased Susceptibility to oxidation of serum derived from Septic patients. 2003. The 36th Annulal Meeting of the Israel Society for Clinical Laboratory Sciences. Tel-Aviv, January 23-24.

[24] Offen, D., A. Hochman, S. Gorodin, I. Ziv, A. Shirvan, A. Barzilai, and E. Melamed. Oxidative stress and neuroprotection in Parkinson's disease: implications from studies on dopamine-induced apoptosis Adv Neurol; 1999: 80: 265-9.

[25] Mytilineou, C., S. K. Han, and G. Cohen. Toxic and Protective Effects of L-Dopa on Mesencephalic Cell-Cultures Journal of Neurochemistry, 1993; 6: 1470-1478.

[26] Offen, D., I. Ziv, A. Barzilai, S. Gorodin, E. Glater, A. Hochman, and E. Melamed. Dopamine-melanin induces apoptosis in PC12 cells; possible implications for the etiology of Parkinson's disease Neurochem Int. 1997: 3: 207-16.

[27] Offen, D., I. Ziv, H. Sternin, E. Melamed, and A. Hochman. Prevention of dopamine-induced cell death by thiol antioxidants: possible implications for treatment of Parkinson's disease Exp Neurol., 1996; 141:32-39.

[28] Du G., Mouithys-Mickalad A., Sluse FE. Generation of superoxide anion by mitochondria and impairment of their functions during anoxia and reoxygenation in vitro; Free Rad Biol Med. 1998: 25: 1066 –74.

[29] Mason RB, Pluta RM, Walbridge S., Wink DA., Oldfield EH., Boock RJ. Production of reactive oxygen species after reperfusion in vitro and in vivo: protective effect of nitric oxide. J Neurosurg., 2000; 93: 99-107.

[30] Sasaki H., Ray PS., Zhu L., Galang N., Maulik N. Oxidative stress due to hypoxia/reoxygenation induced angiogenic factor VEGF in adult rat myocardium: possible role of NfkappaB. Toxicology, 2000; 30: 27-35.

[31] Halliwell B. and John M.C. Gutteride. Free radicals in Biology and Medicine. Third Edition.1999. The chemistry of free radials and related " reactive species" p.98

[32] Reznick AZ., Klein I., Eiserich JP., Cross E., Nagler RM. Inhibition of oral peroxidase activity by cigarette smoke: in vivo and in vitro studies. Free Rad Biol Med., 2003; 34: 101-108.

[33] Nagler RM., Lischinsky S., Diamond E., Drigues N., Klein Y., Reznick AZ. Effect of cigarette smoke on salivary proteins and enzyme activities. Arch. Biochem. Biophys., 2001; 379:229-236.

Frontiers in Neurodegenerative Disorders and Aging:
Fundamental Aspects, Clinical Perspectives and New Insights
T. Özben and M. Chevion (Eds.)
IOS Press, 2004

The Role of Insulin/IGF-1 Signaling Pathway in Aging and Cancer

Vladimir N. Anisimov
Department of Carcinogenesis and Oncogerontology, N.N. Petrov Research Institute of Oncology, Pesochny-2, St.Petersburg 197758, Russia, e-mail: aging@mail.ru

Abstract: Studies in mammals have led to the suggestion that hyperglycemia and hyperinsulinemia are important factors both in aging and in the development of cancer. Insulin/insulin-like growth factor 1 (IGF-1) signaling molecules that have been linked to longevity include DAF-2 and InR and their homologues in mammals, and inactivation of the corresponding genes followed by the increase in life span in nematodes, fruit flies and mice. It is possible that the life-prolonging effect of caloric restriction are due to decreasing IGF-1 levels. A search of pharmacological modulators of insulin/IGF-1 signaling pathway mimetic effects of life span extending mutations or calorie restriction could be a perspective direction in regulation of longevity. Some old and new observations suggest that antidiabetic biguanides could be promising candidates for both the life span extension and the prevention of cancer.

1. Introduction

The potential link between aging and insulin/IGF-1 signaling has attracted substantial attention during last years, on the basis of evidence including age-related increase in incidence of insulin resistance and type 2 diabetes in accelerated aging syndromes and life span extension by caloric restriction in rodents. Concomitant reduction in plasma insulin and plasma glucose levels, which implies increases sensitivity to insulin, emerges as a hallmark of increased longevity [17,18,128]. Hyperglycemia is an important aging factor involved in generation of advanced glycosylation endproducts (AGEs) [53,55,132]. There are evidence that hyperinsulinemia favors accumulation of oxidized protein by reducing its degradation as well as facilitates protein oxidation by increasing steady-state level of oxidative stress [55,144]. Untreated diabetics with elevated glucose levels suffer many manifestations of accelerated aging, such as impaired wound healing, obesity, cataracts, vascular and microvascular damage [39]. It was shown that centenarians have a preserved glucose tolerance and sensitivity to insulin as well as lower degree of oxidative stress as compared to aged persons [16,109]. The IGF-1 play a critical role in both cell cycle control and apoptosis, two functions involved in regulation of growth as well as tumorigenesis [74,86].

It is important to stress that hyperinsulinemia is an important factor not only in aging but also in the development of cancer [30,38,39,65]. It is evident that the incidence of both total and fatal tumors decreases in the oldest groups of male and female mice [7,112]. The analysis of data on tumor incidence in *ad libitum* and calorie restricted mice [89,90] shows the same. This result corresponds to observations on a decrease in cancer incidence in centenarians [24,104,111,125].

In organisms ranging from yeast to rodents, both calorie restriction and mutations in insulin/IGF-1 signaling pathway extend life span [17,28,91,117,128,141]. The both approaches have some side effects. For example, calorie restriction increases the level of serum glucocorticoids and decreases resistance to infection [95,96,126] whereas genetic modifications on insulin/IGF-1 signaling pathway cause obesity, dwarfism and cardiopulmonary lesions [91]. Reviewing the available data on the benefits and adverse effects of calorie restriction and genetic modifications Longo and Finch [91] suggested three categories of drugs which may have potential to prevent or postpone age-related diseases and extend life span: drugs that (1) stimulate dwarf mutations and therefore decrease pituitary production of GH; (2) prevent IGF-1 release from the liver, or (3) decrease IGF-1 signaling by the action on either extracellular or intracellular targets. The concept of calorie restriction mimetics is now being intensively explored [66,100,139]. Calorie restriction mimetics involves interventions that produce physiological and anti-aging effects similar to calorie restriction. The comparison of the effects of genetic and pharmacological modifications of insulin/IGF-1 signaling pathway on the longevity in carcinogenesis in mammals reviewed in this chapter have shown the critical role of insulin regulation in aging and cancer.

2. Insulin/IGF-1 signaling pathway and longevity in worms

The intensive investigations in *C. elegans* since 1990's, which have identified insulin signaling components including *daf-2*, *age-1* and *daf-16* as the genes whose mutations lead to life span extension shed new light on molecular mechanisms underlying aging [80,82,88,142]. In *C. elegans*, whole-genome analysis of gene expression during chronological aging has shown that coordinate expression changes in several functional gene groups, including increased expression of insulin-like genes [92]. Three of 12 insulin-related genes have been analysed and insulin homolog, *ins-2* expression was highest in young adult at day 4 and then decreased starting at day 7 until the end of life. *ins-17* and *ins-18* expression levels were 3-folds higher at day 16-19 relative to day 3, and this was similar to the expression level of *ins-2,* whereas *ins-7* expression decreased by 3.3-fold throughout life of worms. At the same time genes of the insulin-like signaling pathway itself (*daf-2* and *age-1*) did not show change in expression during aging. Expression of *sir-2.1* shown a mild increase during days 6-11, followed by a decrease at the end of life. *ins-2* and *ins-18* are thought to antagonize the *daf-2/age-1* insulin-signaling pathway [110]. Lund et al. [92] suggested that increased expression of *ins-2* and *ins-18* in old worms would lead to decreased insulin signaling, increased expression of dauer genes, and increased resistance to late life stressors.

It was shown that mutation in age-1 or daf-23 which encodes catalytic subunit-p110 of PI3-kinase of insulin-like growth factor signal transduction pathway increases life span up to 70-100% in axenic culture [1,105,110]. age-1 mutants also have elevated levels of superoxide dismutase and catalase activities [133,134]. Mutation in age-2 gene increases life-span by 15-20% [146]. A Gompertz analysis suggests that mutation extends life span by reducing the initial mortality rate. An age-1 age-2 double mutant strain lives longer than either single mutant and exhibits a longer life-span at 25 0C than at 20 0C. It was shown that the mutants exhibits normal motility and reduced fertility [146]. Mutation of homologue of mammalian insulin/ insulin-like growth factor ceinsulin-1 or ins-18 which encodes insulin-like ligand predicted to bind DAF-2 display an increased life span of around 30-40% [79]. Mutation of gene daf-2 encoding insulin-like/IGF-1 tyrosine kinase receptor increases life span more than 100% [81] whereas daf-2 daf 12 a double mutation results in a nearly 300% increase in life span [85]. There are evidences that a mutation of daf-2 also increased expression of SOD-3, the Mn-superoxide dismutase [70]. Mutation of nuclear hormone receptor gene daf-12 modestly shortens mean life span of C.elegans [60,85].

Overexpression of forkhead transcription factor gene *daf-16* increases life-span by 20%, whereas a loss of function allele shortens it [68]. Mutation of *daf-16* suppresses all the phenotypes of *daf-2* and *age-1* mutants, including life span extension, dauer arrest, reduced fertility, and viability defects [51,81,85,130]. Mutation of gene encoding RFX-type transcription factor *daf-19* or *daf-24* increases life span by 50% [13]. Transgenic overexpression of human insulin gene *INS* under an inducible heat shock promoter or gene *ins-1* encoding the insulin-like protein under its own promoter as well as a heat shock promoter increases the life span of *C. elegans* by 25% and also enhances the life span extension of a *daf-2* mutant [110].

3. Insulin/IGF-1 signaling pathway and longevity in fruit flies

In *D. melanogaster*, the mutation modification of genes operating in the signal transduction from insulin receptor to transcription factor *daf-16* (*age*-1, daf-2, CHICO, InR и др.) are strongly associated with longevity [29,36,80,129]. It was demonstrated that FKHR, FKHRL1 and AFX, which are mammalian homologues of daf-16 forkhead transcription factor, function downstream of insulin signaling and akt/PKB under cellular conditions [113,115]. However, it is an open question whether insulin signaling components, including forkhead transcriptional factors, play a critical role in aging and longevity in mammals as well as in *C. elegans* and *D. melanogaster*.

4. Insulin/IGF-1 signaling pathway and longevity in rodents

Daf-2 and InR are structural homologues of tyrosine kinase receptors in vertebrata that includes the insulin receptor and the insulin-like growth factor type 1 receptor (IGF-1R). It was shown that in vertebrates the insulin receptor regulates energy metabolism whereas IGF-1R promotes growth. Although decreased insulin-like signaling appears to increase longevity in *C. elegans* and in *D. melanogaster*, whether the same is true in mammals is unclear. At least three genes ($Pit1^{dw}$, $Prop1^{dw}$, *Ghr*) has been identified in which knockout lead to dwarfism with reduced levels of IGF-1 and insulin and to increased longevity [31,58]. In Snell and Ames dwarf mice, sexual maturation is delayed, and male only few males are fertile, while females are invariably sterile [18]. These mice as well as $Ghr^{-/-}$ knockout mice have significantly reduced glucose levels and fasting insulin levels, decreased tolerance to glucose and increased sensitivity to insulin which appears to be combined with reduced ability to release glucose in response to acute challenge [17,18].

Recently, very strong support for the role of insulin/IGF-1 signaling pathway in the control of mammalian aging and for the involvement of this pathway in longevity of IGF-1 deficient mice was provided by Hsieh et al. [71,72]. It was shown that in the Snell dwarf mice, GH deficiency would lead to reduced insulin secretion and alterations in insulin signaling via InRβ, IRS-1 or IRS-2 and P13K affects genes involved in the control longevity. The authors concluded that the Pit1 mutation may result in physiological homeostasis that favors longevity.

Reduction in both glucose and insulin levels as well as an increase in the sensitivity to insulin are a well-documented response to caloric restriction in rodents and monkey [117,140]. It was shown that improved sensitivity to insulin in caloric restricted animals is specifically related to reducing visceral fat [19]. It is worthy to note that *Ghr*$^{-/-}$ mice have a major increase in the level of insulin receptors [49], while Ames dwarf mice have a smaller increase in insulin receptor and substantially increased amount of insulin receptor substrates IRS-1 and IRS-2 [50]. It is worthy of note that the development of tumors in Ames dwarf mice was postponed and the incidence was reduced as compared to the control [77,97].

The crucial event of the effect of caloric restriction is low levels of insulin and IGF-1 and also an increase insulin sensitivity in rodents [28,141] as well as in monkeys [83,98,101]. Many characteristics of these long-lived mutants and GH-receptor knockout mice resemble those of normal animals exposed to caloric restriction. These characteristics include reduced plasma levels of IGF-1, insulin and glucose, with the consequent reductions in growth and body size, delayed puberty, and significantly increased sensitivity to insulin action.

In a bid to discover whether the IGF-1 receptor might control vertebrate longevity, Holzenberger et al. [69] inactivated the *Igf1r* gene by homologous recombination in mice. It was shown that *Igf1r*$^{-/-}$ mice dead early in the life, whereas heterozygous *Igf1r*$^{+/-}$ mice live on average 26% longer than their wild-type littermates ($p<0.02$). It is worthy of note that long-lived mice do not develop dwarfism, their energy metabolism was normal. Food intake physical activity, fertility and reproduction were also unaffected in *Igf1r*$^{+/-}$. The spontaneous tumor incidence in the aging cohort of *Igf1r*$^{+/-}$ mice was similar to that in wild-type controls. It is very important that these *Igf1r*$^{+/-}$ mice, and mouse embryonic fibroblasts derived from them, were more resistant to oxidative stress than controls. At the molecular level, insulin receptor substrate and the *p52* and *p66* isoforms of *Shc*, both main substrates of IGF-1 receptor, showed decreased tyrosine phosphorylation. *p66*^{Shc} mediated cellular responses to oxidative stress. Two main pathways - the extracellular-signal reulated kinase (ERK)/mitogen-activated protein kinase (MAPK) pathway and the phosphatidylinositol 3-kinase (PI3K)-Akt pathway – were downregulated in *Igf1r*$^{+/-}$ mice.

The extension of longevity was observed in fat-specific insulin receptor knockout (FIRKO) mice [22]. These animals have reduced fat mass and were protected against age-related obesity and its subsequent metabolic abnormalities including deterioration in glucose tolerance, although their food intake was normal. Both male and female FIRKO mice were found to have an increase in mean life span (by 18%) with parallel increases in maximum life span. Extended longevity in FIRKO mice was associated with a shift in the age at which age-dependent increase in mortality risk becomes appreciable and a decreased rate of age-related mortality, especially after 36 months of age. In FIRKO mice, the resistance to obesity, despite normal food intake, suggests that metabolic rate is increased, rather than decreased [23]. The authors believe that decreased fat mass could lead to a decrease in oxidative stress in FIRKO mice. Another possibility is that the increased longevity in these mice is the direct result of altered insulin signaling.

Shimokawa et al. [122] designed a transgenic strain of rats whose GH gene was suppressed by an anti-sense GH transgene. Male rats homozygous for the transgene (*tg/tg*) had a reduced number of pituitary GH cells, a lower plasma concentration of IGF-1, and a dwarf phenotype. Heterozygous rats (*tg/-)* had an intermediate phenotype in plasma IGF-1, food intake, and body weight between *tg/tg* and control (-/-) rats. The life span of *tg/tg* rats was 5 to 10% shorter than -/- rats. In contrast, the life span of *tg/-* rats was 7 to 10% longer than -/- rats.

It was found that tumors caused earlier death in *tg/tg* rats; in contrast, *tg/-* rats had reduced nonneoplastic diseases and a prolonged life span. Immunological analysis revealed a smaller population and lower activity of splenic natural killer cells in homozygous *tg/tg* rats. These results provided evidence that an optimal level of the GH-IGF-1 axis function needs for longevity in mammals.

5. Insulin/IGF-1 signaling pathway and longevity in humans

Recently it was shown that the incidence of mutations in insulin regulatory region (IRE) of APO C-III T-455 C directly correlates with longevity in humans. This is the first evidence showing that mutation located downstream to *daf-16* in the insulin signal transduction system is associated with longevity [3]. It is worth noting that centenarians display lower degree of resistance to insulin and lower degree of oxidative stress as compared with elderly persons before 90 years [16,109]. The authors suggest that centenarians may have been selected for appropriate insulin regulation as well as for the appropriate regulation of tyrosine hydroxylase (TH) gene, whose product is the rate limiting in the synthesis of catecholamines, stress-response mediators. It was shown that catecholamine may increase free radical production through induction of the metabolic rate and autooxidation in diabetic animals [123]. Recent study on aging parameters of young (up to 39) and old (over 70) individuals having similar IGF-1 serum levels provides evidence of important role of this peptide for life potential [119]. Roth et al. [118] analyzed data from the Baltimore Longitudinal Study of Aging and reported that survival was greater in men who maintained lower insulin level.

6. Pharmacological effects on insulin/IGF-1 signaling pathway and longevity

It is clear that the direct translation of genetic manipulations or calorie restriction to humans is generally impractical because major dietary and lifestyle changes, such as 20-40% decrease in calorie intake, are very difficult for most people [103]. It was stressed that new approaches to translation are therefore needed to fulfill the promise of the health benefits of calorie restriction. Agents or interventions that reduce IGF-1 may provide an effective pharmacological mimetic of those effects, which could be readily adopted by a large proportion of the populations [74]. Small-molecule inhibitors of IGF-1 [136] or IGF/IGFBP [27], as well as antisense IGF-1 inhibitor [121] and anti-IGF-1 antibody therapies [64] could be used for the decrease in IGF-1 serum level.

Several years ago, it was suggested to use biguanide antidiabetics as a potential anti-aging treatment [37-39]. The antidiabetic drugs, phenformin (1-phenylethylbiguanide), buformin (1-butylbiguanide hydrochloride) and metformin (N,N-dimethylbiguanide) were observed to reduce hyperglycemia, improve glucose utilization, reduce free fatty acid utilization, gluconeogenesis, serum lipids, insulin, somatomedin, reduce body weight and decrease metabolic immunodepression both in humans and rodents [20,38,39,106,107] (Table 1). Nowadays, phenformin is not used in clinical practice due to it side effects (mainly lactic acidosis) observed in patients with non-compensated diabetes. It is worthy of note that during more than 10-year-long experience of administration of phenformin to patients without advanced diabetes no cases of lactic acidosis or any other side effects have been observed [20,39]. Nevertheless we believe that the analysis of results of long-term administration of this drug as well as another antidiabetic biguanides (buformin and metformin) to non-diabetic animals is seems very important for understanding of links between insulin and longevity.

Buformin was supplemented to nutrient medium in various concentration (from 1.0 to 0.00001 mg/ml) during the larvae stage and over the life span of *C. elegans*. The drug given at the concentration of 0.1 mg/ml increased the mean life span of the nematoda by 23.4% ($p < 0.05$) and the maximum life span by 26.1% as compared to the controls [15].

. The available data on effect of antidiabetic biguanides on life span in mice and rats summarized in the Table 2. Female C3H/Sn mice were kept from the age of 3.5 months at standard *ad libitum* diet were given phenformin 5 times a week orally at a single dose 2 mg/mouse until a natural death [42]. The treatment with phenformin prolonged the mean life span of mice by 21% ($p < 0.05$), the mean life span of last 10% survivors by 28% and the maximum life span by 5.5 months (by 26%) in comparison with the control. At the time of death of the last mice in the control group 42% of phenformin-treated mice were alive (Fig.1A).

Table 1. Effects of antidabetic biguanides [39,106,104]

Effects on metabolic parameters	Effects on homeostatic regulation	Effects on age-related pathology
Reduction of excessive insulin levels after glucose loading in obese and diabetic subjects	An increase in the sensitivity of the hypothalamo-pituitary complex to inhibition by estrogens	Inhibition of the development of atherosclerosis
A decrease in IGF-1 in the serum	A restoration of ovarian function in aged rats	Inhibition of spontaneous tumors development
Inhibition of hepatic gluconeogenesis	An increase in the sensitivity of the hypothalamo-pituitary complex to inhibition by glucocorticoids	Reduction in blood pressure in hypertensive patients
Lowering of blood cholesterol and triglyceride levels	An altered hypothalamic regulation of ingestive behaviors	An increase in blood fibrinolytic activity
An increase in the insulin sensitivity of target cells	Increase dopamine release in mesolimbic structures	An improvement in indices of cellular immunity in humans
An increase in glucose utilization	A lowering of monoamine oxidase activity	A decrease in the immunosuppressive effect of a potent carcinogen, 1,2-dimethylhydrazine
An increase in glucose utilization		
A decrease in cholesterol metabolism in human fibroblasts		
A decrease in the concentration of cholesterol in lymphocytes and platelets		

Phenformin was given 5 times a week to female outbred LIO rats starting from the age of 3.5 month until a natural death in a single dose of 5 mg/rat/day orally [5,6]. Administration of phenformin failed influence the mean life span in rats. At the same time, the mean life span of the last 10% survivors was increased by 10% ($p < 0.005$), and maximum life span was increased by 3 months (+ 10%) in comparison with the controls (Table 2). The treatment with phenformin slightly decreased the body weight of rats in comparison with the control ($p > 0.05$). The disturbances in the estrus function observed in 36 % of 15-16-month old rats of the control group and only in 7% of rats in phenformin-treated group ($p < 0.05$).

Table 2. Effect of antidiabetic biguanides on life span in mice and rats

Species, strain	Treatment	No. of animals	Life span, days			References
			Mean	Last 10% of survivors	Maximum	
C3H/Sn mice	Control	30	450 ± 23.4	631 ± 11.4	643	[42]
	Phenformin	24	545 ± 39.2 (+21.1%)	810 ± 0 ** (+28.4%)	810 (+26%)	
LIO rats	Control	41	652 ± 27.3	885 ± 11.3	919	[5,6]
	Phenformin	44	652 ± 28.7	974 ± 16.2** (+10.1%)	1009 (+9.8%)	
	Control	74	687 ± 19.2	925 ± 22.5	1054	[4]
	Buformin	42	737 ± 26.4 (+7.3%)	1036± 38.9* (+12%)	1112 (+5.5%)	

The difference with control is significant: * - $p < 0.05$; ** $p < 0.01$ (Student's *t* test).

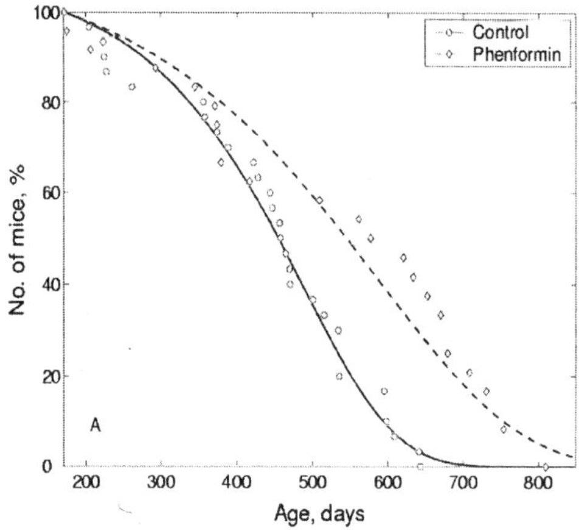

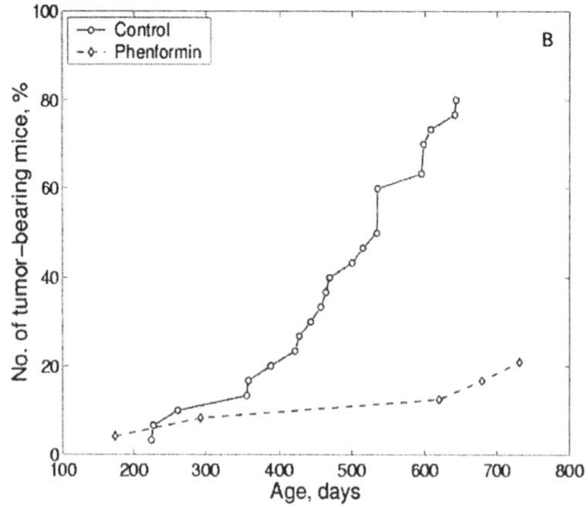

Figure 1. Effect of phenformin on the survival (A) and tumor yield (B) curves in female C3H/Sn mice.

Buformin was given 5 times a week to female LIO rats starting from the age of 3.5 month until a natural death in a single dose of 5 mg/rat/day orally [4]. The treatment slightly increased the mean life span of rats (by 7%; $p > 0.05$). The mean life span of the last 10% survivors increased by 12% ($p < 0.05$) and the maximum life span increased by 2 months (+5.5%) as compared with controls. The body weight of rats treated with buformin was slightly (5.2 to 9.4%) but statistically significantly ($p < 0.05$) decreased in comparison with the control from the age of 12 months to 20 months ($p < 0.05$). At the age of 16-18 months 38% of control rats revealed the disturbances in the estrus cycle persistent estrus, repetitive pseudopregnancies or anestrus), whereas in females treated with buformin these disturbances were observed only in 9% of rats ($p < 0.05$).

Recently it was found that metformin, like buformin and phenformin, significantly increases the life span of rats (G.S. Roth, personal communication).

Several other effects of treatment with antidiabetic biguanides related to reproduction and aging, are known from earlier studies. For example, it decreased hypothalamic threshold of the sensitivity to feedback inhibition by estrogens [10,40], which is one of the most important mechanisms regulating age-related decline and switch-off of the reproductive function [40,73,116,145]. It is worthy of note that another antidiabetic biguanide, metformin, may improve menstrual regularity, leading to spontaneous ovulation, and enhance the induction of ovulation with clomiphene citrate in women with polycystic ovary syndrome [14,108]. The treatment with phenformin also decreased hypothalamic threshold sensitivity to feedback regulation by glucocorticoids and by metabolic stimuli (glucose and insulin) [39,40]. It was recently shown that elements involved in the insulin/IGF-1 signaling pathway are regulated at the expression and/or functional level in the central nervous system. This regulation may play a role in the brain's insulin resistance [57], in the control of ovarian follicular development and ovulation [114], and brain's control of life span [28,99,101]. Antidiabetic biguanides also alleviated age-related metabolic immunodepression [39]. These mechanisms can be involved in geroprotective effect of biguanides (Fig.2). Treatment with chromium picolinate which elevated the insulin sensitivity in several tissues, including hypothalamus, significantly increased the mean life span and decreased the development of age-related pathology in rats [102]. We hypothesized that antidiabetic biguanides and possibly chromium picolinate, have regulate thyrosine hydroxilase and insulin/IGF-1 signaling pathway genes both associated with longevity [32,33,80]. It was shown that the polymorphism at TH-INS locus affects non-insulin dependent type 2 diabetes [76], and is associated with hypothalamic obesity [138], polycystosis ovary syndrome [137], hypertriglyceridemia and atherosclerosis [131].

7. The role of IGF-1 in cancer

It was shown that GF enhances the growth of a variety of cancer cell lines in vitro [87,94,124]. IGF-1 receptors (IGF-1R) overexpressed in many tumors, and IGF-1 acts directly on cells via the IGF-1R or indirectly through its action with other molecules. IGF-1 and p53 appear to function together in a regulatory network. The p53 gene regulates the expression of IGFBP-3 [25], and IGF-1-induced mitogenesis is associated with phosphorylation and translocation of the p53 protein from the nucleus to the cytoplasm [127]. In various animals models, stimulation of IGF-1 level was followed by promoting effect on carcinogenesis [61].

It was discussed in previous sections that in genetically modified mice with low level of IGF-1 the postponement and, in some cases, the decrease in spontaneous tumor development have been observed. In contrast, tissue-specific overexpression of IGF-1 through the keratin 5 promoter increases spontaneous tumor development [34,35] and susceptibility to bladder carcinogenesis [75].

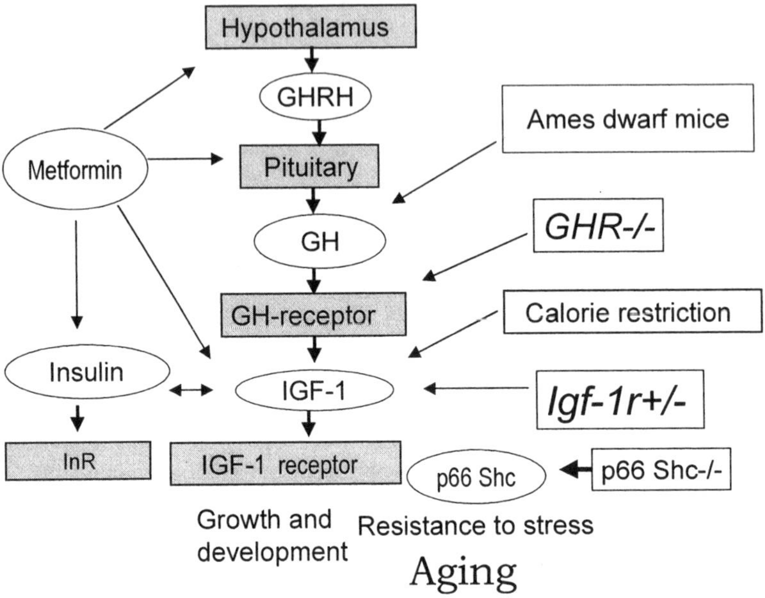

Figure 2. Proposed effects of metformin, calorie restriction and genetic modifications on insulin/IGF-1 signaling pathway in control of aging

There are epidemiological evidence which supports the hypothesis that IGF-1 is involved in human cancer. Clinical conditions associated with high levels of insulin (noninsulin-dependent diabetes mellitus and hypertriglyceridemia) and IGF-1 (acromegaly) are related to increased risk of colon cancer, and increasing circulating levels of nsulin and IGF-1 are related to a higher risk of colonic neoplasia [61,62]. In the studies to investigate whether IGF-1 and/or IGFBP-3 levels are associated with colon cancer risk, it was found that both elevated levels of IGF-1 and decreased levels of IGFBP-3 were associated with an increased risk of developing colon cancer in men [93,148]. A study nested within the Nurses Health Study subsequently found similar results [63]. It was found that elevated serum IGF-1 levels are associated with an increased risk of developing prostatic cancer in men [relative risk (RR): 4.1] [26], breast cancer in premenopausal women (RR: 2.3) but not in postmenopausal women [67]. On the other hand, IGFBP-3 levels were not associated with cancer risk in either group. Another case-control study demonstrated that levels of IGF-1, but not of IGF-2 or IGFBP-3, were linked with lung cancer [148]. The epidemiological association between levels of IGF-1 and IGFBP and the risk of various cancers certainly requires more investigation, particularly additional prospective studies to better establish the temporal nature of any associations. However, when considered together, the multiple human studies reported to date suggest that components of the IGF-1 system are important risk factors in the development of several human cancers [74,78,147,148].

8. Pharmacological modification of insulin/IGF-1 signaling pathway in cancer treatment and prevention

Long-term treatment with phenformin significantly inhibited (by 4.0-fold, $p < 0.01$) the incidence of spontaneous mammary adenocarcinomas in female C3H/Sn mice [42]. The tumor yield curve rise was also significantly slowed down as a result of the treatment (Fig. 1B). The treatment with phenformin was followed by 1.6-fold decrease in total spontaneous tumor incidence in rats [5], whereas total tumor incidence was decreased by 49.5% in buformin-treated rats [4].

The anticarcinogenic effect of antidiabetic biguanides has been demonstrated in several models of induced carcinogenesis (Table 3). Daily oral administration of phenformin or buformin suppressed DMBA-induced mammary tumor development in rats [9,11,45]. Phenformin-treated rats revealed a tendency toward a decrease in serum insulin level. The treatment with phenformin normalised the tolerance to glucose and serum insulin and IGF-1 level in rats exposed to intravenous injections of N-nitrosomethylurea (NMU) and inhibited mammary carcinogenesis in these animals [9]. Treatment of rats with 1,2-dimethylhydrazine (DMH) (once a week during 4 weeks) caused the decrease in the level of biogenic amines, particularly, of dopamine in the hypothalamus, the decrease of glucose tolerance and the increase of the blood level of insulin and triglycerides. The exposure to DMH also caused the inhibition of lymphocyte blastogenic response to phytohemagglutinin and lipopolysaccharide, the decrease in the level of antibody produced against sheep erythrocytes and the decrease in phagocytic activity of macrophages [48]. Administration of phenformin started from the 1st injection of the carcinogen restored all the above mentioned immunological indices and inhibited DMH-induced colon carcinogenesis [12,48]. It is worthy to note that colon 38 adenocarcinoma growth was significantly inhibited in liver-specific IGF-1-deficient mice whereas injections with recombinant human IGF-1 displayed sufficiently promoted the tumor growth and metastazing [143]. A treatment with somatostatin analogue, which reduces circulating IGF-1 levels, retards colonic tumor growth [52].

A decrease of glucose utilisation in the oral glucose tolerance test was found in the 3-month-old female progeny of rats exposed to NMU on the 21st day of pregnancy [2]. The serum insulin level did not differ from the control, but the cholesterol level was higher in offspring of NMU-treated rats as compared with the control. Postnatal treatment with buformin started from the age of 2 months significantly inhibited the development of malignant neurogenic tumors in rats transplancentally exposed to NMU [2]. Similar results have been observed in rats exposed transplacentally to N-nitrosoethylurea (NEU) and postnatally to phenformin [21]. The authors observed the decrease of development of nervous system and renal tumors induced transplacentally with NEU. The treatment with phenformin inhibited also the carcinogenesis induced by a single total-body X-rays irradiation in rats [8].

Table 3. Effect antidiabetic biguanides on carcinogenesis in mice and rats

Species	Drug	Carcinogen	Main target(s)	Effect of treatment	References
Mouse	Phenformin	Spontaneous	Mammary gland	Inhibition	[42]
	Phenformin	MCA	Subcutaneous tissue	Inhibition	[135]
Rat	Buformin	Spontaneous	Total incidence	Inhibition	[4]
	Phenformin	Spontaneous	Total incidence	Inhibition	[5,6]
	Phenformin	DMBA	Mammary gland	Inhibition	[45]
	Phenformin	NMU	Mammary gland	Inhibition	[9]
	Buformin	DMBA	Mammary gland	Inhibition	[11]
	Buformin	NMU, transplacentally	Nervous system	Inhibition	[2]
	Phenformin	NEU, transplacentally	Nervous system, kidney	Inhibition	[21]
	Phenformin	DMH	Colon	Inhibition	[12,48]
	Phenformin	X-rays	Total incidence	Inhibition	[8]
Hamster	Metformin	NBOPA	Pancreas	Inhibition	[120]

Abbreviations: DMH – 1,2-dimethylhydrazine; MCA – 20-methylcholanthrene; NBOPA -N-nitrosobis-(2-oxopropyl)amine; NEU – N-nitrosoethylurea; NMU – N-nitrosomethylurea; X-rays – total-body X-ray irradiation.

Vinnitski and Iakumenko [135] have shown that treatment with phenformin increased the immunological reactivity and inhibited carcinogenesis induced by s.c. administration of 20-methylcholanthrene in BALB/c mice. In high fat-fed hamsters, the treatment with N-nitrosobis-(2-oxopropyl)amine was followed by the development of pancreatic malignancies in 50% of cases, whereas no tumors were found in the hamsters treated with the carcinogen and metformin [120].

Thus, anticarcinogenic effect of antidiabetic biguanides has been demonstarted in relation to spontaneous carcinogenesis in mice and rats, in different models of chemical carcinogenesis in mice, rats and hamsters, and in radiation carcinogenesis model in rats. Phenformin administered orally to mice potentiated the antitumor effect of cytostatic drug cyclophosphamide on transplantable squamous cell cervical carcinoma, hepatoma-22a and Lewis lung carcinoma. Administration of phenformin to rats with transplanted Walker 256 carcinoma enhanced the antitumor effect of hydrazine sulfate [41].

The comparative study of 10-years results of metabolic rehabilitation (included restricted in fat and carbohydrate diet and treatment with antidiabetic biguanides) of cancer patients had shown significant increase in the survival of breast and colorectal cancer patients, the increase in the length of cancer-free period, the decrease in the incidence of metastasis as compared with control patients [20].

It was suggested that antidiabetic biguanides inhibit the metabolic immunodepression, developed in animals exposed to carcinogenic agents which is similar to the immunodepression inherent to normal aging and specific age-related pathology [38,39]. If immunodepression is one of the important factors in carcinogenesis, then the elimination of metabolic immunodepression, which arises in the course of normal aging or under the influence of chemical carcinogens or ionizing radiation, can provide an anticarcinogenic prophylactic effect [6,38,39,48].

Although it is known that free radicals are produced during metabolic reactions, it is largely unknown which factor(s), of physiological or pathophysiological significance, modulate their production in vivo. It has been suggested that hyperinsulinemia may have increase free radicals and therefore promote aging, independent of glycemia [37,39,54-56]. Plasma levels of lipid hydroperoxides are higher, and antioxidant vitamins are lower in individuals who are resistant to insulin-stimulated glucose disposal but otherwise glucose tolerant, nonobese, and normotensive [56]. This finding indicates that enhanced oxidative stress is present before diabetes ensues and therefore cannot simply be explained by overt hyperglycemia. There is substantial evidence supporting the hypothesis that selective resistance to insulin-stimulated (muscle) glucose disposal and the consequential compensatory hyperinsulinemia trigger a variety of metabolic effects, likely resulting in accelerated oxidative stress and aging [39,55].

The anti-diabetics biguanides inhibit fatty acid oxidation, inhibit gluconeogenesis in the liver, increase the availability of insulin receptors, inhibit monoamine oxidase [106,107], increase sensitivity of hypothalamo-pituitary complex to negative feedback inhibition, reduce excretion of glucocorticoid metabolites and dehydroepiandrosterone-sulfate [39]. These drugs have been proposed for the prevention of the age-related increase of cancer and atherosclerosis, and for retardation of the aging process [38,39]. It has been shown that administration of antidiabetic biguanides into patients with hyperlipidemia lowers the level of blood cholesterol, triglycerides, and β-lipoproteins. It also inhibits the development of atherosclerosis, reduces hyperinsulinemia in men with coronary artery disease. It increases hypothalamo-pituitary sensitivity to inhibition by dexamethasone and estrogens, causes restoration of estrous cycle in persistent-estrous old rats, improves cellular immunity in atherosclerotic and cancer patients, lowers blood IGF-1 levels in cancer and atherosclerotic patients with Type IIb hyperlipoproteinemia [43,44,46,47]. Recently it was shown that metformin decreases platelet superoxide anion production in diabetic patients [59].

Table 4. Comparison of characteristics of rodents subjected to normal aging, caloric restriction, genetic modifications or treatment with antidiabetic biguanides

Parameters	Aging	Calorie restriction	Dwarf mice	$GHR^{-/-}$	$Igf1r^{+/-}$	FIRKO	Antidiabetic biguanides
Life span extension	↓	+40-50%	+50%	+46%	+33%	+18%	+20%
Tolerance to glucose	↓	↑	↓	↓	↑↓[a]	= or ↑	↑
Sensitivity to insulin	↓	↑	↑	↑	↑	↑ in fat	↑
Serum level: insulin	↑	↓	↓	↓	=	↓	↓
GH	↓	↓	Absent	↑	ND	↓	↓
IGF-1	↓	↓	↓	↓	↓	↓	↓
Body size	↑	↓	↓	↓	↓	↓	↓
Body fat content	↑	↓	↑	ND	↑↓	↓	↓
Reproductive function	↓	↓[b]	↓[b]	↓[b]	=[b]	ND	↑
Thyroid function	↓	↓	↓	↓	=	ND	↑
Serum corticosterone	↑	↑	=	=	ND	ND	↓
Immune function	↓	↓	= or ↓	ND	ND	ND	↑
Resistance to oxidatve stress	↓	↑	↓	↓	↑	↑	↑
Tumor incidence	↑	↓	= or ↓	=	=	ND	↓

Note: ↓ - decrease; ↑ - increase; = no effect; ND – no available data.

[a] The tolerance to glucose is increased in females but decreased in male.

[b] Reproductive function in relation to normal aging mice.

9. Conclusion

The striking similarities have been described between insulin/IGF-1 signaling pathways in yeast, worms, flies, and mice [80]. Many characteristics of mice that are long lived due to genetic modifications resemble effects of caloric restriction in wild-type (normal) animals (Table 4). Comparison of characteristics of exposed to these endogenous and exogenous influences shows a number of similarities but also some differences. Effects of antidiabetic biguanides seems to be more adequate in the prevention of age-related deteriorations in glucose metabolism and in insulin signaling pathway as well as in such important for longevity parameters as a fertility and a resistance to oxidative stress and tumorigenesis than those induced by caloric restriction and genetic manipulations.

Acknowledgements

This paper was written in the framework of the project "Cancer Rates Over Age, Time, and Place" at the Max-Planck Institute for Demographic Research, Rostock, Germany, and was supported in part by grant # 01-04-07007 from the Russian Foundation for Basic Research. The author is thankful to James W. Vaupel for the opportunity to use the facilities of the Max Planck Institute for Demographic Research to complete this paper.

References

[1] Ailion M, Inoue T, Weaver CI et al. Neurosecretory control of aging in *Caenorhabditis elegans. Proc Natl Acad Sci USA* 1999; 96: 7394-7397.
[2] Alexandrov VA, Anisimov VN, Belous NM et al. The inhibition of the transplacental blastomogenic effect of nitrosomethylurea by postnatal administration of buformin to rats. *Carcinogenesis* 1980; 1: 975-978.
[3] Anisimov SV, Volkova MV, Lenskaya LV et al. Age-associated accumulation of the Apolipoprotein C-III gene T-455C polymorphism C allele in a Russian population. *J Gerontol Biol Sci* 2001; 56A: B27-B32.
[4] Anisimov VN. Effect of buformin and diphenylhydantoin on life span, estrus function and spontaneous tumor incidence in female rats. *Vopr Onkol* 1980; 26(6): 42-48.
[5] Anisimov VN. Effect of phenformin on life span, estrus function and spontaneous tumor incidence in rats. *Farmakol Toksikol* 1982; 45(4): 127.
[6] Anisimov VN. *Carcinogenesis and Aging. Vol. 2.* Boca Raton: CRC Press, 1987.
[7] Anisimov VN. The relationship between aging and carcinogenesis: a critical appraisal. *Crit Rev Oncol Hematol* 2003; 45: 277-304.
[8] Anisimov VN, Belous NM, Prokudina EA. Inhibition by phenformin of the radiation carcinogenesis in female rats. *Exp Onkol* 1982; 4(6): 26-29.
[9] Anisimov VN, Belous NM, Vasilyeva IA, Dilman VM. Inhibitory effect of phenformin on the development of mammary tumors induced by N-nitrosomethylurea in rats. *Exp Onkol* 1980; 2(3): 40-43.
[10] Anisimov VN, Dilman VM. The increase of hypothalamic sensitivity to the inhibition by estrogens induced by the treatment with L-DOPA, diphenylhydantoin or phenformin in old rats. *Bull Exp Biol Med* 1975; 80(11): 96-98.
[11] Anisimov VN, Ostroumova MN, Dilman VM. Inhibition of blastomogenic effect of 7,12-dimethylbenz-(a)anthracene in female rats by buformin, dipheninhydantoin, polypeptide pineal extract and L-DOPA. *Bull Exp Biol Med* 1980; 89: 723-725.
[12] Anisimov VN, Pozharisski KM, Dilman VM. Effect of phenformin on the blastomogenic action of 1,2-dimethylhydrazine in rats. *Vopr Onkol* 1980; 26(8): 54-58.
[13] Apfeld J, Kenyon C. Regulation of lifespan by sensory perception in *Caenorhabditis elegans. Nature* 1999; 402: 804-809.
[14] Awartani KA, Cheung AP. Metformin and polycystic ovary syndrome: a literature review. *J Obstet Gynecol Can* 2002. 24, 393-401.
[15] Bakaev VV. Effect of 1-butylbiguanide hydrochloride on the longevity in the nematoda *Caenorhabditis elegans. Biogerontology* 2002; 3(Suppl 1): 23-24.
[16] Barbieri M, Rizzo MR, Manzella D et al. Glucose regulation and oxidative stress in healthy centenarians. *Exp Gerontol* 2003; 38: 137-143.
[17] Bartke A, Chandrashekar V, Dominici F et al. Insulin-like growth factor 1 (IGF01) and aging: controverses and new insights. *Biogerontology* 2003; 4: 1-8.
[18] Bartke A, Turyn D. Mechanisms of prolonged longevity: mutants, knock-outs, and caloric restriction. *J*

Anti-Aging Med 2001; 4: 197-203.
[19] Barzilai N, Gupta G. Interaction between aging and syndrome X: new insights on the pathophysiology of fat distribution. *Ann NY Acad Sci* 1999; 892: 58-72.
[20] Berstein LM, Evtushenko TP, Tsyrlina EV et al. Comparative study of 5- and 10-year-long results of the metabolic rehabilitation of cancer patients. In: Hanson KP, Dilman VM (Eds). *Neuroendocrine System, Metabolism, Immunity and Cancer (Clinical Aspects)*. St. Petersburg: NN Petrov Research Institute of Oncology Publ, 1992, pp 102-112.
[21] Bespalov VG, Alexandrov VA. Influence of anticarcinogenic agents on the transplacental carcinogenic effect of N-nitroso-N-ethylurea. *Bull Exp Biol Med* 1985; 100: 73-76.
[22] Bluher M, Kahn BB, Kahn CR. Extended longevity in mice lacking the insulin receptor in adipose tissue. *Science* 2003; 299: 572-574.
[23] Bluher M, Michael MD, Peroni OD et al. Adipose tissue selective insulin receptor knockout protects against obesity and obesity-related glucose intolerance. *Dev Cell* 2002; 3: 25-38.
[24] Bordin P, Da Gol PG, Peruzzo P et al. Causes of death and clinical diagnostic error in extreme aged hosptalized people: a retrospective clinical-necropsy survey. J Gerontol Med Sci 1999; 54A:M554-M559.
[25] Buckbinder L, Talbott R, Velasco-Miguel S et al. Induction of the growth inhibitor IGF–binding protein 3 by p53. *Nature* 1995; 377: 646–649.
[26] Chan JM, Stampfer MJ, Giovannucci E et al. Plasma insulin-like growth factor–I and prostate cancer risk: a prospective study. Science 1998; 279: 563–566.
[27] Chen C, Zhu YF, Liu XJ et al. Discovery of a series of nonpeptide small molecules that inhibit the binding of insulin-like growth factor (IGF) to IGF-binding proteins. *J Med Chem* 2001; 44: 4001–4010.
[28] Chiba T, Yamaza H, Higami Y, Shimokawa I. Anti-aging effects of caloric restriction: Involvement of neuroendocrine adaptation by peripheral signaling. *Microsc Res Tech* 2002; 59: 317-324.
[29] Clancy DJ, Gems D, Harshman LG et al. Extension of life-span by loss of CHICO, a Drosophila insulin receptor substrate protein. *Science* 2001; 292: 104-106.
[30] Colangelo LA, Gapstur SM, Gann PH et al. Colorectal cancer mortality and factors related to the insulin resistance syndrome. *Cancer Epidemiol Biomarkers Prev* 2002; 11: 385-391.
[31] Coschigano KT, Clemmons D, Bellush LL, Kopchick JJ. Assessment of growth parameters and life span of GHR/BP gene-disrupted mice. *Endocrinology* 2000; 141: 2608-2613.
[32] De Benedictis G, Carotenuto L, Carrieri G et al. Gene/longevity association studies at four autosomal loci (REN, THO, PARP, SOD2). *Eur J Human Gen* 1998; 6: 534-541.
[33] De Benedictis G, Tan Q, Jeune B et al. Recent advances in human gene-longevity association studies. *Mech Ageing Dev* 2001; 122: 909-920.
[34] DiGiovanni J, Bol DK, Wilker E, et al. Constitutive expression of insulin-like growth factor–1 in epidermal basal cells of transgenic mice leads to spontaneous tumor promotion. *Cancer Res* 2000; 60: 1561–1570.
[35] DiGiovanni J, Kiguchi K, Frijhoff A et al. Deregulated expression of insulin-like growth factor 1 in prostate epithelium leads to neoplasia in transgenic mice. *Proc Natl Acad Sci USA* 2000; 97: 3455–3460.
[36] Dillin A, Crawford DK, Kenyon C. Timing requirements for insulin/IGF-1 signaling in *C. elegans*. *Science* 2002; 298: 830-834.
[37] Dilman VM. Age-associated elevation of hypothalamic threshold to feedback control and its role in development, aging and disease. *Lancet* 1971; 1: 1211-1219.
[38] Dilman VM. Ageing, metabolic immunodepression and carcinogenesis. *Mech Ageing Dev* 1978; 8: 153-173.
[39] Dilman VM. *Development, Aging and Disease. A New Rationale for an Intervention.* Chur: Harwood Academic Publ, 1994.
[40] Dilman VM, Anisimov VN. Hypothalamic mechanisms of ageing and of specific age pathology – I. Sensitivity threshold of hypothalamo-pituitary complex to homeostatic stimuli in the reproductive system. *Exp Gerontol* 1979; 14: 161-174.
[41] Dilman VM, Anisimov VN. Potentiation of antitumor effect of cyclophosphamide and hydrazine sulfate by treatment with the antidiabetic agent, 1-phenylethylbiguanide (phenformin). *Cancer Lett* 1979; 7: 357-361.
[42] Dilman VM, Anisimov VN. Effect of treatment with phenofromin, dyphenylhydantoin or L-DOPA on life span and tumor incidence in C3H/Sn mice. *Gerontology* 1980; 26: 241-245.
[43] Dilman VM, Berstein LM, Ostroumova MN et al. Metabolic immunodepression and metabolic immunotherapy: an attempt of improvement in immunologic response in breast cancer patients by correction of metabolic disturbances. *Oncology* 1982; 39: 13-19.
[44] Dilman VM, Berstein LM, Yevtushenko TP et al. Preliminary evidence on metabolic rehabilitation in

cancer patients. *Arch Geschwulstforsch* 1988; 58: 175-183.
[45] Dilman VM, Berstein LM, Zabezhinski MA et al. Inhibition of DMBA-induced carcinogenesis by phenformin in the mammary gland of rats. *Arch Geschwulstforsch* 1978; 48: 1-8.
[46] Dilman VM, Bobrov JF, Ostroumova MN et al. Hypothalamic mechanisms of ageing and of specific age pathology – III. Sensitivity threshold of hypothalamo-pituitary complex to homeostatic stimuli in energy system. *Exp Gerontol* 1979; 14: 217-224.
[47] Dilman VM, Ostroumova MN, Tsyrlina EV. Hypothalamic mechanisms of ageing and of specific age pathology – II. Sensitivity threshold of hypothalamo-pituitary complex to homeostatic stimuli in adaptive homestasis. *Exp Gerontol* 1979; 14: 175-181.
[48] Dilman VM, Sofronov BN, Anisimov VN et al. Phenformin elimination of the immunodepression caused by 1,2-dimethylhydrazine in rats. *Vopr Onkol* 1977; 23(8): 50-54.
[49] Dominici FP, Arosegui Diaz G, Bartke A et al. Compensatory alterations of insulin signal transduction in liver of growth hormone receptor knockout mice. *J Endocrinol* 2000; 166: 579-590.
[50] Dominici FP, Hauck S, Argention DP et al. Increased insulin sensitivity and upregulation of insulin receptor, insulin receptor substrate (ISR)-1 and IRS-2 in liver of Ames dwarf mice. *J Endocrinol* 2002; 173: 81-94.
[51] Dorman JB, Albinder B, Shroyer T, Kenyon C. The *age-1* and *daf-2* genes function in a common pathway to control the lifespan of *Caenorhabditis elegans. Genetics* 1995; 141: 1399-1406.
[52] Dy DY, Whitehead RH, Morris DL. SMS 201.995 inhibits in vitro and in vivo growth of human colon cancer. *Cancer Res* 1992; 52: 917-923.
[53] Elahi D, Muller DC, Egan JM et al. Glucose tolerance, glucose utilization and insulin secretion in aging. *Novartis Found Symp* 2002; 242: 222-242.
[54] Facchini FS, Hua N, Abbasi F, Reaven GM. Insulin resistance as a predictor of age-related diseases. *J Clin Endocrinol Metab* 2001; 86: 3574-3578.
[55] Facchini FS, Hua NW, Reaven GM, Stoohs RA. Hyperinsulinemia: the missing link among oxidative stress and age-related diseases? *Free Radicals Biol Med* 2000; 29: 1302-1306.
[56] Facchini FS, Humphreys MH, Abbasi F et al. Relation between insulin resistance and plasma concentrations of lipid hydroperoxides, carotenoids, and tocopherols. *Am J Clin Nutr* 2000; 72: 776-779.
[57] Fernandes ML, Saad MJ, Velloso LA. Effect of age on elements of insulin-signaling pathway in central nervous system of rats. *Endocrine* 2001;16: 227-234.
[58] Flurkey K, Papaconstantinou J, Miller RA, Harrison DE. Life-span extension and delayed immune and collagen aging in mutant mice with defects in growth hormone production. *Proc Natl Acad Sci USA* 2001; 98: 6736-6741.
[59] Gargiulo P, Caccese D, Pignatelli P et al. Metformin decreases platelet superoxide anion production in diabetic patients. *Diabetes Metab Res Rev* 2002; 18: 156-159.
[60] Gems D, Sutton AJ, Sundermeyer ML et al. Two pleiotropic classes of *daf-2* mutation affect larval arrest, adult behavior, reproduction and longevity in *Caenorhabditis elegans. Genetics* 1998; 150: 129-155.
[61] Giovannucci E. Insulin, insulin-like growth factors and colon cancer: a review of the evidence. *J Nutr* 2001; 131: 3109S-3120S.
[62] Giovannucci E, Pollak M, Liu Y et al. Nutritional Predictors of Insulin-like Growth Factor I and Their Relationships to Cancer in Men. *Cancer Epidemiol Biomarkers Prev* 2003; 12: 84-89.
[63] Giovannucci E, Pollak MN, Platz EA et al. A prospective study of plasma insulin-like growth factor–1 and binding protein–3 and risk of colorectal neoplasia in women. *Çancer Epidemiol Biomarkers Prev* 2000; 9: 345–349.
[64] Granerus M, Engstrom W. Effects of insulin-like growth factor–binding protein 2 and an IGF–type I receptor-blocking antibody on apoptosis in human teratocarcinoma cells in vitro. *Cell Biol Int* 2001; 25: 825–828.
[65] Gupta K, Krishnaswamy G, Karnad A, Peiris AN. Insulin: a novel factor in carcinogenesis. *Am J Med Sci* 2002; 323: 140-145.
[66] Hadley EC, Dutta C, Finkelstein J et al. Human implications of caloric restriction's effect on laboratory animals: An overview of opportunities for research. *J Gerontol Ser A* 2001; 56A (Special issue I): 5-6.
[67] Hankinson SE, Willett WC, Colditz GA et al. Circulating concentrations of insulin-like growth factor–I and risk of breast cancer. Lancet 1998; 351: 1393–1396.
[68] Henderson ST, Johnson TE. *daf-16* integrates developmental and environmental inputs to mediate aging in the nematode *Caenorhabditis elegans. Curr Biol* 2001; 11: 1975-1980.
[69] Holzenberger M, Dupond J, Ducos B et al. IGF-1 receptor regulates lifespan and resistance to oxidative stress in mice. *Nature* 2003; 421: 182-187.

[70] Honda Y, Honda S. The *daf-2* gene network for longevity regulates oxidative stress resistance and Mn-superoxide dismutase gene expression in *Caenorhabditis elegans*. *FASEB J* 1999; 13: 1385-1393.
[71] Hsieh CC, DeFord JH, Flurkey K et al. Implications for the insulin signaling pathway in Snell dwarf mouse longevity: a similarity with the *C. elegans* longevity paradigm. *Mech Ageing Dev* 2002; 123: 1229-1244.
[72] Hsieh CC, DeFord JH, Flurkey K et al. Effects of the Pit1 mutation on the insulin signaling pathway: implications on the longevity of the long-lived Snell dwarf mouse. *Mech Ageing Dev* 2002; 123: 1245-1255.
[73] Hung AJ, Stanbury MG, Shanabrough M et al. Estrogen, synaptic plasticity and hypothalamic reproductive aging. *Exp Gerontol* 2003; 38: 53-59.
[74] Hursting SD, Lavigne JA, Berrigan D et al. Calorie restriction, aging, and cancer prevention: mechanisms of action and applicability to humans. *Annu Rev Med* 2003; 54: 131-152.
[75] Hursting SD, Lavigne JA, Perkins SN et al. Susceptibility of BK5.IGF-1 transgenic mice to p-cresidine–induced bladder carcinogenesis. *Proc Annu Meet Am Assoc Cancer Res* 2002: 168.
[76] Huxtable SJ, Saker PJ, Haddad L et al. Analysis of parent-offspring trios provides evidence for linkage and association between the insulin gene and type 2 diabetes mediated exclusively through paternally transmitted class III varable number tandem repeat allels. *Diabetes* 2000; 49: 126-130.
[77] Ikeno Y, Bronson RT, Hubbard GB et al. Delayed occurrence of fatal neoplastic diseases in Ames dwarf mice: correlation to extended longevity. *J Gerontol A Biol Sci Med Sci* 2003; 58: B291-B296.
[78] Kaaks R, Lukanova A. Energy balance and cancer: the role of insulin and insulin-like growth factor-I. *Proc Nutr Soc* 2001; 60: 91-106.
[79] Kawano T, Ito Y, Ishiguro M et al. Molecular cloning and characterization of a new insulin/IGF-like peptide of the nematode *Caenorhabditis elegans*. *Biochem Biophys Res Commun* 2000; 273: 431-436.
[80] Kenyon C. A conserved regulatory system for aging. *Cell* 2001; 105: 165-168.
[81] Kenyon C, Chang J, Gensch E et al. A *C. elegans* mutant that lives twice as long as wild type. *Nature* 1993; 366: 461-464.
[82] Kimura KD, Tissenbaum HA, Liu Y, Ruvkun G. daf-2, an insulin receptor-like gene that regulates longevity and diapause in *Caenorhabditis elegans*. *Science* 1997; 277: 942-946.
[83] Lane MA, Tilmont EM, De Angelis H et al. Short-term calorie restriction improves disease-related markers in older male rhesus monkeys (Macaca mulatta). *Mech Ageing Dev* 2000; 112: 185-196.
[84] Lane MA, Mattison J, Ingram DK, Roth GS. Caloric restriction and aging in primates: Relevance to humans and possible CR mimetics. *Microsc Res Tech* 2002, 59: 335-338.
[85] Larsen PL, Albert PS, Riddle DL. Genes that regulate both development and longevity in *Caenorhabditis elegans*. *Genetics* 1995; 139: 1567-1583.
[86] Le Roith D, Bondy C, Yakar S et al. The somatomedin hypothesis: 2001. *Endocrine Rev* 2001; 22: 53-74.
[87] Le Roith D, Baserga R, Helman L, Roberts CT. Insulin-like growth factors and cancer. *Ann Intern Med* 1995; 122: 54–59.
[88] Lin K, Dorman JB, Rodan A, Kenyon C. *daf-16*: An HNF-3/forkhead family member that can function to double the life-span of *Caenorhabditis elegans*. *Science* 1997; 278: 1319-1322.
[89] Lipman RD, Dallal GE, Bronson RT. Lesion biomarkers of aging in B6C3F1 hybrid mice. *J Gerontol Med Sci* 1999; 54A: 466-477.
[90] Lipman RD, Dallal GE, Bronson RT. Effect of genotype and diet on age-related lesions in ad libitum fed and calorie-restricted F344, BN, and BNF3F1 rats. *J Gerontol Med Sci* 1999; 54A: 478-491.
[91] Longo VD, Finch CE. Evolutionary medicine: from dwarf model systems to healthy centenarians? *Science* 2003; 299: 1342-1346.
[92] Lund J, Tedesco P, Duke K et al. Transcriptional profile of aging in *C. elegans*. *Curr Biol* 2002; 12: 1566-1573.
[93] Ma J, Pollak MN, Giovannucci E et al. Prospective study of colorectal cancer risk in men and plasma levels of insulin-like growth factor (IGF)–I and IGF–binding protein–3. *J Natl Cancer Inst* 1999; 91: 620–625.
[94] Macaulay VM. Insulin-like growth factors and cancer. *Br J Cancer* 1992; 65: 311–320.
[95] Masoro EJ. Caloric restriction and ageing: an update. *Exp Gerontol* 2000; 35: 299-305.
[96] Masoro EJ. Subfield history: Caloric restriction, slowing aging, and extending life. *Science's SAGE KE*, 2003, ns2 (26 February 2003) http://Sageke.sciencemag. org/cgi/content/full/ sageke;2003/8/re2.
[97] Mattison JM, Wright C, Bronson RT et al. Studies of aging in Ames dwarf mice: effects of caloric restriction. J. Amer Aging Assoc 2000; 23: 9-16.
[98] Mattson JA, Lane MA, Roth GS, Ingram DK. Calorie restriction in rhesus monkeys. *Exp Gerontol* 2003; 38: 35-46.

[99] Mattson MP. Brain evolution and lifespan regulation: conservation of signaling trnsduction pathways that regulate energy metabolism. *Mech Ageing Dev* 2002; 123: 947-953.

[100] Mattson MP, Duan W, Lee J et al. Progress in the development of caloric restriction mimetic dietary supplements. *J Anti-Aging Med* 2001; 4: 225-232.

[101] Mattson MP, Duan W, Maswood N. How does the brain control lifespan? *Ageing Res Rev* 2002; 1: 155-165.

[102] McCarty MF. Longevity effect of chromium picolinate – 'rejuvenation' of hypothalamic function? *Medical Hypotheses* 1994; 3: 253-265.

[103] McGuire MT, Wing RR, Klem ML, Hill JO. Behavioral strategies of individuals who have maintained long-term weight losses. *Obes Res* 1999; 7: 334–341.

[104] Miyaishi O, Ando F, Matsuzawa K et al. Cancer incidence in old age. *Mech Ageing Dev* 2000; 117: 47-55.

[105] Morris JZ, Tissenbaum HA, Ruvkun G. A phosphatidylinositol-3-OH kinase family member regulating longevity and diapause in *Caenorhabditis elegans*. *Nature* 1996; 382: 536-538.

[106] Muntoni S. Inhibition of fatty acid oxidation by biguanides: implication for metabolic physiopathology. *Adv Lipid Res* 1974; 12: 311-377.

[107] Muntoni S. Metformin and fatty acids. *Diabetes Care* 1999; 22: 179-80.

[108] Nestler JE, Stovall D, Akhther N et al. Strategies for the use of insulin-sensitizing drugs to treat infertility in women with polycystic ovary syndrome. *Fertil Steril* 2002; 77: 209-215.

[109] Paolisso G, Gambardella A, Ammendola S et al. Glucose tolerance and insulin action in healthy centenarians. *Am J Physiol* 1996; 270: E890-E-896.

[110] Pierce SB, Costa M, Wisotzkey R et al. Regulation of DAF-2 receptor signaling by human insulin and *ins-1*, a member of the unusually large and diverse *C. elegans* insulin gene family. *Genes Dev* 2001; 15: 672-686.

[111] Pompei F, Wilson R. Age distribution of cancer: the incidence turnover at old age. *Human Ecol Risk Assesment* 2001; 7: 1619-1650.

[112] Pompei F, Polkanov M, Wilson R. Age distribution of cancer in mice: the incidence turnover at old age. *Toxicol Industr Health* 2001; 17: 7-16.

[113] Ramaswamy S, Nakamura N, Sansal I et al. A novel mechanism of gene regulation and tumor suppression by the transcription factor FKHR. *Cancer Cell* 2002; 2: 81-91.

[114] Richards JS, Russell DL, Ochsner S et al. Novel signaling pathways that control ovarian follicular development, ovulation, and luteinization. *Recent Prog Horm Res* 2002; 57: 195-220.

[115] Richards JS, Sharma SC, Falender AE, Lo YH. Expression of FKHR, FKHRL1, and AFX genes in the rodent ovary: evidence for regulation by IGF-I, estrogen, and the gonadotropins. *Mol Endocrinol* 2002; 16: 590-599.

[116] Rossmanith WG Neuroendocrinology of aging in the reproductive system: gonadotropin secretion as an example. In Kumar A, Mukhopadhayay AK (Eds). *Follicular Gowrth, Ovulation and Fertilization: Molecular and Clinical Basis.* New Dehli: Narosa Publ. House, 2001, pp.15-25.

[117] Roth GS, Ingram DK, Lane MA. Calorie restriction in primates: will it work and how will we know? *J Am Geriatr Soc* 1999; 46: 869-903.

[118] Roth GS, Lane MA, Ingram DK et al. Biomarkers of caloric restriction may predict longevity in humans. *Science* 2002; 297: 811.

[119] Ruiz-Torres A, Soares de Melo Kirzner M. Ageing and longevity are related to growth hormone/insulin-like growth factor-1 secretion. *Gerontology* 2002; 48: 401-407.

[120] Schneider MB, Matsuzaki H, Harorah J et al. Prevention of pancreatic cancer induction in hamsters by metformin. *Gastroenterology* 2001; 120: 1263-1270.

[121] Scotlandi K, Maini C, Manara MC et al. Effectiveness of insulin-like growth factor I receptor antisense strategy against Ewing's sarcoma cells. *Cancer Gene Ther* 2002; 9: 296–307.

[122] Shimokawa I, Higami Y, Utsuyama M et al. Life span extension by reducing in growth hormone-insulin-growth factor-1 axis in a transgenic rat model. *Am J Pathol* 2002; 160: 2259-2265.

[123] Singal PK, Beamish RE, Dhalla NS. Potential of oxidative pathways of catecholamine in the formation of lipid peroxides and genesis of heart disease. *Adv Exp Biol Med* 1983; 161: 391-401.

[124] Singh P, Dai B, Yallampalli U et al. Proliferation and differentiation of a human colon cancer cell line ($CaCo_2$) is associated with significant changes in the expression and secretion of insulin-like growth factor (IGF) IGF-II and IGF binding protein–4: role of IGF-II. Endocrinology 1996; 137: 1764–1774.

[125] Smith DWE. Cancer mortality at very old ages. *Cancer* 1996; 77: 1376-1373.

[126] Sun D, Muthukumar AR, Lawrence RA, Fernandes G. Effects of calorie restriction on polymicrobial pertonits induced by cecum ligation and puncture in young C57Bl/6 mice. *Clin Diagn Lab Immunol* 2001;

8: 1003-1011.
[127] Takahashi K, Suzuki K. Association of insulin-like growth-factor-I–induced DNA synthesis with phosphorylation and nuclear exclusion of p53 in human breast cancer MCF-7 cells. *Int J Cancer* 1993; 55: 453–458.
[128] Tatar M, Bartke A, Antebi A The endocrine regulation of aging by insulin-like signals. *Science* 2003; 299: 1346-1351.
[129] Tatar M, Kopelman A, Epstein D et al. A mutant Drosophila insulin receptor homolog that extends life-span and impairs neuroendocrine function. *Science* 2001; 292: 107-110.
[130] Tissenbaum HA, Ruvkun G. An insulin-like signaling pathway affects both longevity and reproduction in *Caenorhabditis elegans. Genetics* 1998; 148: 703-717.
[131] Tybaierg-Hansen A, Gerdes IU, Overgaard K et al. Polymorphysm in 5' flanking region of human insulin gene. Relationships with atherosclerosis, lipid levels and age in three samples from Denmark. *Arteriosclerosis* 1990; 10: 372-378.
[132] Ulrich P, Cerami A. Protein glycation, diabetes, and aging. *Recent Prog Horm Res* 2001; 56: 1-21.
[133] Vanfleteren JR. Oxidative stress and aging in *Caenorhabditis elegans. Biochem J* 1993; 292: 605-608.
[134] Vanfleteren JR, de Vreese A. The gerontogenes *age-1* and *daf-2* determine metabolic rate potential in aging *Caenorhabditis elegans. FASEB J* 1995; 9: 1355-1361.
[135] Vinnitski VB, Iakimenko VA. Effect of phenformin, L—DOPA and para-chlorophenylalanine on the immunological reactivity and chemical carcinogenesis in BALB/c mice. *Vopr Onkol* 1981; 27(6): 45-50.
[136] Vogt A, Rice RL, Settineri CE et al. Disruption of insulin-like growth factor–1 signaling and down-regulation of cdc2 by SC-αα δ9, a novel small molecule antisignaling agent identified in a targeted array library. *J Pharmacol Exp Ther* 1998; 287: 806–813.
[137] Waterworth DM, Bennett ST, Gharani N et al. Linkage and association of insulin gene VNTR regulatory polymorphysm with polycystic ovary syndrome. *Lancet* 1997; 349: 986-990.
[138] Weaver JU, Kopelman PG, Hitman GA. Central obesity and hyperinsulinemia in women are associated with polymorphism in the 5' flanking region of the human insulin gene. *Eur J Clin Invest* 1992; 22: 265-270.
[139] Weindruch R, Keenan KP, Carney JM et al. Caloric restriction mimetics: metabolic intervention. *J Gerontol Biol Sci* 2001; 56A (Special Issue 1): 20-33.
[140] Weindruch R, Sohal RS. Caloric intake and aging. *The New Engl J Med* 1997; 337: 986-994.
[141] Weindruch R, Walford R. *The Retardation of Aging and Disease by Dietary Restriction.* Springiefld, Ill: CC Thomas. 1988
[142] Wolkov CA, Kimura KD, Lee MS, Ruvkun G. Regulation of *C. elegans* life-span by insulin-like signalling in the nervous system. *Nat Genetics* 2000; 290: 147-150.
[143] Wu Y, Yakar S, Zhao L et al. Circulating insulin-like growth factor-1 levels regulate colon cancer growth and metastasis. *Cancer Res* 2002; 62: 1030-1035.
[144] Xu L, Bard MZ. Enhanced potential for oxidative stress in hyperinsulinemic rats: imbalance between hepatic peroxisomal hydrogen peroxide production and decomposition due to hyperinsulinemia. *Horm Metab Res* 1999; 31: 278-282.
[145] Yaghmaie F, Garan SA, Massaro M, Timiras PS. A comparison of estrogen receptor-alpha immunoreactivity in the arcuate hypothalamus of young and middle-aged C57BL6 female mice. *Exp Gerontol* 2003; 38: 220.
[146] Yang Y, Wilson DL. Characterization of a life-extending mutation in *age-2*, a new aging gene in *Caenorhabditis elegans. J Gerontol* 1999; 54: B137-B142.
[147] Yu H, Rohan T. Role of the insulin-like growth factor family in cancer development and progression. *J Natl Cancer Inst* 2000; 92: 1472–1489.
[148] Yu H, Spitz MR, Mistry J et al. Plasma levels of insulin-like growth factor–I and lung cancer risk: a case-control analysis. *J Natl Cancer Inst* 1999; 91: 151–156.

Frontiers in Neurodegenerative Disorders and Aging: Fundamental Aspects, Clinical Perspectives and New Insights
T. Özben and M. Chevion (Eds.)
IOS Press, 2004

Diabetes and the Brain: Advanced Ageing?

Geert Jan Biessels[1, 2] and Willem Hendrik Gispen [1]
Department of Medical Pharmacology (1), Department of Neurology (2) Rudolf Magnus Institute for Neurosciences, University Medical Centre Utrecht, The Netherlands

Abstract: Diabetes mellitus is associated with moderate cognitive deficits and neurophysiological and structural changes in the brain, a condition that may be referred to as diabetic encephalopathy. Diabetes increases the risk of dementia, particularly in the elderly. The emerging view is that the diabetic brain features many symptoms that are best described as "accelerated brain ageing". The clinical characteristics of diabetic encephalopathy are discussed, as well as behavioural (e.g. spatial learning) and neurophysiological (e.g. hippocampal synaptic plasticity) findings in animal models. Animal models can make a substantial contribution to our understanding of the pathogenesis, which shares many features with the mechanisms underlying brain ageing. By unravelling the pathogenesis, targets for pharmacotherapy can be identified. This may allow treatment or prevention of this diabetic complication in the future. This manuscript of the lecture is largely based on excerpts of recent reviews written by the authors [1,2,3]

1 Introduction

Diabetes mellitus is a heterogeneous metabolic disorder characterised by hyperglycaemia resulting from defective insulin secretion, resistance to insulin action, or both [4]. Type 1 diabetes is the consequence of an auto immune-mediated destruction of pancreatic ß-cells, leading to insulin deficiency. Patients require insulin treatment for survival. Type 2 diabetes is characterised by insulin resistance and relative, rather than absolute, insulin deficiency. Type 2 diabetes usually occurs in obese individuals and is associated with hypertension and dyslipidaemia. Treatment aims to reduce insulin resistance (diet, exercise, and drug therapy) and to stimulate insulin secretion.

Diabetes mellitus is often associated with (severe) complications such as cardiovascular disease, the "diabetic foot", kidney failure, retinopathy and peripheral and autonomic neuropathy. Although proper metabolic control reduces the development of these complications, it is not sufficient to prevent them completely [5]. In this review we discuss the neurological complications of diabetes, focussing on the brain. In particular, we explore underlying pathogenetic mechanisms, highlighting the possible interaction of diabetes and ageing.

2. Diabetes and the brain

2.1 Encephalopathy?

In recent years evidence is emerging that diabetes affects the central nervous system [6,7]. Both acute and chronic metabolic and vascular disturbances can impair the functional and structural integrity of the brain in diabetic patients. For example, diabetes increases the risk for stroke and stroke outcome is worse in diabetic patients [8,9]. In addition, hyper- and hypo glycaemic episodes may result in acute cerebral dysfunction [6,10]. The consequences of these acute insults to the brain are well recognised. We did, in contrast, know much less of the functional and structural cerebral alterations that develop more insidiously and tend to be subtler. Recent studies now show that long term effects of diabetes on the brain are manifested at the structural, neurophysiological and neuro-psychological level and the emerging view is that the diabetic brain features many symptoms that are best described as accelerated brain ageing.

2.2 Structural changes

There is only a limited amount of data from brain autopsy studies. In an early study of young (<40 years of age) type 1 diabetic patients with severe and widespread diabetic angiopathy Reske-Nielsen and co-workers [11] observed diffuse degenerative abnormalities of brain tissue. They considered these degenerative changes to be so pronounced that they implied a dual pathogenesis: "ischaemia caused by an angiopathy and a primary diabetic abnormality of the brain tissue". An increased frequency in the occurrence of ischaemic brain lesions among diabetic patients compared to age matched controls was confirmed by an autopsy study by Peress et al [12].

More recently, neuroimaging techniques, such as magnetic resonance imaging and computed tomography, have provided data on structural changes in the brain that may be more relevant to the general population of diabetic patients. Cerebral atrophy, as manifested by widened sulci and/or enlarged lateral ventricles, appears to be more pronounced in diabetic patients than in age matched controls [13,14,15]. As atrophy is one of the hallmarks of brain ageing [16], the radiological appearance of the brain in diabetic patients has been considered to reflect a process of accelerated ageing. In addition to the global subcortical and cortical atrophy there is a tendency for an increased occurrence of white matter hyper-intensities on magnetic resonance imaging studies [14,17], possibly related to the ischaemic lesions that were observed in the autopsy.

2.3 *Electrophysiological changes*

Measurements of the latencies of evoked potentials have been widely used to examine the functional integrity of the central nervous system in diabetic patients [18]. Increases in the latencies of these evoked potentials provide a central equivalent of reduced conduction velocity in peripheral nerves. The latencies of both central and peripheral components of the brainstem auditory evoked potential are affected in type 1 as well as in type 2 diabetic patients [19,20,18]. Likewise, the latency of the P100 wave of the visual evoked potential, which is thought to be generated in the visual cortex [21], is increased [22,21]. P100 latencies correlate positively with the duration of diabetes and HbA1 levels [23] and can be improved by intensive insulin treatment [22].

Event related potentials are a valuable tool for the quantification of changes in cognitive resources in normal ageing and conditions associated with cognitive decline [24,25]. The P300 wave is a positive deflection in the human event- related potential that is thought to result from neural activity associated with attentional and memory processes [24]. It is most commonly elicited in an "oddball" paradigm in which a subject is instructed to detect an occasional "target" stimulus in a regular train of standard stimuli [24]. The P300 latency increases markedly with age [25], but more so in diabetic patients [26,27], which may be a neurophysiological manifestation of impairment of higher brain functions.

2.4 Cognition

As early as in the 1920's it was recognised that diabetes mellitus may affect cognition [28]. Numerous studies have since reported cognitive deficits in both type 1 and type 2 diabetic patients. In adult type 1 diabetic patients modest reductions in mental efficiency have been reported repeatedly, particularly involving learning and memory, problem solving and mental and motor speed [29]. Severe deficits occur only in few patients [30]. The pattern of impairments across different cognitive domains is rather inconsistent among studies, probably due to the subtle nature of the deficits, but also to the heterogeneity of the populations studied. In addition, the exposure to the two extremes of blood glucose levels, severe hypoglycaemia on the one hand and chronic hyperglycaemia on the other, varies between patients. Chronic hyperglycaemia and repeated episodes of severe hypoglycaemia may both adversely affect the brain [31,32,33], albeit through different mechanisms, thus leading to different cerebral deficits.

Compared to type 1 diabetes, neuropsychological studies in type 2 diabetic patients have provided more consistent results. Moderate degrees of cognitive impairment have been reported, particularly in tasks involving verbal memory or complex information processing [34,7]. Basic attentional processes, motor reaction time and immediate memory appear to be relatively unaffected [34]. Risk factors for cognitive dysfunction in type 2 diabetes are chronic hyperglycaemia, dyslipidaemia and the presence of peripheral neuropathy [34]. Hypoglycaemic episodes do not appear to be a prime determinant, as cognitive deficits also occur in subjects with impaired glucose tolerance and in newly diagnosed type 2 diabetic patients who had not yet been treated with glucose lowering drugs [35,36].

2.5 Dementia

There is an increasing body of evidence to support a relation between especially type 2 diabetes and dementia in old age [37,38,39]. The Rotterdam study is a community based prospective cohort study in which chronic disorders of the elderly are under investigation [38]. The relative risk for developing dementia was doubled in diabetic patients [38], suggesting that diabetes may contribute to the to the clinical syndrome of dementia in a substantial proportion of all dementia patients. In the Honolulu-Asia Aging Study brain autopsy data have become available from a proportion of the participants of a prospective cohort study that was initiated in the late 60’s [37]. These autopsy data confirm the increased risk of both vascular dementia and Alzheimer disease in diabetic patients.

In an extensive review of the literature, Stewart and Liolitsa [7] conclude that there is a cross-sectional and prospective association between type 2 and cognitive impairment, probably both for memory and executive functions. Their review confirms the elevated risk of dementia in type 2 diabetes patients, albeit with strong interactions with other risk factors.

3. Cognition and synaptic plasticity in experimental ageing and diabetes

Animal models have been widely used to explore the connection between age-related memory deficits and changes in the anatomy and physiology of the brain [40]. Although aged rodents can learn and retain new information, they exhibit slower learning and rapid forgetting. Spatial learning in a Morris water maze, for example, is much slower than in young adult control rats [41,42]. In view of the crucial role of the hippocampus in certain types of learning and memory, several groups have studied the functional and structural integrity of the hippocampus in aged rodents. One aspect of hippocampal function, synaptic plasticity, has attracted particular attention, as plastic changes in synaptic strength are assumed to be involved in learning and memory [43,44]. Long-term potentiation (LTP) and depression (LTD) are two forms of activity-dependent synaptic plasticity that have been studied extensively. In LTP, brief high-frequency afferent activity leads to a long-lasting increase in the strength of synaptic transmission, whereas in LTD prolonged low-frequency activity results in a persistent reduction in synaptic strength. Both processes are triggered by an increase in the level of postsynaptic intracellular calcium concentration $[Ca^{2+}]_i$ [45,44,43]. LTP is triggered by a brief increase of $[Ca^{2+}]_i$ with relatively high magnitude, whereas a prolonged modest rise of $[Ca^{2+}]_i$ induces LTD [45]. A complex pattern of changes in synaptic plasticity has been observed in hippocampal slices of aged rodents, including an increase in the threshold for LTP induction and a decrease in the threshold for LTD induction [40,46]. These changes have been related to alterations in $[Ca^{2+}]_i$ homeostasis in neurones of aged animals [40,47].

Animal models have also been used to examine the relation between memory deficits and changes in synaptic plasticity in diabetes. The most commonly used method for induction of diabetes is an intravenous or intraperitoneal injection of the ß-cytotoxic agent streptozotocin (STZ). STZ-diabetic rodents are hypoinsulinaemic, but do not require insulin treatment to survive. Blood glucose levels typically are 20-25 mmol/l (normal 5 mmol/l). Like diabetic patients, STZ-diabetic rats develop end-organ damage affecting the eyes, kidneys, heart, blood vessels, and peripheral and central nervous system.

Studies into cognitive functioning in STZ-diabetic rodents have used several learning tasks. STZ-diabetes does not disturb operant behaviour for food reward [48]. Retention of passive avoidance in rats and mice is reported to be facilitated [49,50], but not invariably [51]. In more complex learning tasks, such as an active avoidance T-maze, or a Morris water maze, diabetic rodents consistently displayed performance deficits [50,52,53,54]. The development of the deficits was dependent on the duration of STZ diabetes [52,53]. Subcutaneous implantation of insulin pellets at the onset of diabetes, so that blood glucose levels decreased from about 25 mmol/l to about normal (7 mmol/l), completely prevented the learning deficit. If, however, this insulin-treatment was started 10 weeks after diabetes onset, when learning is already impaired, there was only partial improvement [53]. Control experiments showed that these performance deficits were not due to sensorimotor impairments [52,53].

Learning deficits in STZ-diabetic rats develop in association with distinct changes in synaptic plasticity in hippocampal slices, which appear to be dependent on diabetes duration and severity [3]. A deficit in the expression of N-methyl-D-aspartate (NMDA)-dependent LTP in the CA1 field was shown to develop gradually and reach a maximum at 12 weeks after diabetes induction [55,56,52]. At this time point, NMDA-dependent LTP in the dentate gyrus and NMDA-independent LTP in the CA3 field are also impaired [56]. Insulin treatment prevents the development of the changes in LTP but is less effective against existing LTP deficits [53]. In contrast to LTP, expression of LTD is enhanced in the CA1 field following low-frequency stimulation of slices from diabetic rats [56]. This enhancement of LTD appears to be dependent on the stimulus frequency [3].

A number of studies have tried to pinpoint the mechanisms underlying the alterations in hippocampal synaptic plasticity in STZ-diabetic rats and have been discussed before [1,2]. Age-related changes in cognition and synaptic plasticity have often been linked to alterations in glutamatergic neurotransmission [46,57]. The density of NMDA binding sites in the hippocampus, for example, is markedly reduced in aged rodents [57]. Hence we were interested in the efects of diabetes on postsynaptic glutamate receptors in the hippocampus. In Sprague-Dawley rats, after 6-8 weeks STZ-diabetes, the affinity of glutamate for AMPA, but not for NMDA-receptors, was reported to be decreased [58]. The reduced affinity for AMPA was associated with reduced levels of the GluR1 subunit of the AMPA receptor [58], whereas the level of GluR2 and 3 in the hippocampus and cortex was unaffected [58] . After 12 weeks of STZ-diabetes the levels of the NMDA receptor subunits NR1 and NR2A were not changed, but there was a marked decrease (-40%) in NR2B [59]. Furthermore, the phosphorylation of the NR2A/B subunits by Ca^{2+}/calmodulin-dependent protein kinase II was reduced in diabetes [59]. It was suggested that these NMDA receptor related changes underlie the LTP deficits [59]. The recent finding that over-expression of NR2B in the forebrains of non-diabetic transgenic mice facilitates induction of LTP and enhances learning abilities [60] supports this suggestion.

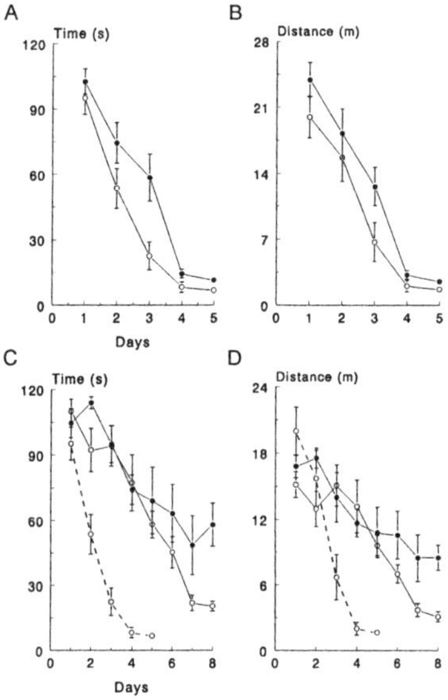

Figure 1: Effects of STZ-diabetes and ageing on spatial learning in a Morris water maze. **A, B** Young-adult (5 months) rats were tested after 8 weeks of streptozotocin-diabetes. The maze consisted of a large circular black

pool (210 cm diameter, 50 cm height), which was placed in a darkened room. A curtain that obscured visual cues surrounded the maze. Rats were trained on 5 consecutive days, 3 trials per day. Latencies (A) and swimming distances (B) to reach the platform were measured. Young adult diabetic rats (♦, n=9) performed significantly worse than age-matched non-diabetic controls (✌, n=9): latencies ANOVAR(day1-5): F(1, 16) = 5.77, P< 0.05; swimming distance ANOVAR(day3-5): F(1, 16) = 4.77, P< 0.05. The possible involvement of sensorimotor dysfunction in the performance deficit of diabetic rats was carefully excluded using adapted versions of the maze [53,52] **C, D** Aged (2 years) rats were also tested after 8 weeks of streptozotocin-diabetes. Rats were trained on 8 consecutive days, 3 trials per day. Latencies (C) and swimming distances (D) to reach the platform were measured. Aged diabetic rats (♦, n=7) performed significantly worse than age-matched non-diabetic controls (✌, n=6): latencies ANOVAR(day1-8): F(1, 11) = 3.66, P=0.08. ANOVAR(day 6-8): F(1, 11) = 5.33, P< 0.05; swimming distance ANOVAR(day1-8): F(1, 11) = 5.29, P< 0.05. Note the difference in comparison to the latencies and distances swum by the young-adult non-diabetic animals (interrupted line). Data are mean ± S.E.M. Adapted from Kamal et al.[41], with permission.

As both ageing and diabetes affect cognition, synaptic plasticity and glutamatergic neurotransmission in rats, it is conceivable that the effects of diabetes and ageing interact. This was examined in a recent study (Figs. 1, 2), which used an experimental protocol in which each of the two conditions in isolation produces only moderate deficits. Rats were examined after 2 months of STZ-diabetes, which produces half-maximal deficits in synaptic plasticity in young-adult rats [56]. Aged rats were examined at 2 years of age, when they have developed moderate changes in synaptic plasticity due to ageing alone. In aged rats (24 months) the diabetic deficit in water maze performance was larger than expected from the effect in young-adult rats (Fig. 1). Likewise, the impairment of hippocampal LTP and enhancement of LTD was accentuated by the combination of the two conditions (Fig. 2), suggesting that there is an interaction between ageing and diabetic cerebral dysfunction [41].

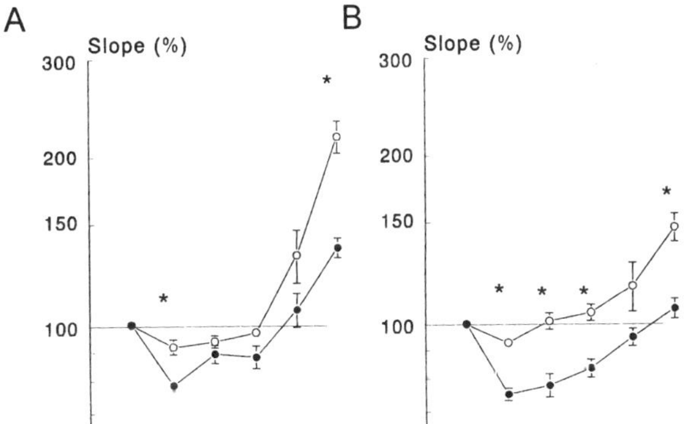

Figure 2: Effects of STZ-diabetes and ageing on hippocampal synaptic plasticity. The same animals from which the behavioural data are depicted in Fig. 1 were used. One to two weeks after the water maze, LTP was measured in the CA1-field of the hippocampus in vitro. The baseline slope of the field excitatory postsynaptic potential (fEPSP) was recorded for 15 minutes. Next, a conditioning stimulus was applied to the afferent fibres of CA1 field, consisting of 900 pulses, given at different frequencies (from 0.05 to 100 Hz). High-frequency stimulation (HFS; 100 Hz for 1 s, and 50 Hz for 2 s) was applied at intervals of 10 sec. Low frequency stimulation (LFS) was given as a single train of 900 stimuli at 10 Hz (for 1.5 min), 5 Hz (for 3 min) or 1Hz (for 15 min). The change in slope (expressed as % of baseline) was measured at 30 minutes after the conditioning stimuli. **A.** Hippocampal slices from young-adult animals: LFS induced depression of the fEPSP, whereas HFS induced potentiation. In comparison to controls (✌, n=8 at each frequency), expression of long-term depression at 1 Hz stimulation was significantly enhanced in diabetic slices (♦, n=8), whereas expression of long-term potentiation at 100 Hz

stimulation was significantly impaired (*: P<0.05; t-test). **B.** Hippocampal slices from aged animals. In comparison to controls (☿, n=8), expression of LTD was significantly enhanced in diabetic slices (♦, n=7) after 1, 5 and 10 Hz stimuli (*: P<0.05; t-test), whereas expression of LTP after100 Hz stimulation was significantly impaired (*: P<0.05). Note the difference in comparison to the frequency curve in hippocampal slices from the young-adult non-diabetic animals Data are mean ± S.E.M. Adapted from Kamal et al.[41], with permission.

In a further study we examined whether CA1 pyramidal neurons from streptozotocin-induced diabetic rats display an increased slow afterhyperpolarization, often considered as a hallmark of neuronal ageing. We found no differences in resting membrane potential, input resistance, membrane time-constant, and action potential amplitude and duration between CA1 pyramidal neurons from streptozotocin-induced diabetic and age-matched control rats. During a train of action potentials, however, there is an increased broadening of the action potentials in diabetic animals, so-called "spike broadening". The amplitude of the slow afterhyperpolarization elicited by a train of action potentials is indeed increased in diabetic animals[61]. Interestingly, when the slow afterhyperpolarization is elicited by a Ca(2+) spike, there is no difference between control and diabetic rats. This indicates that the increased slow afterhyperpolarization in diabetes is likely to be due to an increased Ca(2+) influx resulting from the increased spike broadening. These data underscore the notion that the diabetic brain at the neuronal level shares key- properties with brain ageing.

4. Ageing and diabetes: shared pathogenetic mechanisms?

The aforementioned clinical and experimental data clearly show that diabetes can affect the brain and that the effects of diabetes and ageing on the brain may interact. The underlying mechanisms, however, are still mostly unclear and subject of current research and speculation. As will be discussed below, some authors emphasise the common feature of advanced glycated end products and reduced anti-oxidant defence in the brains of type 2 diabetes and Alzheimer patients. In addition, an extremely interesting lead emerges, suggesting that sporadic Alzheimer disease may reflect the "brain type" of type 2 diabetes mellitus [62]. In this concept hyperinsulinaemia, brain glucose utilisation and insulin signal transduction in the brain play an interconnected role in the pathophysiology. Clinical and experimental studies indeed show that altered glucose regulation impairs learning and memory [63] and defects in insulin action, both in the periphery and the brain, have recently been implicated in the pathogenesis of sporadic Alzheimer's disease [64,65,66]. Ryan and Geckle [67] come to the conclusion that the increased risk of cognitive dysfunction in elderly type 2 patients is the consequence of a synergistic interaction between diabetes related metabolic derangements and structural and functional cerebral changes due to the normal ageing process. In an excellent review Klein and Waxman [68] also point to the important molecular changes that occur in the brain as end-organ damage resulting from diabetes. Here we discuss some of the pathogenic mechanisms that seem to be common to both ageing and diabetes related changes in brain function.

4.1 Oxidative stress

A common theory for ageing and for the pathogenesis of Alzheimer's disease relates cell death to oxidative stress mediated by free radicals [69,70]. Accumulation of damaged, oxidised, dysfunctional proteins seems to result from a combination of an age-related increase in the rate of oxygen free radical-mediated damage and a loss of the ability to degrade oxidised proteins

[71]. Indeed, increased levels of oxidised proteins and reduced activity of antioxidant enzymes have been demonstrated in the brains of aged individuals with and without Alzheimer's disease [72,73].

Diabetes is associated with increased oxidative stress, as reflected in an increased presence of lipid peroxidation products [74,75]. Like in ageing increased oxidative stress appears to be the result of increased formation of reactive oxygen species (ROS), reductions in ROS scavengers or both. Increased ROS production in diabetes is a consequence of the process of glucose auto-oxidation. This process, in which glucose is oxidised in the presence of free metal ions, leads to superoxide and hydroxyl radical release, and finally causes protein oxidation [76,77]. The activity of ROS scavenging compounds, like glutathione, catalase and superoxide dismutase may be affected by diabetes [78,79], but experimental data are not always consistent, and highly depend on the duration of diabetes and the organ studied [80]. Decreases in ROS scavenging compounds may be due to direct effects of diabetes on scavenger production or activity. For example, enhanced protein glycation may be responsible for the reduced enzymatic antioxidant activity of superoxide dismutase [81]. Attenuation of glutathione levels may be related to an increased polyol pathway activity, as this leads to a depletion of NADPH, which is necessary for the enzymatic reduction of oxidised glutathione [82]. On the other hand, local decreases in endogenous ROS scavenging compounds may be due to increased consumption by ROS. For example, a local endoneurial deficit in the reduced form of glutathione has been attributed to the generation of increased amounts of hydrogen peroxide [83].

Increased concentration of lipid peroxidation by-products has been demonstrated in the brain of diabetic rats [84,85]. The activity of superoxide dismutase and catalase, enzymes involved in the antioxidant defence of the brain, appears to be decreased in STZ-diabetic rats [85,86], whereas in type 2 diabetic mice increased brain superoxide dismutase activity has been reported [87].

4.2 Non-enzymatic protein glycation: accelerated AGEing

Glucose irreversibly modifies long-lived macromolecules by forming advanced glycation end products (AGEs), as a function of glucose concentration and time [88,89]. The glycation reaction is a post-translational modification process occurring between free reducing sugars and free amino groups of proteins. Amadori products, the first stable products of the reaction, can consequently be transformed in AGEs, irreversible adducts of the Maillard reaction [88,89]. AGEs tend to accumulate in the brain during ageing [90,91], and the accumulation of AGEs has been implicated in the pathogenesis of Alzheimer's disease [70,92]. The formation of AGEs may affect neuronal function through various mechanisms [89,88], including modification of functionally important proteins like tubulin and Na^+, K^+-ATPase [93]. The formation of AGEs is also associated with the increased production of ROS [77,70], thus linking the pathophysiological model of non-enzymatic glycation to oxidative stress. In addition, increased circulating levels of AGEs and glycation of basement membranes of vessel walls may affect vascular function, as endothelial oxidative damage and endothelial dysfunction have been observed in the presence of AGEs [94]. Furthermore, AGEs may be responsible for the quenching of the vasodilating compound nitric oxide [95].

In tissues affected by diabetic complications the amounts of AGEs are generally increased, leading to structural changes in the extracellular matrix, as well as to modifications to cell membranes and intracellular components [Review [88,89]]. Increased levels of AGEs have been reported in central and peripheral nervous tissue from diabetic animals, but the number of studies is still limited [96,97,98].

4.3 Adverse effects of insulin?

Recent data implicate insulin itself in the pathogenesis of age-related memory decline and diabetic encephalopathy [64,3,99]. Insulin was long considered to be incapable of crossing the blood brain barrier but insulin and its receptor are now known to be present in the brain [100]. Although widely distributed, the insulin receptor is concentrated in specific brain regions including the olfactory bulbs, limbic system, hypothalamus and hippocampus, whereas insulin itself is particularly abundant in the hypothalamus and olfactory bulb [99]. The physiological function of insulin in these regions remains largely unknown. Although glucose uptake by the brain is considered to be mainly insulin-insensitive [101], insulin does affect cerebral glucose utilisation to some extent [99,102], analogous to its role in the periphery. In addition, brain insulin does seem to play a role in the regulation of food intake and body weight [103], and it may act as a "neuromodulator", influencing the release and re-uptake of neurotransmitters [104] and probably also learning and memory [105,99].

Impairments in the insulin signalling pathway in the periphery and in the brain have been implicated in Alzheimer's disease, diabetes and ageing [3,62,66]. Ageing is associated with reductions in the level of both insulin and its receptor in the brain [66]. In Alzheimer's disease this age-related reduction in insulin cerebral levels appears to be accompanied by functional disturbances of the insulin receptor [66], leading to the qualification of Alzheimer's disease as "an insulin-resistant brain state" [62]. In elderly non-demented, non-diabetic individuals chronic hyperinsulinemia is associated with cognitive decline, even after adjustment for possible confounding factors like cardiovascular disease and glucose levels [35,106]. In contrast to the apparent negative association between chronic hyperinsulinemia and cognitive functioning, acute insulin administration, while keeping glucose at fasting levels, actually improves memory in individuals with Alzheimer's disease, as well as in healthy controls [107].

Which mechanisms underlie the potential adverse effects of defective cerebral insulin signalling? Some suggest that disturbances in cerebral glucose metabolism are involved [62]. Links may also exist with the formation of AGEs and oxidative stress [71]. Degradation of oxidised molecules is mainly mediated by the proteasome, a large intracellular multienzymatic proteolytic complex [108]. Binding of insulin degrading enzyme to the proteasome increases its activity [109]. Insulin degrading enzyme is a metallo-endopeptidase that is also involved in the extra-cellular degradation of amyloid beta-protein [110]. Beta-amyloid, the main substance of senile plaques, has been implicated in the pathology of Alzheimer's disease and has been shown to induce apoptosis in vitro [111,112]. In vitro, insulin inhibits insulin degrading enzyme activity and proteasomal function competitively [110,113,114] impairing protein turnover, thereby facilitating the gradual accumulation of oxidised proteins. Recent studies support the significance of these in vitro findings for the in vivo situation [115,116]. An alternative route through which hyperinsulinaemia may favour the accumulation of oxidised-proteins was recently demonstrated in Caenorhabditis elegans. In this species a family of transcription factors has been described that is a target of insulin mediated signalling [117]. These transcription factors increase the defence against oxidative stress [118], decrease oxidative stress [119] and increase life-span [120]. Insulin inactivates these transcription factors, eliminating these effects [121].

Diabetes and its treatment with insulin are likely to affect cerebral insulin levels and insulin signalling. It is difficult however, to separate these "direct" effects of alterations in insulin homeostasis on the brain from the consequences of the accompanying alterations in peripheral and central glucose homeostasis, which in themselves can affect the brain. For example, in the type 2 diabetic population, those individuals who are treated with insulin appear to be at the highest risk of developing dementia[38]. Does this observation just reflect the severity of diabetes in this subgroup of patients, or could it be related to insulin treatment itself? This ambiguous role of insulin should form a focus of future research.

5. Conclusion

We have reviewed herein clinical and experimental data on the effects of diabetes on the brain and have explored the hypothesis that effects of diabetes and ageing on the brain may interact. Due to the ageing of the western population the prevalence of diabetes and the combination of diabetes and advanced age is expected to increase considerably. Diabetes appears to be an important risk factor for significant cognitive decline and dementia in the elderly. The challenge for the next decades will be to unravel the complex interaction between the mechanisms of ageing and diabetes. Further insight into this interaction may lead to the development of preventive measures or treatment strategies that may be of relevance to the growing population of diabetic patients and to the elderly in general. Preliminary studies in experimental models of diabetes and ageing provide evidence that treatment aimed at the pathogenetic factors described above may be fruitful.

Acknowledgements

The research described in this review was supported by grant 96125H from the Dutch Diabetes Foundation. The research of Geert Jan Biessels is also supported by grant 2000D030 from the Dutch Heart Association.

References

[1] Artola A, Kamal A, Ramakers GM, Gardoni F, Di Luca M, Biessels GJ, Cattabeni F, Gispen WH (2002) Synaptic plasticity in the diabetic brain: advanced aging? Prog Brain Res 138: 305-314
[2] Biessels GJ, Van der Heide LP, Kamal A, Bleys RL, Gispen WH (2002) Ageing and diabetes: implications for brain function. Eur J Pharmacol 441: 1-14
[3] Gispen WH,Biessels GJ (2000) Cognition and synaptic plasticity in diabetes mellitus. Trends Neurosci 23: 542-549
[4] Gavin JR, III, Alberti KGMM, Davidson MB et al. (1997) Report of the Expert Committee on the Diagnosis and Classification of Diabetes Mellitus. Diabetes Care 20: 1183-1197
[5] The Diabetes Control and Complications Study Group (1993) The effect of intensive treatment of diabetes on the development and progression of long-term complications in insulin-dependent diabetes mellitus. N Engl J Med 329: 977-986
[6] Biessels GJ, Kappelle AC, Bravenboer B, Erkelens DW, Gispen WH (1994) Cerebral function in diabetes mellitus. Diabetologia 37: 643-650
[7] Stewart R,Liolitsa D (1999) Type 2 diabetes mellitus, cognitive impairment and dementia. Diabet Med 16: 93 112
[8] Bell DS (1994) Stroke in the diabetic patient. Diabetes Care 17: 213-219
[9] Mankovsky BN, Metzger BE, Molitch ME, Biller J (1997) Cerebrovascular disorders in patients with diabetes mellitus. J Diabetes Complic 10: 228-242
[10] Cryer PE, Fisher JN, Shamoon H (1994) Hypoglycemia. Diabetes Care 17: 734-755

[11] Reske-Nielsen E, Lundbaek K, Rafaelsen OJ (1965) Pathological changes in the central and peripheral nervous system of young long-term diabetics. Diabetologia 1: 233-241
[12] Peress NS, Kane WC, Aronson SM (1973) Central nervous system findings in a tenth decade autopsy population. Prog Brain Res 40: 473-483
[13] Soininen H, Puranen M, Helkala EL, Laakso M, Riekkinen PJ (1992) Diabetes mellitus and brain atrophy: a computed tomography study in an elderly population. Neurobiol Aging 13: 717-721
[14] Araki Y, Nomura M, Tanaka H, Yamamoto H, Yamamoto T, Tsukaguchi I (1994) MRI of the brain in diabetes mellitus. Neuroradiology 36: 101-103
[15] Lunetta M, Damanti AR, Fabbri G, Lombardo M, Di Mauro M, Mughini L (1994) Evidence by magnetic resonance imaging of cerebral alterations of atrophy type in young insulin-dependent diabetic patients. J Endocrinol Invest 17: 241-245
[16] Manolio TA, Kronmal RA, Burke GL, Poirier V, O'Leary DH, Gardin JM, Fried LP, Steinberg EP, Bryan RN (1994) Magnetic resonance abnormalities and cardiovascular disease in older adults. The Cardiovascular Health Study. Stroke 25: 318-327
[17] Ylikoski A, Erkinjuntti T, Raininko R, Sarna S, Sulkava R, Tilvis R (1995) White matter hyperintensities on MRI in the neurologically nondiseased elderly. Analysis of cohorts of consecutive subjects aged 55 to 85 years living at home. Stroke 26: 1171-1177
[18] Di Mario U, Morano S, Valle E, Pozzessere G (1995) Electrophysiological alterations of the central nervous system in diabetes mellitus. Diabetes Metab Rev 11: 259-278
[19] Donald MW, Williams Erdahl DL, Surridge DHC, Monga TN, Lawson JS, Bird CE, Letemendia FJJ (1984) Functional correlates of reduced central conduction velocity in diabetic subjects. Diabetes 33: 627-633
[20] Khardori R, Soler NG, Good DC, DevlescHoward AB, Broughton D, Walbert J (1986) Brainstem auditory and visual evoked potentials in type 1 (insulin-dependent) diabetic patients. Diabetologia 29: 362-365
[21] Parisi V,Uccioli L (2001) Visual electrophysiological responses in persons with type 1 diabetes. Diabetes Metab Res Rev 17: 12-18
[22] Ziegler O, Guerci B, Algan M, Lonchamp P, Weber M, Drouin P (1994) Improved visual evoked potential latencies in poorly controlled diabetic patients after short-term strict metabolic control. Diabetes Care 17: 1141-1147
[23] Moreo G, Mariani E, Pizzamiglio G, Colucci GB (1995) Visual evoked potentials in NIDDM: A longitudinal study. Diabetologia 38: 573-576
[24] Picton TW (1992) The P300 wave of the human event-related potential. J Clin Neurophysiol 9: 456-479
[25] Anderer P, Pascual-Marqui RD, Semlitsch HV, Saletu B (1998) Differential effects of normal aging on sources of standard N1, target N1 and target P300 auditory event-related brain potentials revealed by low resolution electromagnetic tomography (LORETA). Electroencephalogr Clin Neurophysiol 108: 160-174
[26] Mooradian AD, Perryman K, Fitten J, Kavonian GD, Morley JE (1988) Cortical function in elderly non-insulin dependent diabetic patients. Behavioral and electrophysiologic studies. Arch Intern Med 148: 2369-2372
[27] Pozzessere G, Valle E, de-Crignis S et al. (1991) Abnormalities of cognitive functions in IDDM revealed by P300 event-related potential analysis. Comparison with short-latency evoked potentials and psychometric tests. Diabetes 40: 952-958
[28] Miles WR,Root HF (1922) Psychologic tests applied in diabetic patients. Arch Intern Med 30: 767-777
[29] Ryan CM (1988) Neurobehavioral complications of type I diabetes. Examination of possible risk factors. Diabetes Care 11: 86-93
[30] Gold AE, Deary IJ, Jones RW, O'Hare JP, Reckless JP, Frier BM (1994) Severe deterioration in cognitive function and personality in five patients with long-standing diabetes: a complication of diabetes or a consequence of treatment? Diabet Med 11: 499-505
[31] Wredling R, Levander S, Adamson U, Lins PE (1990) Permanent neuropsychological impairment after recurrent episodes of severe hypoglycaemia in man. Diabetologia 33: 152-157
[32] Langan SJ, Deary IJ, Hepburn DA, Frier BM (1991) Cumulative cognitive impairment following recurrent severe hypoglycaemia in adult patients with insulin-treated diabetes mellitus. Diabetologia 34: 337-344
[33] Ryan CM,Williams TM (1993) Effects of insulin-dependent diabetes on learning and memory efficiency in adults. J Clin Exp Neuropsychol 15: 685-700
[34] Strachan MWJ, Deary IJ, Ewing FME, Frier BM (1997) Is type II diabetes associated with an increased risk of cognitive dysfunction? A critical review of published studies. Diabetes Care 20: 438-445

[35] Kalmijn S, Feskens EJM, Launer LJ, Stijnen T, Kromhout D (1995) Glucose intolerance, hyperinsulinaemia and cognitive function in a general population of elderly men. Diabetologia 38: 1096-1102
[36] Vanhanen M, Koivisto K, Karjalainen L, Helkala EL, Laakso M, Soininen H, Riekkinen P (1997) Risk for non-insulin-dependent diabetes in the normoglycaemic elderly is associated with impaired cognitive function. NeuroReport 8: 1527-1530
[37] Peila R, Rodriguez BL, Launer LJ (2002) Type 2 diabetes, APOE gene, and the risk for dementia and related pathologies: The Honolulu-Asia Aging Study. Diabetes 51: 1256-1262
[38] Ott A, Stolk RP, Van Harskamp F, Pols HA, Hofman A, Breteler MM (1999) Diabetes mellitus and the risk of dementia: The Rotterdam Study. Neurology 53: 1937-1942
[39] Leibson CL, Rocca WA, Hanson VA, Cha R, Kokmen E, O'Brien PC, Palumbo PJ (1997) Risk of dementia among persons with diabetes mellitus: a population-based cohort study. Am J Epidemiol 145: 301-308
[40] Foster TC (1999) Involvement of hippocampal synaptic plasticity in age-related memory decline. Brain Res Brain Res Rev 30: 236-249
[41] Kamal A, Biessels GJ, Duis SEJ, Gispen WH (2000) Learning and hippocampal synaptic plasticity in streptozotocin-diabetic rats: interaction of diabetes and ageing. Diabetologia 43: 500-506
[42] Pitsikas N,Algeri S (1992) Deterioration of spatial and nonspatial reference and working memory in aged rats: protective effect of life-long calorie restriction. Neurobiol Aging 13: 369-373
[43] Bliss TV,Collingridge GL (1993) A synaptic model of memory: long-term potentiation in the hippocampus. Nature 361: 31-39
[44] Malenka RC,Nicoll RA (1999) Long-term potentiation--a decade of progress? Science 285: 1870-1874
[45] Yang SN, Tang YG, Zucker RS (1999) Selective induction of LTP and LTD by postsynaptic [Ca2+]i elevation. J Neurophysiol 81: 781-787
[46] Barnes CA (1994) Normal aging: regionally specific changes in hippocampal synaptic transmission. Trends Neurosci 17: 13-18
[47] Landfield PW (1994) Increased hippocampal Ca2+ channel activity in brain aging and dementia. Hormonal and pharmacologic modulation. Ann N Y Acad Sci 747: 351-364
[48] Kaleeswari R, Thombre DP, Chakrabarty AS (1986) Acute effect of streptozotocin induced diabetes on bar pressing for food reward in albino rats. Indian J Physiol Pharmacol 30: 319-321
[49] Bellush LL,Rowland NE (1989) Stress and behavior in streptozotocin diabetic rats: biochemical correlates of passive avoidance learning. Behav Neurosci 103: 144-150
[50] Flood JF, Mooradian AD, Morley JE (1990) Characteristics of learning and memory in streptozocin-induced diabetic mice. Diabetes 39: 1391-1398
[51] Mayer G, Nitsch R, Hoyer S (1990) Effects of changes in peripheral and cerebral glucose metabolism on locomotor activity, learning and memory in adult male rats. Brain Res 532: 95-100
[52] Biessels GJ, Kamal A, Ramakers GM, Urban IJ, Spruijt BM, Erkelens DW, Gispen WH (1996) Place learning and hippocampal synaptic plasticity in streptozotocin-induced diabetic rats. Diabetes 45: 1259-1266
[53] Biessels GJ, Kamal A, Urban IJ, Spruijt BM, Erkelens DW, Gispen WH (1998) Water maze learning and hippocampal synaptic plasticity in streptozotocin-diabetic rats: effects of insulin treatment. Brain Res 800: 125-135
[54] Popovic M, Biessels GJ, Isaacson RL, Gispen WH (2001) Learning and memory in streptozotocin-induced diabetic rats in a novel spatial/object discrimination task. Behav Brain Res 122: 201-207
[55] Chabot C, Massicotte G, Milot M, Trudeau F, Gagne J (1997) Impaired modulation of AMPA receptors by calcium-dependent processes in streptozotocin-induced diabetic rats. Brain Res 768: 249-256
[56] Kamal A, Biessels GJ, Urban IJA, Gispen WH (1999) Hippocampal synaptic plasticity in streptozotocin-diabetic rats: impairment of long-term potentiation and facilitation of long-term depression. Neuroscience 90: 737-745
[57] Segovia G, Porras A, Del Arco A, Mora F (2001) Glutamatergic neurotransmission in aging: a critical perspective. Mech Ageing Dev 122: 1-29
[58] Gagne J, Milot M, Gelinas S, Lahsaini A, Trudeau F, Martinoli MG, Massicotte G (1997) Binding properties of glutamate receptors in streptozotocin- induced diabetes in rats. Diabetes 46: 841-846
[59] Di Luca M, Ruts L, Gardoni F, Cattabeni F, Biessels GJ, Gispen WH (1999) NMDA receptor subunits are modified transcriptionally and post-translationally in the brain of streptozotocin-diabetic rats. Diabetologia 42: 693-701

[60] Tang YP, Shimizu E, Dube GR, Rampon C, Kerchner GA, Zhuo M, Liu G, Tsien JZ (1999) Genetic enhancement of learning and memory in mice. Nature 401: 63-69
[61] Kamal A, Ramakers GM, Biessels GJ, Gispen WH (2003) Effects of a phorbol ester and cyclosporin A on hippocampal synaptic plasticity in streptozotocin-induced-diabetic rats: reduced sensitivity to phorbol esters. Neurosci Lett 339: 45-48
[62] Hoyer S (1998) Is sporadic Alzheimer disease the brain type of non-insulin dependent diabetes mellitus? A challenging hypothesis. J Neural Transm 105: 415-422
[63] Messier C,Gagnon M (1996) Glucose regulation and cognitive functions: Relation to Alzheimer's disease and diabetes. Behav Brain Res 75: 1-11
[64] Gasparini L, Netzer WJ, Greengard P, Xu H (2002) Does insulin dysfunction play a role in Alzheimer's disease? Trends Pharmacol Sci 23: 288-293
[65] Vanhanen M,Soininen H (1998) Glucose intolerance, cognitive impairment and Alzheimer's disease. Curr Opin Neurol 11: 673-677
[66] Frolich L, Blum-Degen D, Bernstein HG et al. (1998) Brain insulin and insulin receptors in aging and sporadic Alzheimer's disease. J Neural Transm 105: 423-438
[67] Ryan CM,Geckle MO (2000) Circumscribed cognitive dysfunction in middle-aged adults with type 2 diabetes. Diabetes Care 23: 1486-1493
[68] Klein JP,Waxman SG (2003) The brain in diabetes: molecular changes in neurons and their implications for end-organ damage. Lancet Neurology 2: 548-554
[69] Beckman KB,Ames BN (1998) The free radical theory of aging matures. Physiol Rev 78: 547-581
[70] Smith MA, Sayre LM, Monnier VM, Perry G (1995) Radical AGEing in Alzheimer's disease. Trends Neurosci 18: 172-176
[71] Facchini FS, Hua NW, Reaven GM, Stoohs RA (2000) Hyperinsulinemia: the missing link among oxidative stress and age- related diseases? Free Radic Biol Med 29: 1302-1306
[72] Troni W, Carta Q, Cantello R, Caselle MT, Rainero I (1984) Peripheral nerve function and metabolic control in diabetes mellitus. Ann Neurol 16: 178-183
[73] Gsell W, Conrad R, Hickethier M et al. (1995) Decreased catalase activity but unchanged superoxide dismutase activity in brains of patients with dementia of Alzheimer type. J Neurochem 64: 1216-1223
[74] Jennings PE, Jones AF, Florkowski CM, Lunec J, Barnett AH (1987) Increased diene conjugates in diabetic subjects with microangiopathy. Diabet Med 4: 452-456
[75] Rosen P, Nawroth PP, King G, Moller W, Tritschler HJ, Packer L (2001) The role of oxidative stress in the onset and progression of diabetes and its complications: a summary of a Congress Series sponsored by UNESCO-MCBN, the American Diabetes Association and the German Diabetes Society. Diabetes Metab Res Rev 17: 189-212
[76] Wolff SP,Dean RT (1987) Glucose autoxidation and protein modification. Biochem J 245: 243-250
[77] Wolff SP, Jiang ZY, Hunt JV (1991) Protein glycation and oxidative stress in diabetes mellitus and ageing. Free Radic Biol Med 10: 339-352
[78] Wohaieb SA,Godin DV (1987) Alterations in tissue antioxidant systems in the spontaneously diabetic (BB Wistar) rat. Can J Physiol Pharmacol 65: 2191-2195
[79] Mukherjee B, Mukherjee JR, Chatterjee M (1994) Lipid peroxidation, glutathione levels and changes in glutathione-related enzyme activities in streptozotocin-induced diabetic rats. Immunol Cell Biol 72: 109-114
[80] Van Dam PS, Van Asbeck BS, Erkelens DW, Marx JJM, Gispen WH, Bravenboer B (1995) The role of oxidative stress in neuropathy and other diabetic complications. Diabetes Metab Rev 11: 181-192
[81] Adachi T, Ohta H, Hirano K, Hayashi K, Marklund SL (1991) Non-enzymic glycation of human extracellular superoxide dismutase. Biochem J 279: 263-267
[82] Costagliola C (1990) Oxidative state of glutathione in red blood cells and plasma of diabetic patients: in vivo and in vitro study. Clin Physiol Biochem 8: 204-210
[83] Ikebuchi M, Kashiwagi A, Asahina T, Tanaka Y, Takagi Y, Nishio Y, Hidaka H, Kikkawa R, Shigeta Y (1993) Effect of medium pH on glutathione redox cycle in cultured human umbilical vein endothelial cells. Metabolism 42: 1121-1126
[84] Mooradian AD,Smith TL (1992) The effect of experimentally induced diabetes mellitus on the lipid order and composition of rat cerebral microvessels. Neurosci Lett 145: 145-148
[85] Kumar JS,Menon VP (1993) Effect of diabetes on levels of lipid peroxides and glycolipids in rat brain. Metabolism 42: 1435-1439
[86] Makar TK, Rimpel-Lamhaouar K, Abraham DG, Gokhale VS, Cooper AJL (1995) Antioxidant defense systems in the brains of type II diabetic mice. J Neurochem 65: 287-291

[87] Huang WC, Juang SW, Liu IM, Chi TC, Cheng JT (1999) Changes of superoxide dismutase gene expression and activity in the brain of streptozotocin-induced diabetic rats. Neurosci Lett 275: 25-28
[88] Singh R, Barden A, Mori T, Beilin L (2001) Advanced glycation end-products: a review. Diabetologia 44: 129-146
[89] Brownlee M (2000) Negative consequences of glycation. Metabolism 49: 9-13
[90] Kimura T, Takamatsu J, Ikeda K, Kondo A, Miyakawa T, Horiuchi S (1996) Accumulation of advanced glycation end products of the Maillard reaction with age in human hippocampal neurons. Neurosci Lett 208: 53-56
[91] Mrak RE, Griffin ST, Graham DI (1997) Aging-associated changes in human brain. J Neuropathol Exp Neurol 56: 1269-1275
[92] Yan SD, Chen X, Fu J et al. (1996) RAGE and amyloid-β peptide neurotoxicity in Alzheimer's disease. Nature 382: 685-691
[93] Garner MH, Bahador A, Sachs G (1990) Nonenzymatic glycation of Na,K-ATPase. Effects on ATP hydrolysis and K+occlusion. J Biol Chem 26739: 15058-15066
[94] Wautier JL, Wautier MP, Schmidt AM et al. (1994) Advanced glycation end products (AGEs) on the surface of diabetic erythrocytes bind to the vessel wall via a specific receptor inducing oxidant stress in the vasculature: a link between surface-associated AGEs and diabetic complications. Proc Natl Acad Sci U S A 91: 7742-7746
[95] Bucala R, Tracey KJ, Cerami A (1991) Advanced glycosylation products quench nitric oxide and mediate defective endothelium-dependent vasodilatation in experimental diabetes. J Clin Invest 87: 432-438
[96] Vlassara H, Brownlee M, Cerami A (1983) Excessive non enzymatic glycosylation of peripheral and central nervous system myelin components in diabetic rats. Diabetes 32: 670-674
[97] Pekiner C, Cullum NA, Hughes JN, Hargreaves AJ, Mahon J, Casson IF (1993) Glycation of brain actin in experimental diabetes. J Neurochem 61: 436-442
[98] Ryle C, Leow CK, Donaghy M (1997) Nonenzymatic glycation of peripheral and central nervous system proteins in experimental diabetes mellitus. Muscle Nerve 20: 577-584
[99] Schulingkamp RJ, Pagano TC, Hung D, Raffa RB (2000) Insulin receptors and insulin action in the brain: review and clinical implications. Neurosci Biobehav Rev 24: 855-872
[100] Havrankova J, Schmechel D, Roth J, Brownstein M (1978) Identification of insulin in rat brain. Proc Natl Acad Sci U S A 75: 5737-5741
[101] Kumagai AK (1999) Glucose transport in brain and retina: implications in the management and complications of diabetes. Diabetes Metab Res Rev 15: 261-273
[102] Duelli R, Schrock H, Kuschinsky W, Hoyer S (1994) Intracerebroventricular injection of streptozotocin induces discrete local changes in cerebral glucose utilization in rats. Int J Dev Neurosci 12: 737-743
[103] Schwartz MW, Baskin DG, Kaiyala KJ, Woods SC (1999) Model for the regulation of energy balance and adiposity by the central nervous system. Am J Clin Nutr 69: 584-596
[104] Sauter A, Goldstein M, Engel J, Ueta K (1983) Effect of insulin on central catecholamines. Brain Res 260: 330-333
[105] Zhao W, Chen H, Xu H, Moore E, Meiri N, Quon MJ, Alkon DL (1999) Brain insulin receptors and spatial memory. Correlated changes in gene expression, tyrosine phosphorylation, and signaling molecules in the hippocampus of water maze trained rats. J Biol Chem 274: 34893-34902
[106] Stolk RP, Breteler MMB, Ott A, Pols HAP, Lamberts SWJ, Grobbee DE, Hofman A (1997) Insulin and cognitive function in an elderly population - The Rotterdam Study. Diabetes Care 20: 792-795
[107] Craft S, Asthana S, Newcomer JW et al. (1999) Enhancement of memory in Alzheimer disease with insulin and somatostatin, but not glucose. Arch Gen Psychiatry 56: 1135-1140
[108] Pacifici RE, Salo DC, Davies KJ (1989) Macroxyproteinase (M.O.P.): a 670 kDa proteinase complex that degrades oxidatively denatured proteins in red blood cells. Free Radic Biol Med 7: 521-536
[109] Hamel FG, Bennett RG, Duckworth WC (1998) Regulation of multicatalytic enzyme activity by insulin and the insulin- degrading enzyme. Endocrinology 139: 4061-4066
[110] Qiu WQ, Walsh DM, Ye Z et al. (1998) Insulin-degrading enzyme regulates extracellular levels of amyloid beta- protein by degradation. J Biol Chem 273: 32730-32738
[111] Forloni G (1993) beta-Amyloid neurotoxicity. Funct Neurol 8: 211-225
[112] Watt JA, Pike CJ, Walencewicz-Wasserman AJ, Cotman CW (1994) Ultrastructural analysis of beta-amyloid-induced apoptosis in cultured hippocampal neurons. Brain Res 661: 147-156
[113] Hamel FG, Bennett RG, Harmon KS, Duckworth WC (1997) Insulin inhibition of proteasome activity in intact cells. Biochem Biophys Res Commun 234: 671-674

[114] Bennett RG, Hamel FG, Duckworth WC (2000) Insulin inhibits the ubiquitin-dependent degrading activity of the 26S proteasome. Endocrinology 141: 2508-2517

[115] Farris W, Mansourian S, Chang Y et al. (2003) Insulin-degrading enzyme regulates the levels of insulin, amyloid beta-protein, and the beta-amyloid precursor protein intracellular domain in vivo. Proc Natl Acad Sci U S A 100: 4162-4167

[116] Cook DG, Leverenz JB, McMillan PJ et al. (2003) Reduced hippocampal insulin-degrading enzyme in late-onset Alzheimer's disease is associated with the apolipoprotein E-epsilon4 allele. Am J Pathol 162: 313-319

[117] Ogg S, Paradis S, Gottlieb S, Patterson GI, Lee L, Tissenbaum HA, Ruvkun G (1997) The Fork head transcription factor DAF-16 transduces insulin-like metabolic and longevity signals in C. elegans. Nature 389: 994-999

[118] Johnson TE, Cypser J, de Castro E, de Castro S, Henderson S, Murakami S, Rikke B, Tedesco P, Link C (2000) Gerontogenes mediate health and longevity in nematodes through increasing resistance to environmental toxins and stressors. Exp Gerontol 35: 687-694

[119] Honda Y,Honda S (1999) The daf-2 gene network for longevity regulates oxidative stress resistance and Mn-superoxide dismutase gene expression in Caenorhabditis elegans. FASEB J 13: 1385-1393

[120] Lin K, Dorman JB, Rodan A, Kenyon C (1997) daf-16: An HNF-3/forkhead family member that can function to double the life-span of Caenorhabditis elegans. Science 278: 1319-1322

[121] Kops GJ,Burgering BM (1999) Forkhead transcription factors: new insights into protein kinase B (c- akt) signaling. J Mol Med 77: 656-665

Frontiers in Neurodegenerative Disorders and Aging:
Fundamental Aspects, Clinical Perspectives and New Insights
T. Özben and M. Chevion (Eds.)
IOS Press, 2004

Role of Hypothetical Nuclear Organelles – Redusomes – in Morphogenesis, Aging and Cancer

Alexey Olovnikov
Inst. Biochem. Physics of RAS,
Chernyakhovskogo 5 - 94, Moscow 125319 Russia
olovnikov@dol.ru

Abstract: The role of the postulated perichromosomal organelles – redusomes – in individual development and in oncogenesis is examined. Also considered are the possible mechanisms of the shortening of linear DNA molecules and their biological role as applied to a redusomal DNA and telomeres.

1. Redusomes are hypothetical nuclear organelles

In present communication, basic questions related to the so-called redusome loss hypothesis of aging [3] are considered. Redusomes are hypothetical nuclear organelles. It is postulated that time-dependent developmental changes and aging (temporal events) are supervised by chronomeres, whereas morphogenesis (spatial events) is directed by printomeres. Both, chronomeres and printomeres, have the generic name - redumeres. Redumere is a linear DNA molecule. Redusome is the redumere covered with proteins. Redusomes are located at special chromosomal nests, in general at the subtelomeric regions of chromosomes. These organelles are the somatically inherited "perichromosomal" particles that are created and expressed during individual development. Redusomes gradually diminish in size due to the shortening of their DNA. Owing to this putative peculiarity, an ability to shrink, they were designated as redusomes. Each redusome has its own *ori* for replication, as well as promoter for transcription, but it has no centromere. Hence redusomes are distributed in mitoses among sister cells only due to the behavior of chromosomes that serve as specific carriers for redusomes. Transcripts from redumeres (rdsRNAs) belong to a fraction of small nuclear RNAs, namely to the two subfractions, microRNAs and fountain RNAs (fRNAs). These transcripts participate in chromatin configuration and modulation of chromosomal structural genes expression. As to fRNAs, they interact with the so-called fions (complementary sites in chromosomal DNA located mainly in the vicinity of structural genes), whereas the complex of fRNA-fion, interacting, in its turn, with a closed channel in the inner nuclear membrane, activates the channel for a short time interval and, in this way, provides the gene or corresponding chromosomal region with a portion of the proper ion, e.g., Ca^{2+} or Zn^{2+}, depending on the specificity of corresponding fRNA, fion and ion channel [3]. Controllable changes in the local level of Ca^{2+} can help in repackings of chromosomal structure, thus changing the gene activity. All these rdsRNAs are presumably at the top of a regulatory pyramid in eukaryotic cells, being engaged in modulation of the activity of various structural genes.

In spite of the fact that the main part of telomere-related predictions [2-4] were successfully confirmed (DNA end underreplication of linear DNA molecules; the notion that many prokaryotic genomes are circular in order to avoid DNA shortening; prediction of existence of a telomerase; explanation of correlation of telomere shortening with the number of cell doublings already performed by somatic cells that divide and age in vitro), I state now that the telomere model of cell aging should be rejected, since a telomere-shortening-dependent signal of cellular senescence does not exist. The telomere model of aging should be replaced by the redusome loss hypothesis.

2. Redusomes Should Originate Through the Stage of Reverse Transcription

Stage of reverse transcription in redusomal DNA synthesis is required to avoid possibility of uncontrolled firing of *ori* that could lead to a DNA branching, which would put obstacles in the way of correct segregation of replicating DNA molecules. That is why the endogenous reverse transcriptases may play an important role in the creation of redusomes, which are organelles that presumably participate in some key developmental events (see below). This is in concordance with presence of extrachromosomal DNAs which may occur to be the intermediates of a process of redumere creation in a variety of cells. A reverse transcriptase (RT) activity was found in early cleavage stage of murine embryos. Developmental arrest was induced when anti-RT antibody was microinjected in one blastomere of 2-cell embryos [5]. Elements with open-reading translation frames homologous to retroviral RNA-dependent DNA polymerases (reverse transcriptases) are widely presented in eukaryotic genomes [6-9]. Extrachromosomal circular DNA was found in various eukaryotes from yeast to humans. It is heterogeneous in size and composed of sequences that are homologous to chromosomal sequences; rev. in [10-12]. Among circular molecules of extrachromosomal DNA, there are sequences that are homologous to tandem repeated genes [11]; redusomal DNA should also contain the repeated sequences. In *Drosophila*, extrachromosomal circular DNA molecules (size ranges from <1 kb to > 20 kb) comprising up to 10 % of the total repetitive DNA content were revealed, for example, throughout the fruit fly's life cycle. In various animals, the extrachromosomal DNA populations were shown to contain centromeric heterochromatin sequences, as well as circular multimers of tandemly repeated sequences coded for Stellate, histones, rDNA; they contain telomeric repeats, etc. [12-15]. The extrachromosomal circular DNA molecules are among the earliest features of cellular differentiation in the early development of mice [14]. Extrachromosomal circular DNA has been considered as the substrate that could somehow reflect instability of chromosomal sequences during aging or altered patterns of gene expression, as well as a participant of developmental events [10-18]. Such DNAs were observed in the senescent fibroblasts where they may be involved, as suggested by several authors, upon a terminal differentiation [18]. Also described was the developmentally regulated formation of extrachromosomal circular DNA molecules, which occured *de novo* in preblastula *Xenopus laevis* embryos [14]. At the cleavage stage, before mid-blastula transition, Cohen et al. detected double- and single-stranded linear molecules and a circular DNA. The above molecules with molecular masses of several hundreds of base pairs up to 12 kbp had genomic sequences. The biological significance of the production of an extrachromosomal circular DNA is difficult to address [14]. Nevertheless, it seems reasonable to propose here that cells could use their ability to synthesize an extrachromosomal DNA for the fabrication of intermediates of redusomal DNA using reverse transcription. It should be emphasized that a linearized DNA is necessary for a redusome, whereas circular forms of DNA molecules could exist only as corresponding transitory forms. A curvilinear form possibly helps this DNA at the stage of docking in the chromosomal nest. Then DNA should be subjected to processing, including linearization and the enzymatically controlled treatment of its newly formed free termini, which should be then completed with a chromosomal DNA to protect them from nucleases. Protection of redusomal DNA overhang is similar to the protection of the telomere overhang inserted into DNA double helix with the d-loop formation. The redusomal DNA terminus is also able to form a d-loop, however the redusomal overhang makes a d-loop with another DNA molecule, namely with a chromosomal DNA, whereas telomere overhang, as is known, makes a d-loop with its own molecule. The redusome-chromosome d-loop is formed between the 3' overhang of an acromere (acromere is a redusomal analog of a telomere) and a homologous segment of the double-stranded DNA of a chromosomal nest. Having become perichromosomal, a former extrachromosomal pre-redusomal DNA should be linearized. It forms, probably, a parallel quadruplex with the corresponding sites of chromosomal DNA. It is pertinent to note that the bimolecular parallel quadruplexes, in which the direction of cooperating strands coincides, were shown to be more stable in comparison with the anti-parallel-stranded quadruplexes [19-20]. Being located within a nest and covered with the necessary proteins, redumere, or redusomal DNA, becomes a base of a mature redusome.

It is likely that the most convenient target for the pre-redusomal DNA landing on a chromosome is the single-stranded segment of DNA prepared in a chromosomal nest beforehand. Later, after hybridization with the complementary sites of the pre-redusomal DNA (for example, in a form of the intermediate triplexes), they should be repaired up to the usual double-stranded chromosomal DNA region. For a successful landing, it is not necessary for the whole acceptor area of a chromosomal nest to be transformed into a single-stranded form. For this purpose, it is enough to form a series of single-stranded docking-sites (probably, about some tens of nucleotides in length) separated by usual double-stranded stretches. After the beginning of the landing mission, the arising complex, in the course of the DNA repair synthesis of corresponding single-stranded sites of the chromosomal DNA, is capable to form a series of quadruplexes (replacing the former triplexes) between the redusomal and chromosomal DNA. The process of quadruplex creation is coupled, however, with a certain risk, because intermolecular interactions of DNA molecules can be a source of some unscheduled recombination. To avoid this, i.e. to prevent recombination of the redusomal DNA with the protoredusomal DNA of a chromosome, some enzymes of the RecQ helicases' family could apparently be exploited. Mutants on these enzymes are capable to provoke unscheduled transposition at yeast [21]. It is known that an abnormal activity of the WRN and BLM mutant proteins of this family is a progeria-provoking factor [22,23]. The WRN gene encodes a 3'-5' DNA helicase, or WRN protein; WRN is able to promote the ATP-dependent translocation of Holliday junctions, an activity that is also exhibited by BLM [24]. A progeria-provoked activity of these mutant proteins could be caused, as one can suggest, by the deterioration, in any way, of the activity of redusomes. It seems pertinent to state here that a normal WRN protein apparently should help the correct formation of the above-mentioned intermolecular triplexes and quadruplexes, temporarily and locally dissociating the non-optimally bound segments of the just-now-landed pre-redusomal DNA molecule and helping to create the optimal quadruplex structures along redumere and its specific chromosomal DNA target. Thus, the RecQ helicases are necessary for the appropriate mutual adjustment of both sides of forming quadruplexes, functioning as the "molecular accoucheurs" assisting during a "redusome delivery".

3. Printomeres as a Basis of Regulatory Morphogenesis

Printomeres, or redusomal DNA molecules, operating in dividing cells, are especially important in embryonal organogenesis helping to convert the information of nuclear DNA into three-dimensional multicellular structures of a developing creature (a "printomere mechanism of interpretation of positional information"). When interpreting their Wolpertian positional information, the cells of a morphogenetic field receive, (as one can suggest, with the help of printomeres) a certain imprinting of cells' positions. Here the name of such structures comes from; they could be named as "imprintomeres", but a shorter term, a "printomere", seems more convenient. Printomeres help a cell to somatically inherit its new state. Some of the genes in printomeres could code for mRNAs, which are translated into corresponding regulatory proteins, whereas their other genes code for small RNAs that can quantitatively modify the structural genes's activity and participate in control of chromatin repackings.

As to a principle of interpretation by cells of their positional information with the help of printomeres, cells occupying different positions on the axis of a morphogen concentration gradient should accept the different states of differentiation or determination. As mentioned above, an important role in this process is played by chromosomal originals of printomeres, or protoprintomeres. The choice by the morphogen of adequate protoprintomeres for their activation can be realized in the following way. Let us assume that a certain chromosome of all identical cells of a morphogenetic field have two protoprintomeres, which may be conditionally designated as resistant (R) and sensitive (S) ones; they are compacted with participation of lipid-containing factors, or so to say lipid-containing "seals". Let us also assume that these seals can be an object of burnout caused by free radicals and that they can be treated, with different results, by free radicals generated in cells when these cells were exposed to opposite, high and low, levels of a surrounding morphogen. Near the source of a morphogen, there is a high level of free radicals in a cell (or any other factor which is capable to destroy the seal and unpack protoprintomeres); here, both R and S protoprintomeres occur to be unpacked to give rise to proper active printomeres. However, on the opposite side of the same morphogenetic field, cells will be able to unpack only the protoprintomere S, which is very sensitive even to the low level of the "burning trough" factor. Similar binar choice may be made also by some protoprintomeres of some other chromosomes of the same cell. As a result, cells located near the source of morphogen concentration gradient and near the opposite pole of the morphogenetic field, will obtain distinctly different sets of printomeres, and due to that circumstance cells will obtain distinct cytophenotypes. Such kind of a process can take place in various morphogenetic fields, with their different morphogens and with diverse orientations of axes of morphogen concentration gradients. Recurring cycles of creation and expression of novel sets of printomeres (or, in a broader term, redumeres) are the basis of any regulative morphogeneses, as well as the source of robustness of these developmental events. This is a pivotal way to create three-dimensional multicellular organs, starting only from the linearly encoded DNA information. This solution may be an answer to the most long-standing enigma of embryology - how the 3D forms are properly arising in the individual development, and why in development a part is a function of the whole. Thus, the printomere mechanism ensures, at last, the solution of the long-standing problem of equifinality of embryonic development, the oldest problem of the developmental biology.

Printomeres, playing a pivotal role in the course of estimation and interpretation of positional information of cells, could simultaneously be indispensable participants of the mechanism of cellular differentiation. As Andrews rightly noted, little was understood of the key mechanisms that controlled the differentiation of stem cells, and current concepts about this operation are inadequate [25]. The redusomal mechanism of differentiation, as it seems, could fill this gap.

4. Role of Chronomeres and Scrupting in Measurement of Biological Time in Higher Animal Organisms

The organism needs this life-span clock in order to arrange the time-table for the proper deployment of many key developmental events occuring in its growth and mature state, such, e.g., as pubertat, menopause, etc. The key role in this device, namely the life-span clock, is played by short DNA molecules, or so-called chronomeres. They are located in nondividing neuroendocrine and neurotrophic cells of a brain. Chronomere, like a printomere of dividing cell, is a copy of a minute segment of a chromosomal DNA. Sequences of chronomeres, like other redusomal DNA, are indistinguishable from respective segments of a chromosomal DNA. The size of a nascent chronomere is, possibly, about 10-15 thousand pairs of nucleotides. The chronomere is covered by proteins (in this form it can be designated as chronosome) and lies in a special cavity, or the so-called nest (that is also like printosome) , between chromatin folds of the chromosomal segment that gave birth to it. Periodically hormonal bursts, following in an animal organism one after another at a certain frequency, interfere into the chronomeres' monotonous transcription activity. These hormonal storms last not long, possibly for about 10 minutes. The length of calm periods of corresponding infradian biological rhythms, which depends on the species, may be, for example, about a month or two weeks, at least for long-lived animal species; for more details see in [1]. At the peak of hormonal bursts that lasts those several minutes, RNA-polymerase molecules rush along the chronomere extremely fast. This leads to creating enormous mechanical stress near the terminus of a chronomeric DNA molecule, which is fixed at chromosomal DNA, probably in the d-loop (like d-loop that, as is already known, can protect the telomere's overhang). This structure is formed by interaction of redusomal DNA terminus and chromosomal DNA double helix. The "hypertranscription"-related torsional stress literally tears up the chronomere tip from its chromosomal nest. The released terminus immediately interacts with proteins, which protect it from unscheduled attacks of nucleases and slowly (possibly during an hour or more) restore the fastening of terminus, resuming its position in the chromosomal nest again. The process was designated as scrupting because it permits tran<u>scr</u>iption-dependent <u>rupt</u>ure of DNA and, hence, it leads to the DNA shortening.

In some more details, scrupting is the truncation of a linear redusomal DNA, which is transcribed at an especially high rate; this occurs only on relatively rare peaks of infradian hormonal rhythms, that are designated as T-rhythms (as rhythms involved into the temporal control of individual development). DNA molecules shorten during those rare events when the irrepairing terminal breaches create. The end gap arises under condition of high torsional mechanical strain, which is created when the transcriptional machinery is approaching most closely the very terminus of a redusomal DNA, which is tightly immobilized on the chromosomal DNA. This torsional stress induces disengagement of the 3' overhang of the redusome DNA from its immobilized state. Such event is accompanied either with mechanical disruption of 3' overhang (and, hence, immediate DNA shortening) or only with the extrication from d-loop (and from other contacts with a chromosomal DNA), which is then supplemented with the controlled enzymatic truncation of disengaged terminus, though the first variant is more probable. Accessory proteins assist to restore an immobilized state of the redusome terminus that should be fastened again at the chromosomal DNA. An essential step in the process of scrupting is a stage of an enzymatic stripping of the 5' end at the butt of redusomal DNA double helix (straightway after the transcription-dependent truncation). It leads to enlarging the length of free 3' overhang of a redumere, but, of course, not the length of redumere itself. This procedure is required to provide the possibility of recommencing the effective fastening of redusomal DNA terminus within d-loop at chromosomal DNA. The increase in the size of the terminal breach (which has just now been transcription-dependently diminished) is necessary in order to guarantee the possibility for the free 3' overhang of a redusome to touch a chromosomal DNA and to establish an intermolecular construction with it.

So, chronomeres shorten owing to the scrupting in a stepwise manner and lose their genes, whose products (untranslatable small RNAs and some possible redusomal mRNAs) are necessary for maintenance of a normal hormonal and neurotrophic activity of the CNS that controls individual development and maintenance of body functioning. Therefore, each loss of each chronomeric gene occurring in a coordinated manner in many neurons is a click of a lifelong clock that controls the life span of an animal organism and duration of its aging. Regular and consecutive losses of repeated genes from chronomeres are perceived by cells of the brain's life-long clock as a flow of biological time. Some, though probably rare, types of chronomeres contain genes encoding certain regulatory proteins; the loss of these genes can be a very important factor in the control of biological time during individual development. The intrinsic assessment of the flow of biological time performed with the participation of chronomeres is necessary for a timely beginning of the appropriate events of individual development, such as puberty, menopause, etc. Continuation of shortening of redusomal DNA molecules in organism, which already has achieved its physiological maturity, is responsible both for cellular senescence and the aging of organism as a whole.

There are several ways to intervene into the capability of the organism to evaluate the course of biological time and, hence, to change its biological age. Among potential genetic engineering tools useful for protecting chronomeres or restoring their shortened termini, one can use vectors that carry a telomerase activity together with those RNAs that help it to recognize the chronomere terminal repeats. This is a way of protection of chronomeres' termini in the already mature brain. Other approach can be based on tissue-specific vectors that code directly for chronomeric RNAs. Too early application of such techniques could prematurely stop the normal course of the individual development of a young organism, but being applied in a mature organism, they can protect it from corresponding age-related decline.

5. Fork-Dependent DNA End Underreplication as a Novel Mechanism of Underreplication of Telomeres and Redumeres in Dividing Cells

The inability of conventional DNA polymerases to replicate the very end of a linear DNA should lead to a continuous shortening of any replicating linear DNA molecules, telomeric DNA including [2]. As to a shortening of redusomal DNA in dividing cells, it should occur like telomere truncation. In addition to the two earlier predicted by me mechanisms of marginotomy (the DNA end underreplication of nowadays), namely a role of a "dead zone" in polymerase between its catalytic active center and the edge of polymerase molecule, as well as a role of the length of an eliminated terminal RNA primer [2,3], the additional mechanisms of DNA shortening, which are equally applicable for telomeres and redumeres, are under consideration in the present communication. They are based on the peculiarities of the work of a replisome. I propose here to apply the notion of a dead zone to the replication fork as the highly organized complex of proteins, RNAs and DNA operating at the replication fork area as a single whole.

DNA replication requires, as is known, an RNA primer for the beginning of DNA synthesis, and this is equally true for the lagging strand synthesis and the leading strand synthesis; therefore, the removing of terminal RNA primers is an important cause of incomplete replication both for leading and lagging strands. As DNA replication on the leading strand does need an initiating RNA primer, the leading strand should receive a terminal breach with 3' overhang due to the elimination of this terminal RNA primer. In addition, a dead zone between the rear end of DNA primase and its catalytic center can, and even must, make its own small contribution to the DNA end underreplication. Both of these effects, namely "primer-dependent" and "polymerase-dead-zone-dependent" variants of DNA end underreplication, should affect the length of the DNA replicas on the both replicating DNA strands. At the start of replication of a leading strand (that is near the 3' end of its template), terminal underreplication of the DNA is not very small, it is approximately equal to the sum of primer's length and the primase's dead zone length. Nearby the 5' end of the same template, the DNA polymerase, creating the leading strand, could come nearer to the end of the template. As to the possibility to replicate here the last nucleotides, one can take into account the following. Though polymerases of replicative synthesis need a complementary strand to provide a replica, the polymerase of DNA repair synthesis, unlike that, could partly compensate this inability of replicative polymerase. For this reason, polymerase of DNA repair synthesis, which is able to operate on a single strand of DNA, could complete, at least in part, the 5' end of a growing leading strand.

Measuring a telomere length in a single cell allows estimation of the telomere length of specific chromosome arms from metaphase cell preparations. In comparison with granulocytes, monocytes, CD8 and CD4 T lymphocytes and natural killer cells, approximately 1.3 kb longer telomeres were found in B lymphocytes [26]. This indicates the ability of telomerase, together with other factors, to modify the length of telomeres in a cell-specific manner. It is known that G-rich telomeric DNA 3' overhang is able to form the d-loop, displacing one strand of DNA double helix through interacting with its another strand [27], and a weak telomerase activity could probably elongate the very small 3' overhang before its subsequent protection in d-loop. An additional variant of creation of 3' overhang, at the expense of the work of 5' terminal exonucleolysis, is also plausible.

In addition to the above consideration, primase can introduce some element of stochasticity into the magnitude of DNA end underreplication. This can take place inasmuch as the length of a terminal RNA primer is not strictly fixed. Moreover, primase can begin the synthesis of RNA at various sites, generating, so to say, the «primase-dependent» stochasticity. Nevertheless, consideration of possible mechanisms of DNA end underreplication is not closed with this. Below one can find its additional novel aspect.

It is necessary to take into account that the replicative complex should permanently assemble and disassemble. This brings fundamentally important distinction into the processes deploying at the start and finish of replication of the linear DNA molecule, including telomeric and redusomal DNA. It is predicted here that the most essential contribution to the total effect of replicative shortening of a linear DNA should be mediated by the advancement of the replication fork on the margin of a template. Most important events that happen in the course of the lagging-strand synthesis occur on the background of the regular assemblage and dismantling of replisoma. Especially important are two actions, namely the onset and the termination of the replication fork propulsion. Putting the cart before the horse, the predicted effect could be designated as "the replication fork-dependent DNA end underreplication", or simply "fork shortening". The essence of the presumptive effect of DNA shortening caused by the terminal replisoma's dismantling consists in the following. Progression of the replication fork demands, as is known, participation of the dynamically looping of the template, which is used for the lagging-strand synthesis. This dynamic loop, however, cannot be created when a replication fork is approaching the 3' terminus of this template. Because of this, already at a very big distance (possibly, a hundred or more nucleotides) from 3' end of the template of the lagging strand template, the replisome complex must perform its final dismantling. Because of this, a big portion of 3' terminus of this template remains underreplicated, resulting in a heavy shortening of the lagging replica at its 5' end. As a result, a very long 3' overhang is forming here. The originated terminal breach cannot be healed, because the lagging strand does not contain here a free 3' end, whereas its free 5' terminus cannot be extended even by the DNA repair polymerase. Such is the crucial situation, when a disassembling replisome strives to create the very end of the 5' terminal portion of the growing lagging strand.

Certain restrictions (concerning just the activity of a replication fork) are typical also for the onset of DNA replication at the opposite end of the DNA double helix, that is near the 3' end of the template of leading strand. An initiating assembling of the replication fork on the butt of double helix requires an untwisting of the strands of a helix, liberating the termini from corresponding protective complexes and, therefore, making them more vulnerable to nucleases. During this procedure, the 5' terminus of the template of the lagging strand is compelled (in order to configure the replication fork complex) to make some dynamic pirouettes in space, conceivably remaining unprotected from nucleases for a longer time interval as compared to 3' terminus of the template for the leading strand. This permits some additional nucleolytic attacks on the 5' tail of the lagging strand template, contributing in its nucleolytic truncation, and, thus, potentially, leading to the increasing of the length of 3' overhang at this region of a nascent DNA double helix.

6. RETE as a Novel Mechanism Responsible for Phenomenology Heretofore Referred as ALT of Telomere Maintenance in the Absence of Telomerase

The chromosomal nests for redusomes are, apparently, located most often in subtelomeric regions of chromosomes. It should be noted that a normal process of the redusome forming may be disturbed in case of pathology. One of the forms of such pathology consists in the deletion in a chromosomal DNA at the boundary in-between the chromosomal protoredumere and telomere. In this case, a transcript, which is necessary as a template for the synthesis of extrachromosomal (pre-redusomal) intermediate, will be transcribed not only from protoredumere, but also from a telomeric DNA. As a consequence of that, an unusual extrachromosomal intermediate containing subtelomere and telomere-derived repeats will be synthesized. These superfluous telomere repeats will be able to serve as the source of extension of all telomeres of a nucleus in the course of the following intermolecular recombinations, even in the cells that are devoid of telomerase activity. Just this very thing, as is supposed here, should take place in immortal cancer cells with no detectable telomerase. To put it differently, the proposed process can be a genuine base of ALT (alternative lengthening of telomeres in absence of telomerase). This phenomenon of telomere maintenance is typical for approximately 10% of cancer cells [28-30]; the problem was reviewed in [31-32]. Reasoning from the essence of the above statement, one can now rename ALT as the "RETE" mechanism, since a novel term refers to and explains the kernel of the early unsolved problem. It is coined, using the letters from expression: "redumere-elongation-dependent telomere extension". The considered phenomenon is characterized by such features as a great heterogeneity of telomere size (ranging from undetectable to abnormally long) within individual cells, and a presence of special PML bodies that contain extrachromosomal telomeric DNA, telomere-specific binding proteins, and proteins involved in DNA recombination and replication [33]. Among various examples, one can note the characterization of the telomeric structures, in which the survivor mTER(-/-) mouse embryonic stem cell lines showed amplification of the same tandem arrays of telomeric and nontelomeric sequences at most of the chromosome ends [34]. Apparently, an excess of telomeric repeats that were formed upon the activity of a pathologically changed protoredumere is able to serve for the termini of all chromosomes, protecting them by RETE from telomere erosion. Probably, all non-telomerase cases of immortality of mammalian cells may be explained on the basis of RETE as a novel mechanism of telomere extension.

Thus, redusomes can play important roles in normal individual development and oncogenesis.

Acknowledgement

This study was supported by the Russian Foundation for Basic Research, grant 04-04-49600.

References

[1] Olovnikov AM. Redusomal hypothesis of aging and of the control of biological time during individual development. Biochemistry (Moscow). 2003, 68: 2-33; <protein.bio.msu.su / biokhimiya / contents / v68 / ToC6801.htm>.
[2] Olovnikov AM. Principle of marginotomy in template synthesis of polynucleotides. Dokl Akad Nauk SSSR. 1971, 201: 1496-9.
[3] Olovnikov AM. The immune response and the process of marginotomy in lymphoid cells. Vestnik Akad Med Nauk SSSR. 1972, 27: 85-7.
[4] Olovnikov AM. A theory of marginotomy. The incomplete copying of template margin in enzymic synthesis of polynucleoties and biological significance of the phenomenon. J Theor Biol. 1973, 41: 181-90.
[5] Pittoggi C, Sciamanna I, Mattei E, Beraldi R, Lobascio AM, Mai A, Quaglia MG, Lorenzini R, Spadafora C. Role of endogenous reverse transcriptase in murine early embryo development. Mol Reprod Dev. 2003, 66: 225-36.
[6] Ivanov VA, Il'in IuV. Reverse transcriptase and its biological role. Mol Biol (Moscow) 1995, 29: 258-80.
[7] Simpson GR, Patience C, Lower R, Tonjes RR, Moore HD, Weiss RA, Boyd MT. Endogenous D-type (HERV-K) related sequences are packaged into retroviral particles in the placenta and possess open reading frames for reverse transcriptase. Virology. 1996, 222: 451-6.
[8] Dhellin O, Maestre J, Heidmann T. Functional differences between the human LINE retrotransposon and retroviral reverse transcriptases for in vivo mRNA reverse transcription. EMBO J. 1997, 16: 6590-602.
[9] Menendez-Arias L. Molecular basis of fidelity of DNA synthesis and nucleotide specificity of retroviral reverse transcriptases. Prog Nucleic Acid Res Mol Biol. 2002, 71: 91-147.
[10] Stanfield S, and Helinski D R. Small circular DNA in Drosophila melanogaster. Cell. 1976, 9: 333-345.
[11] Pont G, Degroote F, Picard G. Some extrachromosomal circular DNAs from Drosophila embryos are homologous to tandemly repeated genes. J Mol Biol. 1987, 195: 447-51.
[12] Cohen S, Yacobi K, Segal D. Extrachromosomal circular DNA of tandemly repeated genomic sequences in Drosophila. Genome Res. 2003, 13: 1133-45.
[13] Cohen S, Mechali M. Formation of extrachromosomal circles from telomeric DNA in Xenopus laevis. EMBO Rep. 2002, 3: 1168-74.
[14] Cohen S, Menut S, Mechali M. Regulated formation of extrachromosomal circular DNA molecules during development in Xenopus laevis. Mol Cell Biol. 1999, 19: 6682-9.
[15] Yamagishi H, Kunisada T, Iwakura Y, Nishimune Y, Ogiso Y, Matsushiro A. Emergence of the extrachromosomal circular DNA complexes as one of the earliest signals of cellular differentiation in the early development of mouse embryo. Dev Growth Differ. 1983, 25: 563-9.
[16] Gaubatz JW. Extrachromosomal circular DNAs and genomic sequence plasticity in eukaryotic cells. Mutat Res. 1990, 237: 271-92.
[17] Yamagishi H. Role of mammalian circular DNA in cellular differentiation. Bioessays. 1986, 4: 218-21.
[18] Macieira-Coelho A. The last mitoses of the human fibroblast proliferative life span, physiopathologic implications. Mech Ageing Dev. 1995, 82: 91-104.
[19] Shchelkina AK, Borisova OF, Livshits MA, Jovin TM. Parallel-stranded DNA with natural base sequences. Mol Biol (Moscow) 2003, 37: 255-65.
[20] Borisova OF, Shchelkina AK, Il'icheva IA, Pozmogova GE. Conformational polymorphism and

extensibility of DNA quadruplexes formed from d (GT) n repeats. Mol Biol (Mosk.) 2001, 35: 860-7.
[21] Bryk M, Banerjee M, Conte D Jr, Curcio MJ. The Sgs1 helicase of Saccharomyces cerevisiae inhibits. The Sgs1 helicase of Saccharomyces cerevisiae inhibits retrotransposition of Ty1 multimeric arrays. Mol Cell Biol. 2001, 21: 5374-88.
[22] M. Fossel, Cells, Aging, and Human Disease. Oxford University Press, Oxford. 2003.
[23] VN. Anisimov, Molecular and Physiological Mechanisms of Aging (in Russian), Nauka, Sanct-Petersbourg, 2003.
[24] Constantinou A, Tarsounas M, Karow JK, Brosh RM, Bohr VA, Hickson ID, West SC. Werner's syndrome protein (WRN) migrates Holliday junctions and co-localizes with RPA upon replication arrest. EMBO Rep. 2000, 1: 80-4.
[25] Andrews PW. From teratocarcinomas to embryonic stem cells. Philos Trans R Soc Lond B Biol Sci. 2002, 357: 405-17.
[26] Martens UM, Brass V, Engelhardt M, Glaser S, Waller CF, Lange W, Schmoor C, Poon SS, Landsdorp PM. Measurement of telomere length in haematopoietic cells using in situ hybridization techniques. Biochem Soc Trans. 2000, 28: 245-50.
[27] Griffith JD, Comeau L, Rosenfield S, Stansel RM, Bianchi A, Moss H, de Lange T. Mammalian telomeres end in a large duplex loop. Cell. 1999, 97: 503-14.
[28] Herbert BS, Wright WE, Shay JW. Telomerase and breast cancer. Breast Cancer Res. 2001, 3: 146-9.
[29] Shay JW, Wright WE. Telomerase: a target for cancer therapeutics. Cencer Cell. 2002, 2: 257-65.
[30] Shay JW. Aging and cancer: are telomeres and telomerase the connection? Mol Med Today. 1995, 1: 378-84.
[31] Reddel RR. Alternative lengthening of telomeres, telomerase, and cancer. Cancer Lett. 2003, 194: 155-62.
[32] Reddel RR, Bryan TM, Murnane JP. Immortalized cells with no detectable telomerase activity. Biochemistry (Moscow). 1997, 62: 1254-62.
[33] Henson JD, Neumann AA, Yeager TR, Reddel RR. Alternative lengthening of telomeres in mammalian cells. Oncogene. 2002, 21: 598-610.
[34] Niida H, Shinkai Y, Hande MP, Matsumoto T, Takehara S, Tachibana M, Oshimura M, Landsorp PM, Furuichi Y. Telomere maintenance in telomerase-deficient mouse embryonic stem cells: characterization of an amplified telomeric DNA. Mol Cell Biol. 2000, 20: 4115: 27.

Frontiers in Neurodegenerative Disorders and Aging:
Fundamental Aspects, Clinical Perspectives and New Insights
T. Özben and M. Chevion (Eds.)
IOS Press, 2004

Oxidative Stress and Antioxidants in Aging

Tomris Özben

Akdeniz University Medical Faculty Department of Biochemistry 07058 Antalya TURKEY

Abstract: In accordance with the present state of scientific knowledge, the excessive production of free radicals in the organism, and the imbalance between the concentrations of these and the antioxidant defenses, may be related to processes such as aging and several diseases. Aging is associated with changes in physical characteristics and decline of many physiological functions. The aging process has been described by various theories, in particular the free radical theory of aging has received widespread attention. It has been proposed that the oxidative stress or damage induced by free radicals is related to aging. Oxidants and antioxidants have a clear function in the cellular physiology. When this delicate balance changes, many biochemical and cellular reactions are altered. The free radical hypothesis of aging proposes that deleterious actions of oxygen-derived radicals are responsible for the functional deterioration associated with aging. Modification of membrane lipids by the radicals has been produced to play a major role in the process of aging. Although, the relationship between lipid peroxidation and aging has been investigated extensively, the studies have produced conflicting results. To investigate the correlation between the oxidative stress and aging, we have determined the levels of lipid peroxidation expressed as thiobarbituric acid reactive substances and conjugated dien; oxidative protein damage as indicated by carbonyl content and activities of antioxidant enzymes including superoxide dismutase(SOD), catalase (CAT) and glutathione peroxidase(GPx) in a sample of 100 healthy men and women ranging in age from 20 to 70 years. In addition, vitamin E, C levels, reduced glutathione and sulfhydryl content were determined. The oxidation end product of nitric oxide (nitrate) was also studied to investigate any role of nitrogen radicals in aging. Our data shows that there is an age related increase in the concentration of lipid peroxides expressed as MDA and oxidative protein damage as indicated by carbonyl content. We found that aging is not linked to a decline in antioxidant enzymes except GPx. Our data suggests that the level of oxidative stress increase cannot be entirely attributed to a decrease in the activities of antioxidant defense system and probably various factors may contribute to this process

1. Definition of Aging

Aging is an inevitable biological process affecting most of the living organisms. Despite the enormous consequences associated with the aging process, until recently, relatively little systematic effort has been expended on the scientific understanding of this important life process. Since older population in society is increasing, scientists from many disciplines are being urged to investigate this inevitable and important life process. Aging is one of the nature's most complex phenomena. In recent years, research directed toward the basic understanding of biological aging mechanisms and possible aging interventions have provided new insights into the molecular basis and the biological events that contribute to age-related deterioration[1]. Repair of cellular and extracellular constituents in elderly individuals diminish when compared to younger age groups. Environmental factors and injury throughout life that affect the genome and other constituents of the cells and extracellular components contributes to and cause a time dependent increase in this repair deficiency. Aging causes cells to lose theirresistance to injury, hence making the organism more vulnerable to trauma and infection. Individuals age differently depending upon several factors including the condition of the repair system. The contributions of the aging process to aging changes are small early in life but rapidly increase with age due to the exponential nature of the process[2-7].

Byung defines aging as a genetic physiological process associated with morphological and functional changes in cellular and extracellular components aggravated by injury throughout life and resulting in a progressive inbalance of the control regulatory systems of the organism, including the hormonal, autocrine, neuroendocrine, and immune homeostatic mechanisms[1]. Aging can be considered as the product of an interaction between genetic, environmental, and lifestyle factors, which in turn influence longevity that varies between and within species.

Aging is not considered as a disease. Aging contributes to the susceptibility to disease and one dies from a distinct pathological event, not the aging process[2-7]. In order to understand the basic mechanisms involved in biological aging, it must be differentiated from age-related diseases. It is difficult to find a precise definition of aging upon which every gerontologist can agree. Therefore, it is less problematic relying on a set of characteristics. In general, aging is described as a time-dependent functional decline, loading to the cell's incapacity to withstand external and internal challenges. According to this description, aging is the consequence of two independent biological processes: the loss of functionality, and the loss of resistance or adaptability to stress. The causal factors leading to the loss of these two independent biological processes have not been fully elucidated yet. The time-dependent, deleterious processes of aging have not yet been well defined. There is no single adequate molecular explanation for aging currently available. The consensus among researchers broadly views the concept of biological aging as an organism's failure to maintain homeostasis. The progressive loss of functional capacity of organisms leads to failure to maintain homeostasis and resulting in death [8,9]. Aging causes failure of coordinating systems with neural, neuroendocrine and endocrine origine. Informational failure such as loss of DNA and RNA, single strand breaks, base substitution and deletion and transcriptional and translational impairments are commonly seen during aging. Cell lose and mebrane damage, protein alteration, cross-linking, and glycation, oxidative modification of proteins, lipids and carbohydrates occur and contribute to structural damage and modification in aging. Loss of repair capacity and loss of detoxifying process cause accumulation of deleterious substances[8].

Aging is a universal phenomenon that is both obvious and inevitable, yet poorly understood, and under research at the molecular level[8]. To develop a scientific base with respect to the understanding of the phenomenon of aging, a spectrum of new and innovative strategies and approaches are being increasingly applied to modulate the process of aging at the level of cells, tissues, organs and organisms.

2. Free Radical Theory of Aging

According to a recent account from Medvedev, more than 300 theories on aging exist to explain the progressive and deleterious changes characteristic of aging[10]. So far, no theory has been accepted generally and most of them lack sufficient supporting evidence to merit serious consideration and acceptance[9]. Most aging theories fall into two broad categories based on putative casual forces: (1) intrinsic factors, referring to genomic components and genetic processes; and (2) extrinsic factors, encompassing various external environmental influences on the organism. Among these hypotheses, free radical theory of aging, named recently as oxidative stress hypothesis has gathered strong support by many scientists working in the field.

The free radical theory of aging was proposed in November 1954 by Denham Harman which proposes that aging results from imperfect protection against tissue damage brought about by free radicals. Reactive oxygen species(ROS) cause oxidative damage over the lifetime of the subject. It is the cumulative and potentially increasing amount of accumulated damage that accounts for the dysfunctions and pathologies seen in normal aging[11,12,13]. This aging theory is meritorious for having provided modern gerontologists with both a conceptual base and the experimental opportunities necessary to explain the biological basis of senescence and disease[1,14-20]. All the data obtained to show a direct link between senescence and oxidative stress were mostly correlative[9,21]. A major obstacle to accept of the free radical theory has been the poor record of antioxidants in prolonging the life span of animals. Many other variables, such as genetic factors, temperature, activity and nutrition can affect life span, making it a highly complex multi-factorial process.

The new knowledge we have gained in the field of free radical biochemistry over the last decade necessitated an expansion and modification of the free radical theory of aging[16]. Three major features make the revision noteworthy: (1) the source of reactive species responsible for oxidative damage is not limited to oxygen-derived free radicals(mainly superoxide generation by mitochondria). Reactive nitrogen species and reactive aldehydic species contribute to oxidative damage as well. (2) free radical generation is not stoichiometrically coupled to either oxygen consumption or metabolic rate per se; and (3) biological aging is not likely caused by the pathogenicity of disease. In accordance with these new knowledge and data, the oxidative stress hypothesis of aging has replaced the previous free radical theory of aging. The characteristic natures of aging and free radical reactions are compared in Table 1.

Table 1. Characteristics of Aging and Free Radical Processes

	Aging	Free Radicals
Occurrence	Most organisms	All respiring cells
Cellular homeostasis		
1. Structure	Deterioration	Oxidative modification
2. Function	Dysregulation	Alteration
Pathological status	Increase in prevalence	Causative or promoting
Intervention		
1. Dietary restriction	Retardation	Suppression of oxidative stress
2. Antioxidant feeding	Median life span extension	Selective suppression

differention. High intracellular ROS level gives harm to proteins, lipids and DNA and stimulates apoptosis in cells by specific signal pathways. When ROS generation and resulting oxidative stress are higher for the cells to cope with them, cells may undergo apoptosis. Many signal pathways are redox sensitive. Extracellular signalling molecules and ROS induce several signal transduction pathways leading to alteration of gene expression. A complete understanding of cellular responses to oxidative stress might provide useful information on aging and will be beneficial in manipulating and slowing aging process[39]. These future insights will contribute to our understanding how oxidative stress plays a role in both aging and age related disease states.

5. Damage to Macromolecules

Reactive oxygen species (ROS) leak from mitochondria into the cytoplasm where they cause cellular damage by oxidizing a variety of biologically important molecules, including DNA, proteins and lipids. Peroxidation of polyunsaturated fatty acids generates alkanes. Molecular damage resulting from oxidative stress(OS) is cumulative and ultimately lethal. OS also accelerates shortening of telomeres, the mitotic clock in human somatic cells, causes cellular senescence and death[22]. Aging is associated with the accumulation of oxidized forms of cellular constituents.

Age related progressive oxidative modifications of mitochondrial enzymes, coenzymes and mitochondrial membranes increase ROS generation in mitochondria. There are also many metabolic processes leading to direct formation of ROS which may give harm to the enzymes in that metabolic process. The oxidation of enzymes cause conformational change that can affect the affinites for substrates and/or allosteric effectors that serve as regulators of the enzyme activities. In his review, Stadtman reported that aging is associated with substantial decreases in the activities of numerous enzymes[26]. Many of these enzymes are found only in the cytosol where they catalyze important reactions in the metabolism. A change or loss in the activity of an enzyme may have a profound effect on a particular metabolic process and and this may vary between individuals. Individual variations might me a determining factor in aging of individuals[26].

It is widely accepted that cellular levels of oxidatively modifed proteins, lipids and nucleic acids increase during aging. However, the mechanisms underlying these age related modifications of macromolecules are very complex, variable and multifactorial. Individuals age differently depending on their genetic background, physiological state, life-style, physical activity, dietary habits. Therefore age related accumulation of oxidative macromolecule damage vary among individuals. Many factors leading to ROS generation give damage to macromolecules, especially proteins[26]

Oxidative damage to mitochondrial DNA measured as 8-hydroxy-2'-deoxyguanosine(8-oxodG) correlates negatively with maximum life span potential. Such a correlation doesnot exist for nuclear DNA. Oxidative damage to DNA and lipids can be repaired or prevented by several mechanisms[9,40]. It is known that 8-oxodG is repaired both in nucleus and mitochondria. Oxidative damage to mtDNA is higher in short-lived species in comparison to the long-lived ones. On the other hand, oxidized proteins lose their structural and functional integrity. Oxidation products of proteins and lipids may form a undegradable fluorescent pigment called lipofuscin[9,41]. The degree of fatty acid unsaturation of cellular membranes is an interesting area to explore. Unsaturated fatty acids are the cellular macromolecules most sensitive to free radical attack causing lipid peroxidation. Moreover, lipid peroxidation products(MDA, HNE) cause detrimental protein modifications. The degree of fatty acid unsaturation and its correlation with life sppan in differnet species needs to be explored further. Oxidative damage to cellular constituents are subject to control by enzymatic and nonenzymatic antioxidant defenses that can either scavenge ROS or prevent their formation. Cells are also equipped with enzyme systems that can either repair the damage or degrade the damaged molecules to simple non-toxic metabolites[26].

6. Protein Oxidation and Carbonyl Stress

Oxidized protein build up is commonly seen as a hallmark of cellular aging[40]. The role of increased oxidative stress in the development of oxidative protein damage in aging is currently a subject of great interest[11,13,42-46].

The conversion of proteins to protein carbonyl derivatives occur via direct oxidation by ROS[26,40]. Other mechanisms contributing to age-related increase in protein content originate from the formation of protein adducts with carbohydrates and lipid peroxidation products. Glycation, glycoxidation, and conjugation of protein amino acid side chains with lipid peroxidation products(malondialdehyde,MDA;α,β-unsaturated aldehydes,HNE) cause alterations in proteins. These reactions introduce carbonyl groups in proteins. Aldehydes(MDA and HNE) originating from membrane polyunsaturated fatty acid oxidation binds covalently to the side chains of proteins. HNE particularly reacts with cystein, histidine and lysine. Schiff base formation occurs between ε-amino group of lysine and the aldehyde group of HNE leading to the formation of intra and inter-molecular cross-linking of proteins[40]. ε-amino group of lysine residues in proteins react with aldehyde groups of carbohydrates, known as Maillard reaction generating Amadori products. Further oxidation of these products leads to the formation advanced glycation end products(AGEs). AGEs are carboxymethyl-lysine, pyrraline, imidazolone, carboxyethyl-lysine, pentosidine, glyoxal-lysine and methylglyoxal-lysine dimers. Some of these AGEs such as pentosidine, glyoxal-lysine and methylglyoxal-lysine dimers cause cross-linking of proteins[40]. Another protein modification that occurs during aging is spontaneous deamidation of asparagine and glutamine residues in proteins. Ubiquitin-protein conjugates are another protein modification observed to accumulate with age in certain tissues[40].

Almost all amino acids within proteins can be oxidized by ROS, sulfur-containing (cystein and methionine) and aromatic (tyrosine and tryptophan) amino acids being the most susceptible[40,47,48]. Oxidation products of cystein are disulfide bridges and mixed disulfides while methionine is converted to methionine sulfoxide. Within proteins, mixed disulfides and disulfide bridges are reduced by the thioredoxin/ thiredoxin reductase system while methionine sulfoxide can be reversed to methionine by the peptide methionine sulfoxide reductase[40,49-51]. Oxidative protein damage cannot be repaired except for the oxidation of methionine and cysteine[26]. Oxidation of other amino acids mostly generates hydroxyl and carbonyl(oxoacids and aldehydes) groups. These oxidations cause irreversible modifications in proteins. Highly reactive hydroxyl radical OH• attacks the polypeptide backbone of proteins causing cleavage and/or reticulation of proteins. The structure and activity of oxidized proteins have changed profoundly in comparison to their native forms. They are generally less active and their thermal and thermodynamic stability are less than their native forms[40,52]. Oxidized proteins expose hydrophobic residues at their surface. Alteration of secondary and/or tertiary structure has also been reported for oxidized proteins[40,53,54].

Oxidative modification of proteins in vivo may affect a variety of cellular functions. Receptors, signal transduction mechanisms, transport systems, and enzymes are affected by oxidative modifications.. Protein oxidation also contributes to secondary damage to other biomolecules such as, inactivation of DNA repair enzymes, loss of fidelity of DNA polymerases in DNA replication, and the development of new antigens provoking autoimmune responses[11,55]. Alterations in protein conformations can lead to increased aggregation, fragmentation, distortion of secondary and tertiary structure, susceptibility to proteolysis, and diminution of normal function[11,12]. The impairment of important enzymes and the age-related accumulation of damaged protein are believed to affect cellular integrity[40]. Age related increase in protein carbonyls depends on the individuals susceptibilty to oxidative stress and varies widely among individuals[26].

The oxidative damage to proteins is reflected by increase in levels of protein carbonyls(PCO), and decrease in levels of protein thiols(P-SH) [11,42,45,63,64]. The best marker for intracellular oxidative stress dependent cellular damage is the intracellular protein carbonyl content. The unique advantage of the carbonyl measurement as a good marker of oxidative stress is the fact that it covers a much wider range of oxidative damage than other markers[40]. The detection of protein-associated carbonyls is a common method for a general assessment of protein oxidation level in animal tissues and body fluids.[40,65].The other markers such as nitrotyrosine, hydroxylation of aromatic and hydrophobic amino acids are at very low level in comparison to the carbonyl content. Indeed, measurement of PCO has been used as a sensitive assay for oxidative damage to proteins[11,55,66].

Protein-associated carbonyls can be derivatized by treatment of proteins with DNPH. Using the carbonyl content as a general index for the protein oxidation status, a significant increase of oxidized protein with age has been reported in human dermal fibroblasts, human keratinocytes, human erythrocytes, human brain, rat hepatocytes as well as in *Drosophila*[40,67,68]. Although the level of protein carbonyls groups is currently the best overall marker of oxidative stress, the analytical methods to detect the levels of each kind of protein measurement should be developed.

It has already been shown that free radicals cause oxidation of P-SH groups. P-SH groups in proteins may serve an antioxidant function by several mechanisms. P-SH may scavenge oxidants, thus sparing antioxidants and/or cellular constituents from attack [11,64,69]. Therefore, measurement of oxidised and reduced forms of sulfhydryl groups in proteins may be useful as well as protein carbonyl content.

Nitric oxide(NO) is a biologic mediator released by a variety of cells. NO reacts with the superoxide ion resulting in the generation of peroxynitrite ($ONOO^-$), a strong and relatively long-lived oxidizing agent which can attack protein molecules. The major product of $ONOO^-$ attack on proteins is the addition of a nitro group to the ortho position of tyrosine residues to produce nitrotyrosine(NT). $ONOO^-$ may also produce other chemical modifications of proteins including oxidation of thiol residues[11,46,70,71]. Measurement of protein nitrotyrosine content is a useful marker to demonstrate reactive nitrogen species related protein modifications.

7. Proteasome

Except for the oxidation of cysteine and methionine amino acids in proteins, oxidations and alterations of proteins are irreversible rendering organisms incapable to repair ROS mediated protein damage[26,40]. On the otherhand, protein turnover is essential to preserve cell function. The accumulation of damaged proteins is limited due to the degradation of oxidized proteins by various proteases. The main proteolytic system in charge of cytosolic protein degradation is the proteasome. The proteasome is a multi-catalytic proteolytic complex, which recognizes and selectively degrades oxidatively damaged, misfolded, altered and ubiquitinated proteins. In addition to eliminating damaged proteins, Carrard et al. reported that the proteasome is implicated in a broad range of cellular pathways[40,72,73] such as apoptosis[74,75], cell cycle[76], cell differentiation[77], DNA repair[78,79] and degradation of many important rate-limiting enzymes in metabolic pathways.

The 26S proteasome is an essential component of the ubiquitin and ATP-dependent proteolytic pathway. The 20S proteasome catalytic core is a high molecular weight complex of 700 kDa which represents up to 1% of soluble cellular proteins[40,80]. In the cell, this complex constitutes the main non-lysosomal proteolytic machinery implicated in protein degradation. 20 S proteasome degrades oxidized proteins by a ubiquitin-independent pathway[26,53,81-86]. It was reported that excessive oxidation and/or conversion of oxidized proteins to cross-linked derivatives not only renders them resistant to proteolytic degradation by the proteasome, but also inhibits the capacity of the proteasome to degrade oxidized proteins[26,82,86-92].

One of the hypothesis put forward to explain the accumulation of altered proteins is the decrease of proteasome activity with age[40]. It was demonstrated that aging is associated with a decrease in the proteasome activity, and an increase in the level of oxidized proteins[26,93-99]. Indeed, accumulation of altered protein can be explained by increased protein alteration, decreased protein degradation or the combination of both[40].

Formation of inhibitory damaged proteins with age may also influence the proteasome activities. It was observed that in rat myocardiac cells, the age-dependent decline of certain peptidase activities in cytosolic extracts is partially relieved upon purification of the 20S proteasome[40,100]. Treatment of the model protein glucose-6-phosphate dehydrogenase(G_6PD) with HNE was shown to result in the formation of intra-molecular cross-linking. This HNE cross-linked protein is resistant to proteolysis by the 20S proteasome and was shown to act as non-competitive inhibitor of the 20S proteasome[40,90,91] Proteasome inhibition was observed upon cell loading with ceroid pigment or artificial lipofuscin suggesting an implication of such highly oxidized cross-linked proteins in senescence-associated impairment of proteasome function[40,101].

We can conclude that damaged proteins accumulate while protein turnover declines with age. Evidence has also been provided that the activity of proteasome, which is the major cytosolic protein degradation system, is impaired with age. However, events leading to the age related loss of proteasome function have not been yet fully characterized. The age-related decline of proteasome activity appears to be the result of the combined effects of at least: (1) a decreased proteasome expression; (2) structural modifications and/or replacement of proteasome subunits and (3) inhibition by damaged proteins. More research are needed to clarify the mechanisms responsible for the age related decline of the proteasome and to develop strategies to prevent this decline[40].

8. Life Span Extension Studies

In order to conduct life span extension studies, it is essential to identify alterations occurring during aging. Life span extension studies can be grouped on the following topics:

1. Metabolic rate
2. Oxygen consumption
3. Single gen mutations
4. Calori restriction
5. Environmental conditions such as ambient temperature, nutrients, water, etc.
6. Overexpression of antioxidants enzymes
7. Administration of antioxidants

Pearl proposed the rate of energy utilization is a key determinant of the rate of aging[102]. According to Pearl, two variables determine the duration of life: (1) the genetic constitution of the individual, and (2) the average rate of metabolism during life. He proposed that the duration of life varies inversely with the rate of energy utilization. His proposal subsequently was called as the "rate of living" hypothesis. In several experiments, it was demonstrated that life span can be extended if metabolic rate is decreased[102-105]. In some poikilothermic organisms life span was found to be inversely related to their ambient temperature and rate of metabolism or oxygen consumption[9]. In these experiments, lowered rate of metabolism was achieved by a decrease in the ambient temperature, inactivation of some enzymes, decreased level of physical activity and decreased oxygen consumption. All of these experiments resulted in increased life spans[9,102-105]. It is difficult to demonstrate such a relation in homeothermic species in comparison to poikilotherms since their body temperature is stable and their metabolic rate is not easy to modulate[9]. Lyman et al. demonstrated that life spans of Turkish hamster could be extended by induced hibernation[102,106].

There are exceptions such as birds that prevent Pearl's "rate of living" hypothesis to be generally approved by all gerontologists. Birds are relatively long-lived with a high metabolic rate. In spite of their high rates of oxygen consumption, birds produce less ROS in mitochondria. The explanation for this discrepancy lies also in the fact that the relationship between duration of life and rate of metabolism applies only to the same species. Genetic constitution determines the total energy consumed during life which is termed as metabolic potential. On the other hand, metabolic rate is defined as the rate at which energy is consumed which is the determining factor in the length of life. Metabolic potential varies in different phylogenetic groups. Within each species, there is a definite inverse relationship between metabolic rate and species-specific life span[102,107]. Comparative studies of several mammals with different body sizes showed that maximum life span potential was observed in animals with lower metabolic rates and lower oxygen consumption per kg of body the long-lived animals. Larger animals have lower metabolic rates. While metabolic potential remains unaltered, it is possible to manipulate metabolic rate by several means. Since metabolic rate and oxygen consumption are linked closely, this is an evidence of a clear link between rate of living hypothesis and the oxidative stress hypothesis of aging. It can be concluded that the rate of oxygen radical generation in tissues must be lower in long-lived than in short-lived species. It can be concluded that the mitochondrial rate of ROS production correlates better than the metabolic rate with maximum longevity. Species may have longer life spans if their ROS production is lower even if their metabolic rate is higher as in birds.

Some gerontologists believed in the idea that aging is a genetically programmed process and it might be possible to control it by genetic manipulations. Various life span extension studies have focused on single-gene mutations in lower organisms, such as nematodes and insects. Single gen mutation caused a dramalife span extension in *Caenorhabditis elegans* and *Drosophila melanogaster*. In several studies a mutation in the insulin/IGF-signalling pathway have been reported in these organisms[9,108,109]. The best characterized of these is the first longevity mutant identified—*age-1*[23,110]. This gene encodes a phosphatidylinositol-3 kinase[23,111]. The *age-1* mutant has higher levels of both SOD1 and catalase[23,112,113]. This can be interpreted as providing evidence for the free radical theory of aging. Other single-gene mutation studies include a null mutation of the insulin receptor substrate in *D. Melanogaster*, a gen mutation encoding cotransporter of tricarboxylic acid intermediates, another gen mutation encoding a G-protein-coupled receptor. In these studies, life span extensions achieved only in case of loss of vigor and reproductive output. Results of these studies demonstrated that hypometabolism increases length of survival, resistance to stress, enhanced antioxidative capacity and adaptation to adverse conditions[9,114-116].

The two hypotheses of aging, namely oxidative stress theory and rate-of-living theory are interconnected since the metabolic rate is related to the rate of ROS generation. The repair capacity of the organisms and their antioxidative capacity are determing factors in metabolic potential. It was shown that maximum life span in species with similar metabolic potentials are inversely related to mitochondrial ROS production and damage to macromolecules[9,117,118]. It was reported that caloric restriction lowered mitochondrial ROS production and correlated positively with extension of life span[9]. Accumulating evidence shows that calorie restriction is the only intervention known to delay the onset of age-related deficits and increase life-span of mammals[119].

Several studies have been carried out to test the oxidative stress hypothesis of aging by determining if overexpression of antioxidative enzymes resulted in life-span extension[9]. There are conflicting results in literature. It was demonstrated that Cu-Zn SOD, Mn-SOD and catalase overexpression had no effect on the life spans in transgenic *Drosophila melanogaster* [9,120]. In another study, simultaneous overexpression of Cu, Zn-SOD and catalase was found to result in an increase of up to 34% in life span and an attenuation of macromolecular oxidative damage in *D. Melanogaster*[102,121]. Other aging studies include flies transgenic for both the cytosolic or mitochondrial forms of superoxide dismutase (SOD1 and SOD2, respectively)[23,122-124]. The increased expression of these genes in the fly results in increased life span and a resistance to various types of stress. These results are consistent with the free radical theory of aging[23,125]. The life span extension studies in transgenic animals should be evaluated and compared with the life spans of the control strain(s) used vs. those of the robust long-lived strains of the same species[102]. The current data suggests that aging is amenable to pharmacological interdiction, at least in a simple invertebrate, and a therapeutic strategy can be applied to potentially alleviate some of the degenerative changes associated with aging being dependent on the use of proper antioxidant intervention[23,126].

Several studies have been carried out to prove oxidative stress theory of aging and extending life span and slowing aging process by supplementing dietary antioxidants.These studies couldn't provide evidence for relationship between additional intake of low molecular antioxidants such as α-tocopherol, ascorbate and selenium and extension of life span[9,127] In his review, Sohal concluded that the life prolonging effect of antioxidant intake has been demonstrated to be restricted to a single species and cannot be generalized[9]. Under normal conditions, the rate of production of ROS is slow and this might be a reason of increased levels of antioxidants providing no further protection against ROS. Another reason is that the antioxidants may not access to the sites where ROS production take place.

Many studies attempting to therapeutically treat aging with antioxidants largely failed or were not reproducible leading to a considerable loss of enthusiasm for the free radical theory of aging in the early 1990s[23,127]. In 1990s, the popularization of genetic models of aging which were stress resistant with extended life span lead to additional studies which further examined the free radical theory of aging[23,121-124]. Further research was carried out for antioxidants which were effective in genetic models of oxidative stress, and in mammalian aging[23,128,129]. A certain level of oxidant stress may be beneficial to the organisms since it provides a protection against pathogen microorganisms, involves in signal transduction pathways[9,130,131]. Experimental studies showing loss of DNA and protein repair capacity in animals caused shortening of life spans of different species. It can be concluded that ROS production and oxidative damage to macromolecules increase with age and are inversely related to the maximum life span of different species. Experimental studies to extend life span of different species include enhancement of repair mechanisms, reversal of oxidative damage, increase of antioxidant levels which are all promising attempts but we are still far from reaching a clear confirmation of the oxidative stress hypothesis of aging[9].

References

[1] P. Y. Byung. Aging and Oxidative Stress: Modulation by Dietary Restriction. Free Radical Biology & Medicine 21;5 (1996) 651-668.146

[2] Sharma Ramesh. "Theories of Aging: A Perspective." Pages 1-4 in Warner H. et al., Modern Biological Theories of aging. New York: Raven Press 1987.

[3] Timiras Paola S. "Aging and Disease." Pages 23-35 in Timiras, Paola S., ed., Physiological Basis of Aging and Geriatrics, 2nd ed., Boca Raton:CRC Press, 1994.

[4] Forbes William F. "General Concepts of the Association of Aging and Disease." Pages 3-14 in Hammerman , David. Osteoarthritis:Public Health implications for an Aging Population, Baltimore Johns Hopkins University, 1997.

[5] Harman D. The aging process: major risk factor for disease and death. Proc. Natl. Acad. Sci. USA 88. 5360-5363, 1991

[6] Harman D. Free Radical Theory of Aging:History. Free Radicals and Aging ed. by I. Emerit & B. Chance. 1992. Birkhauser Verlag Basel Switzerland.

[7] Denham H. Free Radical Theory of Aging. Mutation Research 275(1992) 257-266.

[8] John M.C. Gutteridge. Ageing and Free Radicals. Medical Laboratory Science 49:313-318, 1992.

[9] R. J. Sohal, R. J. Mockett, W. C. Orr. Mechanisms of Aging: An Appraisal of the Oxidative Stress Hypothesis. *Free Radical Biology & Medicine* 33;5 (2002) 575–586.

[10] MedvedevZ. An attempt at rational classification of theories of ageing. Biol. Rev. 65:375-398, 1990

[11] U. Cakatay, A. Telci, R. Kayali, F. Tekeli, T. Akcay, A. Sivas. Relation of Aging with Oxidative Protein Damage Parameters in the Rat Skeletal Muscle. *Clinical Biochemistry* 36 (2003) 51–55.

[12] D. A. Butterfield, T. Koppal, B. Howard. Et al. Structural and Functional Changes in Proteins Induced by Free Radical-Mediated Oxidative Stress, and Protective Action of the Antioxidants N-tert-butyl-alpha-phenylnitrone, and Vitamin E. Annals of New York Academy of Sciences 854 (1998) 448–462.

[13] E. Carmeli, R. Coleman, A. Z. Reznick. The Biochemistry of Aging Muscle. Experimental Gerontology 37 (2002) 477–489.

[14] Strehler, B.I. a critique of theories of biological aging. In Dietz, A.A., ed. Aging-Its chemistry. Washington, DC.: Am.Assoc. Clin. Chem.; 1980:25-45.

[15] Comfort A. The biology of senescence, 3rd ed. New york: Elsevier; 1979.

[16] Yu, B. P., Yang Y. A critical evaluation of free radical theory of aging: A new proposal of oxidative stress hypothesis. Ann. NY Acad. Sci. 786:1-11, 1996.

[17] Freeman B.A. Biological sites and mechanisms of free radical protection. In:Armstrong, D., Sohal R.,Cutler R.G., Slater T., eds. Free radicals in molecular biology, aging and disease. New York:Raven Press; 1984:43-52.
[18] Boje KM, Arora PK. Microglial-produced nitric oxide and reactive nitrogen oxides mediate neuronal cell death. Brain Res. 587:250-256;1992.
[19] Masters B.S.S. Nitric oxide syntheses: Why so complex? Annu. Rev. Nutr. 14:131-145;1994
[20] Moncada S, Palmer RMJ, Higgs EA. Nitric oxide: Physiology, pathology and pharmacology. Pharm. Rev. 43:109-142;1992.
[21] Kasapoglu M, Ozben T. Alterations of antioxidant enzymes and oxidative stress markers in aging. Experimental Gerontology 36 (2001) 209-220.
[22] M. Phillips, R. N. Cataneo, J. Greenberg, R. Gunawardena, F. Rahbari-Oskoui. Increased Oxidative Stress in Younger as well as in Older Humans. Clinica Chimica Acta 328 (2003) 83–86.
[23] S. Melov. Animal Models of Oxidative Stress, Aging, and Therapeutic Antioxidant Interventions. The International Journal of Biochemistry & Cell Biology 34 (2002) 1395–1400.
[24] A. Boveris. Determination of the Production of Superoxide Radicals and Hydrogen Peroxide in Mitochondria. Methods in Enzymology 105 (1984) 429–435.
[25] B. Chance, H. Sies, A. Boveris. Hydroperoxide Metabolism in Mammalian Organs. Physiology Reviews 59 (3) (1979) 527–605.
[26] E. R. Stadtman. Importance of Individuality in Oxidative Stress and Aging. Free Radical Biology & Medicine. 33,5 (2002) 597–604.
[27] B. Halliwell, J.M.C. Gutteridge. Free Radicals in Biology and Medicine, 3rd Edition, Oxford University Press, Oxford, 1999.
[28] Ho YS, Magnenat JL, Bronson RT, Cao J, Gargano M, Sugawara M, Funk CD. Mice deficient in cellular glutathione peroxidase develop normally and show no increased sensitivity to hyperoxia. J. Biol. Chem. 272 (26) (1997) 16644–16651.
[29] Mirault ME, Tremblay A, Furling D, Trepanier G, Dugre F, Puymirat J, Pothier F. Transgenic glutathione peroxidase mouse models for neuroprotection studies. Ann. N.Y. Acad. Sci. 738 (1994) 104–115.
[30] Esworthy RS, Mann JR, Sam M, Chu FF. Low glutathione peroxidase activity in Gpx1 knockout mice protects jejunum crypts from gamma-irradiation damage. Am. J. Physiol. Gastrointest. Liver Physiol. 279 (2000) G426–G436.
[31] Reaume AG, Elliott JL, Hoffman EK, Kowall NW, Ferrante RJ, Siwek DF, Wilcox HM, Flood DG, Beal MF, Brown RH Jr, Scott RW, Snider WD. Motor neurons in Cu/Zn superoxide dismutase-deficient mice develop normally but exhibit enhanced cell death after axonal injury. Nat. Genet. 13 (1) (1996) 43–47.
[32] Sturtz LA, Diekert K, Jensen LT, Lill R, Culotta VC. A fraction of yeast Cu,Zn-superoxide dismutase and its metallochaperone, CCS, localize to the intermembrane space of mitochondria. A physiological role for SOD1 in guarding against mitochondrial oxidative damage. J. Biol. Chem. 10 (2001) 10.
[33] Yang G, Chan PH, Chen J, Carlson E, Chen SF, Weinstein P, Epstein CJ, Kamii H. Human copper-zinc superoxide dismutase transgenic mice are highly resistant to reperfusion injury after focal cerebral ischemia. Stroke 25 (1) (1994) 165–170.
[34] Yen HC, Oberley TD, Vichitbandha S, Ho YS, St Clair DK. The protective role of manganese superoxide dismutase against adriamycin-induced acute cardiac toxicity in transgenic mice. J. Clin. Invest. 98 (5) (1996) 1253–1260 (published erratum appears in J. Clin. Invest. 99 (5) (1997) 1141).
[35] Carlsson LM, Jonsson J, Edlund T, Marklund SL. Mice lacking extracellular superoxide dismutase are more sensitive to hyperoxia. Proc. Natl. Acad. Sci. U.S.A. 92 (14) (1995) 6264–6268.
[36] Sheng H, Bart RD, Oury TD, Pearlstein RD, Crapo JD, Warner DS. Mice overexpressing extracellular superoxide dismutase have increased resistance to focal cerebral ischemia. Neuroscience 88 (1) (1999) 185–191.
[37] H. Hu, R. J. Forsey, T. J. Blades, M. E.J. Barratt, P. Parmar, J. R. Powell. Antioxidants may Contribute in the Fight Against Ageing: An in Vitro Model. Mechanisms of Ageing and Development. 121 (2000) 217–230.
[38] Y. Artur, B. Herbeth, L. Guemouri, E. Lecomte, C. Jeandel and G. Siest. Age-related variations of enzymatic defenses against free radicals and peroxides. Free Radicals and Aging. edited by I. Emeritt & B. Chance.1992 Birkhauser Verlag Basel/Switzerland.
[39] S. Yoon, C. Yun, A. Chung. Dose Effect of Oxidative Stress on Signal Transduction in Aging. Mechanisms of Ageing and development 123 (2002) 1597-1604.
[40] G. Carrard, A. L. Bulteau, I. Petropoulos, B. Friguet. Impairment of Proteasome Structure and Function in Aging. The International Journal of Biochemistry & Cell Biology 34 (2002) 1461–1474.

[41] Brunk, U. T.; Terman, A. Lipofuscin: mechanisms of age-related accumulation and influence on cell function. *Free Radic. Biol. Med.* **33:**611–619; 2002.
[42] O. Pansarasa, L. Castagna, B. Colombi, J. Vecchiet, G. Felzani, F. Marzatico. Age, and Sex Differences in Human Skeletal Muscle: Role of Reactive Oxygen Species. Free Radical Research. 33 (2000) 287–293.
[43] R. S. Sohal, S. Agarwal, B. H. Sohal. Oxidative Stress and Aging in the Mongolian Gerbil. Mechanisms of Ageing and Development 81 (1995)15–25.
[44] U. Cakatay, A. Telci, R. Kayali, F. Tekeli, T. Akcay, A. Sivas. Relation of Oxidative Protein Damage, and Nitrotyrosine Levels in the Aging Rat Brain. Experimental Gerontology 36 (2001) 221–229.
[45] P. Mecocci, G. Fano, S. Fulle, et al. Age-Dependent Increases in Oxidative Damage To DNA, Lipids, and Proteins in Human Skeletal Muscle. Free Radical Biology and Medicine 26 (1999) 303–308.
[46] B. S. Berlett, E. R. Stadtman. Protein Oxidation in Aging, Disease, and Oxidative Stress. Journal of Biological Chemistry 272 (1997) 20313–20316.
[47] B.S. Berlett, E.R. Stadtman, Protein oxidation in aging, disease, and oxidative stress, J. Biol. Chem. 272 (1997) 2013–20316.
[48] K.J. Davies, Protein damage and degradation by oxygen radicals. I. General aspects, J. Biol. Chem. 262 (1987) 9895– 9901.
[49] J. Nordberg, E.S. Arner, Reactive oxygen species, antioxidants, and the mammalian thioredoxin system, Free Radic. Biol. Med. 31 (2001) 1287–1312.
[50] K.U. Schallreuter, J.M. Wood, Thioredoxin reductase—its role in epidermal redox status, J. Photochem. Photobiol. B 64 (2001) 179–184.
[51] J. Moskovitz, M.B. Yim, P.B. Chock, Free radicals and disease, Arch. Biochem. Biophys. 397 (2002) 354–359.
[52] M.T. Fisher, E.R. Stadtman, Oxidative modification of *Escherichia coli* glutamine synthetase: decreases in the thermodynamic stability of protein structure and specific changes in the active site conformation, J. Biol. Chem. 267 (1992) 1872–1880.
[53] B. Friguet, L.I. Szweda, E.R. Stadtman, Susceptibility of glucose-6-phosphate dehydrogenase modified by 4-hydroxy- 2-nonenal and metal-catalyzed oxidation to proteolysis by the multi-catalytic protease, Arch. Biochem. Biophys. 311 (1994) 168–173.
[54] D.A. Ferrington, H. Sun, K.K. Murray, J. Costa, T.D. Williams, D.J. Bigelow, T.C. Squier, Selective degradation of oxidized calmodulin by the 20S proteasome, J. Biol. Chem. 276 (2001) 937–943.
[55] Evans P, Lyras L, Halliwell B. Measurement of protein carbonyls in human brain tissue. Methods Enzymol 1999;300:145–56. Enzymol 1994;233:182–9.
[56] E.R. Stadtman, R.L. Levine, Protein oxidation, Ann. N. Y. Acad. Sci. 899 (2000) 191–208.
[57] J. Venkatraman, K. Aggarwal, P. Balaram, Helical peptide models for protein glycation: proximity effects in catalysis of the Amadori rearrangement, Chem. Biol. 8 (2001) 611– 625.
[58] H. Vlassara, R. Bucala, L. Striker, Pathogenic effects of advanced glycosylation: biochemical, biologic, and clinical implications for diabetes and aging, Lab. Invest. 70 (1994) 138–151.
[59] D.R. Sell, V.M. Monnier, End-stage renal disease and diabetes catalyze the formation of a pentose-derived crosslink from aging human collagen, J. Clin. Invest. 85 (1990) 380–384.
[60] R.H. Nagaraj, D.R. Sell, M. Prabhakaram, B.J. Ortwerth, V.M. Monnier, High correlation between pentosidine protein cross-links and pigmentation implicates ascorbate oxidation in human lens senescence and cataractogenesis, Proc. Natl. Acad. Sci. U.S.A. 88 (1991) 10257–10261.
[61] R.W. Gracy, K.U. Yuksel, M.L. Chapman, S.D. Dimitrijevich, Isoprotein changes in aging: biochemical basis and physiological consequences, Prog. Clin. Biol. Res. 344 (1990) 787–817.
[62] A.R. Hipkiss, On the struggle between chemistry and biology during aging—implications for DNA repair, apoptosis and proteolysis, and a novel route of intervention, Biogerontology 2 (2001) 173–178.
[63] Niki E. Oxidative stress and aging. Intern Med J 2000;39:324–6.
[64] Dubey A, Forster MJ, Lal H, Sohal RS. Effect of age and caloric intake on protein oxidation in different brain regions, and behavioral functions of the mouse. Arch Biochem Biophys 1996;333:189–97.
[65] R.L. Levine, J.A. Williams, E.R. Stadtman, E. Shacter, Carbonyl assays for determination of oxidatively modified proteins, Methods Enzymol. 233 (1994) 346–357.
[66] Reznick AZ, Packer L. Oxidative damage to proteins: spectrophotometric method for carbonyl assay. Methods Enzymol 1994;233:357–63.
[67] I. Petropoulos, M. Conconi, X. Wang, B. Hoenel, F. Bregegere, Y. Milner, B. Friguet, Increase of oxidatively modified protein is associated with a decrease of proteasome activity and content in aging epidermal cells, J. Gerontol. A Biol. Sci. Med. Sci. 55 (2000) B220–B227.

[68] R.L. Levine, E.R. Stadtman, Oxidative modification of proteins during aging, Exp. Gerontol. 36 (2001) 1495–1502.
[69] Takenaka Y, Miki M, Yasuda H, Mino M. The effect of α-tocopherol as an antioxidant on the oxidation of membrane protein thiols induced by free radicals generated in different sites. Arch Biochem Biophys1991;285:344–50.
[70] Ischiropoulos H, Al-Mehdi AB. Peroxynitrite-mediated oxidative protein modifications. FEBS Lett 1995;364:279–82.
[71] Usmar VD, Halliwell B. Reactive nitrogen species, reactive oxygen species, transition metal ions, and the vascular system. Pharma Res 1996;13:649–62.
[72] S.H. Lecker, V. Solomon, W.E. Mitch, A.L. Goldberg, Muscle protein breakdown and the critical role of the ubiquitin–proteasome pathway in normal and disease states, J. Nutr. 129 (1999) 227S–237S.
[73] A. Ciechanover, A. Orian, A.L. Schwartz, The ubiquitinmediated proteolytic pathway: mode of action and clinical mplications, J. Cell Biochem. Suppl. 34 (2000) 40–51.
[74] H.G. Drexler, Review of alterations of the cyclin-dependent kinase inhibitor INK4 family genes *p15*, *p16*, *p18* and *p19* in human leukemia–lymphoma cells, Leukemia 12 (1998) 845–859.
[75] Y.C. Chang, Y.S. Lee, T. Tejima, K. Tanaka, S. Omura, N.H. Heintz, Y. Mitsui, J. Magae, mdm2 and bax, downstream mediators of the p53 response, are degraded by the ubiquitin–proteasome pathway, Cell Growth Differ. 9 (1998) 79–84.
[76] R.W. King, R.J. Deshaies, J.M. Peters, M.W. Kirschner, How proteolysis drives the cell cycle, Science 274 (1996) 1652–1659.
[77] K. Helin, Regulation of cell proliferation by the E2F transcription factors, Curr. Opin. Genet. Dev. 8 (1998) 28–35.
[78] T.G. Gillette, W. Huang, S.J. Russell, S.H. Reed, S.A. Johnston, E.C. Friedberg, The 19S complex of the proteasome regulates nucleotide excision repair in yeast, Genes Dev. 15 (2001) 1528–1539.
[79] F. Pajonk, W.H. McBride, The proteasome in cancer biology and treatment, Radiat. Res. 156 (2001) 447 - 459.
[80] K. Tanaka, K. Ii, A. Ichihara, L. Waxman, A.L. Goldberg, A high molecular weight protease in the cytosol of rat liver. I. Purification, enzymological properties, and tissue distribution, J. Biol. Chem. 261 (1986) 15197–15203.
[81] Davies, K. J. A.; Lin, S. W. Oxidatively denatured proteins are degraded by an ATP-independent proteolytic pathway in *Escherichia coli. Free Radic. Biol. Med.* **5**:225–236; 1988.
[82] Rivett, A. J. Purification of a liver alkaline protease which degrades oxidatively modified glutamine synthetase: characterization as a high molecular weight cysteine protease. *J. Biol. Chem.* **260**:12600–12606; 1985.
[83] Davies, K. J. A. A secondary antioxidant defense role for proteolytic degradation. In: Simic, M. G.; Taylor, K. A.; Ward, J. F.; Von Sonntag, C., eds. *Oxygen radicals in biology and medicine.* New York: Plenum Press; 1989:575–585.
[84] Pacifici, R. E.; Salo, D. C.; Davies, K. J. A. Macroxyproteinase (M.O.P.): a 670 kDa proteinase complex that degrades oxidatively denatured proteins in red blood cells. *Free Radic. Biol. Med.* **7**:521–536; 1989.
[85] Murakami, K.; Jahnsen, J. H.; Lin, S. W.; Davies, K. J. A. Lens proteosome shows enhanced rates of degradation of hydroxyl radical modified alpha crystallin. *Free Radic. Biol. Med.* **8**:217– 222; 1990.
[86] Grune, T., Reinheckel, T.; Joshi, M.; Davies, K. J. A. Proteolysis in cultured liver epithelial cells during oxidation stress. Role of the multicatalytic proteinase complex, proteosome. *J. Biol. Chem.* **270**:2344–2351; 1995.
[87] Grant, A. J.; Jessup, W.; Dean, R. T. Accelerated endocytosis and incomplete catabolism of radical-damaged protein. *Biochim. Biophys. Acta* **1134**:203–209; 1992.
[88] Grant, A. J.; Jessup, W.; Dean, R. T. Inefficient degradation of oxidized regions of protein molecules. *Free Radic. Res. Commun* **18**:259–267, 1993.
[89] Dean, R. T.; Armstrong, S.; Fu, S.; Jessup, W. Oxidized proteins and their enzymatic proteolysis in eucaryotic cells: a critical appraisal. In: Nohl, H.; Esterbauer, H.; Rice-Evans, C., eds. *Free radicals in the environment, medicine, and toxicology.* London: Richelieu Press; 1994:47–79.
[90] Friguet, B.; Szweda, L. I. Inhibition of the multicatalytic protease (proteosome) by 4-hydroxy-2-nonenal cross-linked proteins. *FEBS Lett.* **405**:21–25; 1997.
[91] Friguet, B.; Stadtman, E. R.; Szweda, L. I. Modification of glucose-6-phosphate dehydrogenase by 4-hydroxy-2-nonenal. Formation of cross-linked protein that inhibits the multicatalytic protease. *J. Biol. Chem.* **269**:21639–21643; 1994.

[92] Bulteau, A. L.; Verbeke, P.; Petropoulos, I.; Chaffotte, A. F.; Friguet, B. Protease inhibition in glyoxal-treated fibroblasts and resistance of glycated glucose-6-phosphate dehydrogenase to 20 S proteasome degradation *in vitro*. *J. Biol. Chem.* **276:**45662–45668; 2001.

[93] Carney, J. M.; Starke-Reed, P. E.; Oliver, C. N.; Landum, R. W.; Cheng, M. S.; Wu, J. F.; Floyd, R. A. Reversal of age-related increase in brain protein oxidation, decrease in enzyme activity and loss of temporal and spatial memory by chronic administration of the spin-trapping compound N-*tert*-butyl-_-phenylnitrone. *Proc. Natl. Acad. Sci. USA* **88:**3633–3636; 1991.

[94] Chondrogianni, N.; Petropoulos, I.; Franceschi, C.; Friguet, B.; Gonos, E. S. Fibroblast cultures from healthy centenarians have active proteasome. *Gerontology* **35:**721–728; 2000.

[95] Conconi, M.; Szweda, L. I.; Levine, R. L.; Stadtman, E. R.; Friguet, B. Age-related decline of rat liver multicatalytic proteinase activity and protection from inactivation by heat-shock 90. *Arch. Biochem. Biophys.* **331:**232–240; 1996.

[96] Shibatani, T.; Nazir, M.; Ward, W. F. Alternation of rat liver 20 S proteasome activities by age and food restriction. *J. Gerontol.Biol. Sci.* **51A:**B316–B322; 1996.

[97] Hayashi, T.; Goto, S. Age-related changes in the 20 S and 26 S proteasome in liver of male rats. *Mech. Aging Dev.* **102:**55–66; 1999.

[98] Petropoulos, L.; Conconi, M.; Wang, X.; Hoenel, B.; Bregegera, F.; Milner, Y.; Friguet, B. Increase in oxidatively modified protein is associated with a decrease of proteasome activity and content in aging epidermal cells. *J. Gerontol.* **55:**B220–B227; 2000.

[99] Bulteau, A.; Petropoulos, I.; Friguet, B. Age-related alterations of proteasome structure and function in aging. *Exp. Gerontol.* **35:**767–777; 2000.

[100] A.-L. Bulteau, L.I. Szweda, B. Friguet, Age-dependent declines in proteasome activity in the heart, Arch. Biochem. Biophys. 397 (2002) 298–304.

[101] N. Sitte, M. Huber, T. Grune, A. Ladhoff, W.D. Doecke, T. Von Zglinicki, K.J. Davies, Proteasome inhibition by lipofuscin/ceroid during postmitotic aging of fibroblasts, FASEB J. 14 (2000) 1490–1498.

[102] Rajindar S. Sohal. Role of oxidative stress and protein oxidation in the aging process. Free Radical Biology and Medicine. Vol 33, No.1, pp 37-44, 2002

[103] Sohal, R. S. The rate of living theory: a contemporary interpretation. In: Collatz, K. G.; Sohal, R. S., eds. *Insect aging.* Heidelberg, Germany: Springer-Verlag; 1986:23–44.

[104] Van Voorhies, W. A.; Ward, S. Genetic and environmental conditions that increase longevity in *Caenorhabditis elegans* decrease metabolic rate. *Proc. Natl. Acad. Sci. USA* **96:**11399–11403; 1999.

[105] Feng, J.; Bussiere, F.; Hekimi, S. Mitochondrial electron transport is a key determinant of life span in *Caenorhabditis elegans. Develop. Cell* **1:**633–644; 2001.

[106] Lyman, C. P.; O'Brian, R. C.; Greene, G. C.; Papafrangos, E. D. Hibernation and longevity in the Turkish hamster *Mesocricetus brandti. Science* **212:**668–670; 1981.

[107] Cutler, R. G. Antioxidants, aging, and longevity. In: Pryor W. A., ed. *Free Radicals in Biology.* New York: Academic Press; 1984: 371–428.

[108] Finch, C. E.; Ruvkun, G. The genetics of aging. *Ann. Rev. Genomics Hum. Genet.* **2:**435–462; 2001.

[109] Tatar, M.; Kopelman, A.; Epstein, D.; Tu, M. T.; Yin, C. M.; Garofalo, R. S. A mutant *Drosophila* insulin receptor homolog that extends life-span and impairs neuroendocrine function. *Science* **292:**107–110; 2001.

[110] T.E. Johnson, Increased life-span of age-1 mutants in *Caenorhabditis elegans* and lower gompertz rate of aging, Science 249 (4971) (1990) 908–912.

[111] T.E. Johnson, et al., Relationship between increased longevity and stress resistance as assessed through gerontogene mutations in *Caenorhabditis elegans*, Exp. Gerontol. 36 (10) (2001) 1609–1617.

[112] P.L. Larsen, Aging and resistance to oxidative damage in *Caenorhabditis elegans*, Proc. Natl. Acad. Sci. U.S.A. 90 (19) (1993) 8905–8909.

[113] J.R. Vanfleteren, Oxidative stress and ageing in *Caenorhabditis elegans*, Biochem. J. 292 (Pt. 2) (1993) 605–608. in ischemic brain injury, J. Pharmacol. Exp. Ther. 284 (1) (1998) 215–221.

[114] Johnson, T. E.; Cypser, E.; de Castro, E.; de Castro, S.; Henderson, S.; Murakami, S.; Rikke, B.; Tedesco, P.; Link, C. Gerontogenes mediate health and longevity in nematodes through increasing resistance to environmental toxins and stressors. *Exp. Gerontol.* **35:**687–694; 2000.

[115] Hermes-Lima, M.; Storey, J. M.; Storey, K. B. Antioxidant defenses and metabolic depression. The hypothesis of preparation for oxidative stress in land snails. *Comp. Biochem. Physiol. B. Biochem. Mol. Biol.* **120:**437–448; 1998.

[116] Sohal, R. S.; Mockett, R. J.; Orr, W. C. Current issues concerning the role of oxidative stress in aging: a perspective. In: Hekimi, S., ed. *The molecular genetics of aging.* Heidelberg: Springer-Verlag; 2000:45–66.

[117] Ku, H.-H.; Brunk, U. T.; Sohal, R. S. Relationship between mitochondrial superoxide and hydrogen peroxide production and longevity of mammalian species. *Free Radic. Biol. Med.* **15:**621– 627; 1994.

[118] Barja, G.; Herrero, A. Oxidative damage to mitochondrial DNA is inversely related to maximum life span in the heart and brain of mammals. *FASEB J.* **14:**312–318; 2000.

[119] Holbrook, N. Ikeyama S. Age-Related Decline in Cellular Response to Oxidative Stress: Links to Growth Factor Signalling Pathways with Common defects. Biochemical Pharmacology 64(2002) 999-1005.

[120] Huang, T. T.; Carlson, E. J.; Gillespie, A. M.; Shi, Y.; Epstein, C. J. Ubiquitous overexpression of CuZn superoxide dismutase does not extend life span in mice. *J. Gerontol.* **55:**B5–B9; 2000.

[121] Orr, W. C.; Sohal, R. S. Extension of life span by overexpression of superoxide dismutase and catalase in *Drosophila melanogaster*. *Science* **263:**1128–1130; 1994.

[122] J. Sun, J. Tower, FLP recombinase-mediated induction of Cu/Zn-superoxide dismutase transgene expression can extend the life span of adult drosophila melanogaster flies (in process citation), Mol. Cell. Biol. 19 (1) (1999) 216–228.

[123] T.L. Parkes, et al., Extension of *Drosophila* lifespan by overexpression of human SOD1 in motorneurons, Nat. Genet. 19 (2) (1998) 171–174.

[124] J. Sun, et al., Induced over-expression of mitochondrial Mn-superoxide dismutase extends the life span of adult *Drosophila melanogaster*, Genetics 161 (2) (2002) 661–672.

[125] K.B. Beckman, B.N. Ames, The free radical theory of aging matures, Physiol. Rev. 78 (2) (1998) 547–581.

[126] S. Melov, et al., Extension of life-span with superoxide dismutase/catalase mimetics, Science 289 (5484) (2000) 1567–1569.

[127] Herbert, V. The antioxidant supplement myth. *Am. J. Clin. Nutr.* **60:**157–158; 1994.

[128] S. Melov, et al., A novel neurological phenotype in mice lacking mitochondrial manganese superoxide dismutase, Nat. Genet. 18 (2) (1998) 159–163.

[129] S. Melov, et al., Lifespan extension and rescue of spongiform encephalopathy in superoxide dismutase 2 nullizygous mice treated with superoxide dismutase-catalase mimetics, J. Neurosci. 21 (21) (2001) 8348–8353.

[130] Babior, B. M.; Kipnes, R. S.; Curnutte, J. T. Biological defense mechanisms. The production by leukocytes of superoxide, a potential bactericidal agent. *J. Clin. Invest.* **52:**741–744; 1973.

[131] Allen, R. G. Oxygen-reactive species and antioxidant responses during development: the metabolic paradox of cellular differentiation. *Proc. Soc. Exp. Biol. Med.* **196:**117–129; 1991.

Protection of Neural Tissues and the Heart By Ischemic-and Drug Induced Preconditioning

Eduard Berenshtein, Shirley Leibowitz, Nu Nu Aye and Mordechai Chevion
**Department of Cellular Biochemistry and Human Genetics, The Hebrew University-Hadassah Schools of Medicine and Dental Medicine, Jerusalem IL-91120, ISRAEL*

Abstract: Preconditioning (PC) is the process of applying a short and non-lethal stress, such as a short ischemia, on a tissue, and thus accomplishing tissue protection against prolonged or more severe (supposedly lethal) form of stress. The prolonged or more intense stress could be identical or different form of insult than the initial stress. The most investigated form of PC is ischemic PC.

1. Neuronal Preconditioning

Indeed, it has been demonstrated that brief, sub-lethal cerebral ischemia induced tolerance of neurons to subsequent longer (and would be) lethal ischemia. In general, PC can be considered as the response of cells/organ to certain types or levels of injury.

Cerebral PC was first demonstrated using the global ischemia model by Kitagawa et al (1, 2). Both common carotid arteries of the gerbil were occluded for 5min, and consistently resulted in delayed neuronal death in the CA1 region of the hippocampus. A single episode of 2min of global ischemic PC was used in order to protect the brain against the prolonged ischemia, as monitored 24h later. The short ischemic PC depleted high-energy phosphates and perturbed protein synthesis, but never caused neuronal necrosis. Two episodes of 2min ischemic PC were given on two consecutive days and exhibited complete protection against neuronal death. Both the *duration* and the *intervals* between the PC cycles were important factors in the success of the protection. Indeed, one or several cycles of 1min ischemia in the same day did not provide protection against the prolonged ischemia.

Cerebral ischemic tolerance can be attained by global or focal ischemia, both of which are capable of protecting against the other form of ischemia. Also, cerebral ischemic protection can be induced by chemical, pharmacological, electrical, and anoxic/ischemic means, clearly demonstrating the cross-tolerance among the various kinds of stress.

The hypothesis of cross tolerance - that hypoxic preconditioning protects against kainic acid (KA)-induced edema formation was examined. Systemic injection of KA to rats causes a *glutamate-driven* status epilepticus that leads to cellular calcium influx and oxidative stress, similar to that seen in ischemia-reperfusion injury. Hypoxia was shown to provide protection against KA-induced status epilepticus. Hypoxic preconditioning markedly attenuated brain edema (3-5). KA-induced brain edema is associated with necrosis in susceptible brain regions (e.g., piriform cortex and hippocampal CA1 and CA3 regions) that results in epileptic seizures. An early cytotoxic edema and a late vasogenic edema associated with necrosis occur in brain regions (i.e., piriform cortex and hippocampal CA1 and CA3 regions) and are extensively involved in seizure activity (3-5).

KA augments the release of glutamate from vesicles in neurons located in the hippocampus and piriform cortex. Excess stimulation of glutamatergic pathways increases intracellular Na^{+} and Ca^{+2} concentrations leading to cytotoxic osmotic swelling of neurons and glia. As neuronal damage progresses to necrosis, a vasogenic edema results from reduced integrity of vessel endothelial walls and collapse of the blood–brain barrier. Adult male rats were exposed to a 9% O_2/91% N_2 atmosphere for 8 h. KA (14 mg/kg, i.p.) was administered on days 1, 3, 7, or 14 later. Regional analysis of edema indicated that the exposure to hypoxia attenuated edema formation in piriform and frontal cortices and hippocampus when KA was given 1, 3, or 7 days later, but not 14 days after hypoxia. This is in accord with that protection by virtue of PC is always restricted to a well-defined time window – seven days in this model. Cycloheximide (2 mg/kg), given 1 h prior to hypoxia, prevented the protective effect of hypoxia on KA-induced edema attenuation, in the piriform cortex and hippocampus. This is also in accord with that the PC initiates a signal that activates cascade of events that include protein synthesis. What is the control of the synthesis of proteins - is it transcriptional or translational? We will address this question in ischemic PC of the heart (see below).

The excitotoxic hypothesis of ischemic neuronal death is based on the neurotoxic effects of high levels of extra-cellular concentrations of glutamate release, as a result of enhanced excitatory synaptic activity, that is related to calcium influx into affected nerve cells. Brief and non-lethal episode of cerebral ischemia did not cause injury that reached the critical levels for initiation of neuronal death, but rather produced the acquired tolerance to subsequent lethal ischemia. In such ischemia-tolerant neurons the elevation of calcium is markedly inhibited after an anoxic/aglycemic episode, as compared with neurons of control animals.

The brain is *more vulnerable* to ischemic events than any other organ. Even brief interruption of cerebral blood flow (5 min, only) leads to neuronal death in corresponding brain regions. This unusual sensitivity reflects the high metabolic rate in brain that varies between different cerebral regions. The *human* brain represents only 2.5% of body weight, but 25% of basal metabolism. In comparison to the 5min of cerebral ischemia, 20-40 min of ischemia is required to achieve cell death in cardiac myocytes or kidney cells.

Central neurons depend almost exclusively on glucose as the energy source. Also, the brain's intrinsic cell-to-cell and intra-cellular signaling mechanisms become harmful under ischemic conditions, accelerating energy failure, enhancing final pathways that underlie ischemic cell death. Moreover, ischemic conditions eventually lead to the production of free radicals, activate catabolic enzymes, enhance membrane failure, and facilitate apoptosis and inflammation.

Two pathophysiological events contribute to neuronal injury following *transient ischemia*: the initiation of infarction during the ischemic phase, and the reversal of maturation in the re-circulation phase. Not only the severity of the initiation phase is important, but also its duration is a crucial factor, both dictating the potential successful rescuing of the tissue by reperfusion.

Early reports showed that HSP70, HO1 and metallo- thionein play important roles in brain protection by PC, indicating that free radicals, protein folding (or mis-folding), and transition metals are involved in the mechanism of tissue injury (6-10).

Hsp70 is a family of molecular chaperones acting together with Hsp40 facilitating protein synthesis, folding, degradation and translocation across membranes. Many proteins of the mitochondrial matrix are synthesized in the cytosol, and then being translocated across the mitochondrial inner membrane. The driving force is mitochondrial Hsp70 (mito HSP70). A minor Hsp70 component in the mitochondrial matrix is also involved in iron homeostasis and the formation of Fe/S centers.

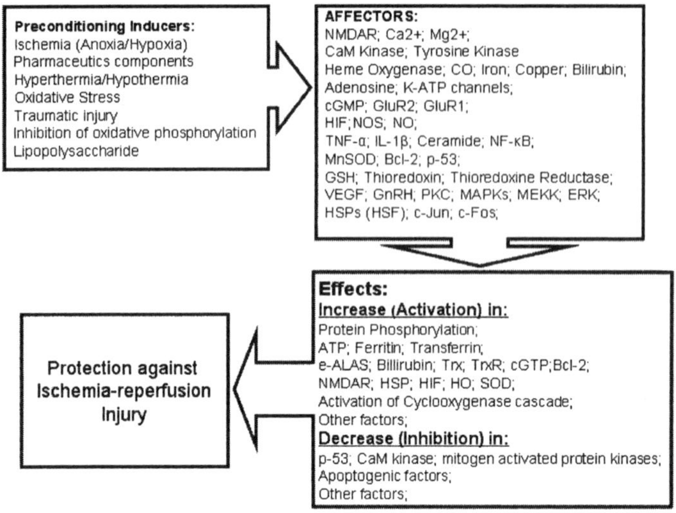

Figure 1.

In a series of studies using human neuroblastoma brain cells (SH-SY5Y cells) it had been shown that applying an insult, in the form of serum deprivation, leads to the production of ·OH and NO radicals (11). A good correlation was found between the level of ·OH production and the degree of damage inflicted on the cells by this mode of oxidative stress that results in apoptosis. ·OH scavengers (like salicylate), but not NOS-inhibitors (like L-NAME or 7-NI) prevented the apoptotic process.

Low concentrations of NO-donors were shown to inhibit oxidative stress-induced neuronal damage both *in vitro* and *in vivo*. Serum deprivation-stress increased the expression of NOS, both the message (within 2h) and the protein (within 12-36 h), as well as the production of NO. The induction of NOS, the excessive production of NO, and the activation of *guanylyl cyclase* played crucial roles in the protection by PC.

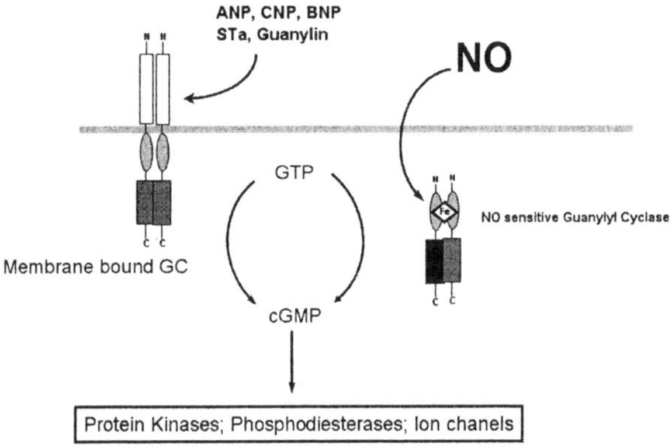

Figure 2.

Andoh, Chiueh and Chock (11) have recently proposed that gene induction and new protein synthesis mediated by the NO-cGMP-PKG signaling is an important pathway that mediates cyto-protection through PC.

Following PC in the form of 2h serum deprivation, a time-dependent increase in NOS1 was observed, and was indicated by enhanced gene expression, protein synthesis, and NO and cGMP production(12, 13)

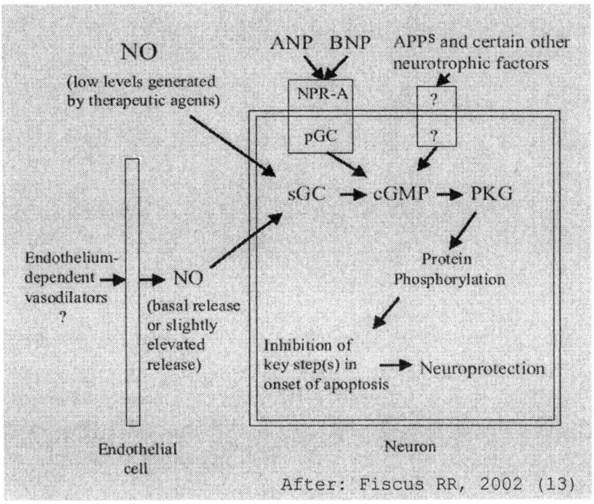

Figure 3.

The PC-induced protection against subsequent stress could be mediated by NO-mediated gene regulation, such as the up-regulation of Bcl-2 and the down-regulation of p66shc (cell-membrane adaptor protein). Bcl-2, like other members of its family, plays a crucial role in life/death decisions made by cells. Indeed, Bcl-2 can bind to cytoplasmic cytochrome c and caspase 9 and prevent the activation of caspase 3, and subsequently Apaf-1 in the mitochondria-mediated apoptotic pathway, inhibiting the apoptosome formation. In several neurologic and neurodegenerative diseases NO production underlies neuronal death following glutamate-mediated excitotoxicity.

The action of p66shc can be visualized by the following mechanisms. Oxidative stress leads to the phosphorylation of p66shc on serine residue. This phosphorylation, in turn, inactivates p66shc, so it can no longer repress oxidative repair functions. Alternatively, phosphorylation activates the p66shc, allowing it to induce apoptosis. For comparison, p53 is activated by oxidative stress or DNA damage to promote apoptosis (14). Knock out of cell-membrane adaptor protein p66shc significantly increased the life span of mice. Likewise, a decrease in the concentration of p66shc led to increased tolerance against oxidative stress.

Interestingly, induction of *de novo* synthesis of Trx was prevented by systemic inhibition of guanylyl cyclase, cGMP, and PKG. Also, inhibition of Trx-reductase (TRT) completely prevented the PC protection. The reduced form of Thioredoxin (Trx) prevented LPO and apoptosis that was caused by ROS. The reduced form of Trx is an omni potent antioxidant, with 2 and 3 orders of magnitude higher activity than that of GSH or GS-NO, respectively.

A commonly used herbicide, paraquat, is structurally similar to the neurotoxic chemical MPP^+, a metabolite of 1-methyl-4-phenyl-1,2,3,6-tetrahydropyridine (MPTP), that in turn, is known to induce Parkinsonism. PC enhanced the tolerance of cells to MPP^+ by 30-fold. Cells transfected with NOS (human NOS-1) were markedly more resistant to the severe MPP^+-induced apoptotic injury (15).

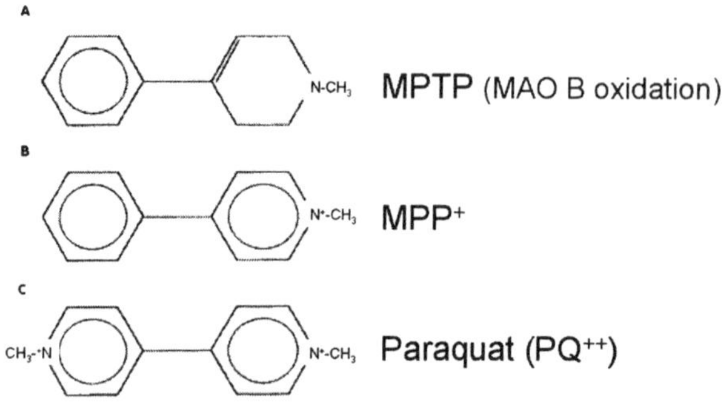

Figure 4.

ERK (also called MAPK) signaling cascades have been shown to play a role in regulating diverse neuronal processes, such as differentiation, synaptic plasticity, and cell death. At the cellular level there are indications that multiple second messengers, such as Ca, cAMP and NO control ERK signaling through small G-proteins (like p21ras or Rap1). Anti-apoptotic activity and protection by ERKs, of certain populations of neurons, against insults have been proposed. Accumulation of lines of evidence has also shown that over-stimulation of ERK signaling cascade could promote neuronal cell death. ERK/MAPK is required for neuronal excitotoxic PC. The events linking the stimulation of glutamate receptor, Ca influx and ERK phosphorylation, to resistance to neuronal excitotoxic damage, may involve ERK-induced phosphorylation and inactivation of pro-apoptotic proteins. The effects of ERK signaling on neuronal survival in PC could stem from the induction of nuclear gene expression. ERKs can translocate to the nucleus, phosphorylate and activate transcription factors, thereby regulating gene transcription (16, 17).

2. Heart ischemic preconditioning - a novel mechanism

The detailed mechanism of myocardial protection via PC is not fully understood, albeit many proposals, including stunning, synthesis of heat-shock proteins, involvement of G-proteins, and nitric oxide production (18-20). The most commonly accepted mechanism of PC is enhanced catabolism of purine nucleotides that forms high level of adenosine, activating PKC and a cascade of steps leading to activation of the MAPK pathway, culminating in affecting ATP-dependent mitochondrial K^+ channels (18, 19, 21, 22).

Tissue injury following ischemia and reperfusion is considered to be mediated by reactive oxygen derived species (ROS) and temporary pools of redox active iron and copper. The role of "free" iron and copper is visualized mainly as causing the conversion of low reactive species, like superoxide radical anion to the highly reactive hydroxyl radicals. The significance of iron in ischemia and reperfusion is supported by studies showing that metal chelation protected post-ischemic tissue, whereas the addition of iron to the perfusate increased the rate of injury (23).

We have previously shown (24, 25) that following myocardial ischemia iron and copper are mobilized from the heart into the coronary flow, in an ischemia-duration-dependent manner, and that the level of mobilized metals well correlated with the degree of heart injury.

While iron and copper ions are found in their 'free state' only in minute concentration within the cell, their total levels are at the micromolar range. In general, a shift in the cellular balance of 'free" and bound iron (and copper) may be harmful to cells due to their high reactivity in producing free radicals. Much of the "free" iron is probably derived from an enhanced catabolism of heme-iron, non-heme-iron and iron-containing proteins (26). Under conditions prevailing in the tissue during an ischemic insult, iron can be mobilized from the major iron storage protein of the heart, i.e. ferritin (27-32).

Ferritin contains up to 4.000-4.500 iron atoms per protein molecule, forming the major iron-storage protein in the cells. During ischemia/ reperfusion iron can be mobilized from ferritin by superoxide radical anion (28, 33) and other small molecules, including adrenergic agents (norepinephrine and epinephrine) (31). The release of iron by epinephrine is significantly enhanced under anaerobic conditions that dominate the ischemic state. Iron release from ferritin can also be mediated by NADH-lipoamide dehydrogenase under aerobic condition (34). The destruction of the ferritin protein-shell seems to be necessary for iron release, *in vivo* (34-38).

Definition of the experimental system and groups: Rat hearts were extracted, prepared for perfusion in the Langendorff configuration as described in 'Methods' (24, 25), and divided into four groups as follows:

Table 1: Group Definition

Group No.	Stabilization (min)	Preconditioning (min)	Ischemia (min)	reperfusion (min)	Comments
I	10	15 (3 episodes)	Variable Duration (18 - 60'; typically 35')	20	PC (+ischemia)
II	10+15+35+20	0	0	0	Normal perfusion
III	10+15	0	D = 18 – 60', typically 35'	20	Ischemia no PC
IV	10	15	----	----	PC alone

PC Hearts (group I) demonstrated a marked and clear protection of their function against the injury following prolonged ischemia (when compared to group III). The residual function after 35min ischemia was 56-78% and 27-49% after 45min.(Table II). Likewise, biochemical parameters of heart tissue (ATP, ADP, AMP, catabolites of adenine nucleotides, ascorbate and urate), following 18, 35 and 60min ischemia, clearly indicated an analogous myocardial protection (data not shown).

Coronary flow fractions (CFF) were collected and analyzed using previously published procedures (24, 25). The first CFFs of reperfusion contained relatively high levels of iron and copper (Table III). The values were dependent on the duration of ischemia, while the concentrations of group I CFFs were always markedly lower (by a factor of 2-5) than the corresponding values of group III. The patterns of mobilization of these metals from the tissue to the CFF were similar to each other, but distinctly different for iron, copper and protein, indicating that this mobilization does not reflect simple necrotic process, but rather a selective one (25).

Table 2: The hemodynamic parameters of hearts following ischemia and reperfusion with or without cardiac preconditioning (CPC). The data represent the recovery values (% of the pre-ischemic value). * = $p \leq 0.05$ – for the CPC group as compared to the control (ischemia/reperfusion group).

Ischemic Duration	Group No.	WI (% Recovery)	DP (% Recovery)
18 min	PC+Ischemia (35')	99 ± 6*	103 ± 5*
	Ischemia 35' no PC	76 ± 6	76 ± 6
25 min	PC+Ischemia (35')	78 ± 11*	79 ± 8*
	Ischemia 35' no PC	4 4± 5	47 ± 4
35 min	PC+Ischemia (35')	56 ± 9*	74 ± 4*
	Ischemia 35' no PC	19 ± 7	21 ± 7
45 min	PC+Ischemia (35')	27 ± 7*	48 ± 4*
	Ischemia 35' no PC	0 ± 0	0 ± 0
52 min	PC+Ischemia (35')	5 ± 2*	25 ± 6*
	Ischemia 35' no PC	0 ± 0	0 ± 0
60 min	PC+Ischemia (35')	4 ± 1*	21 ± 3*
	Ischemia 35' no PC	0 ± 0	0 ± 0

Table 3: The levels of iron, copper and proteins in coronary flow fractions (CFFs) of hearts following ischemia and reperfusion with or without CPC. * = $p \leq 0.05$ – for the CPC group compared to the control group (ischemia and reperfusion without CPC group).

	CFF No.	18min Ischemia		25 min Ischemia		35 min Ischemia		45 min Ischemia	
		Group I	Group III	Group I	Group III	Group I	Group III	Group I	Group III
Cu (ng/ml)	1	2.3±1.6	4.5±1.7	3.0±1.3*	9.5±1.6	7.9±1.1*	11.4±0.7	8.2±0.9*	14.6±1.1
	2	0.6±0.4	0.8±0.4	1.5±0.3	4.1±1.5	4.0±0.4	2.7±0.4	1.5±0.8	3.8±2.1
	5	0.0±0.0	0.5±0.3	0.0±0.0	1.5±0.5	0.4±0.2	1.6±0.8	0.5±0.5	1.5±0.9
Fe (ng/ml)	1	14±3	31±11	15±3*	63±2	25±6*	97±9	28±4*	104±28
	2	8.3±1.0	12.1±4.5	8.7±2.0*	20.7±4.2	9.1±0.5*	31.0±8.9	11.1±1.5*	30.4±6.2
	5	4.2±1.1	4.7±1.9	0.9±0.5*	8.3±1.7	0.6±0.4*	12.1±2.3	1.1±1.1*	7.8±2.4
Protein (μg/ml)	1	26±8	42±1	30±3*	54±2	32±5*	71±6	36±7*	83±11
	2	12±1	28±22	15±5*	38.±5	17±4*	30±0.2	17±4*	34±4
	5	2.5±1.3	13.1±10.6	1.9±1.9*	12.4±1.3	4.6±1.1*	14.3±0.3	3.1±1.0*	11.0±1.8

The total levels of iron and copper, in each CFF, were determined by atomic absorption spectroscopy. In contrast, the redox-active fractions ('free metal' fractions) of these metal ions, that could have played a causative role in the injurious process to the heart, were monitored using a biochemical assay, measuring the ability of added CFF to catalyze the ascorbate-driven conversion of salicylate to its dihydroxybenzoate derivatives (DHBA). Experimentally, HPLC-ECD method (24, 39) was employed (24, 40). Table IV shows the production of 2,5- and 2,3-DHBA that was mediated by the first CFFs, for increasing ischemic duration, with and without PC. This parameter as well, was found to be dependent on the duration of ischemia. This parameter was also markedly lower (by a factor of 2-3) for

CFFs from group I hearts than from group III.

Table 4: Levels of dihydroxybenzoic acids (DHBA) in CFFs of hearts following ischemia and reperfusion with or without CPC. * = p≤0.05 – for the CPC group compared to the control group (ischemia and reperfusion).

Time		18 min		35 min		60 min	
Product	CFF No.	CPC	Control	CPC	Control	CPC	Control
2,5-DHBA	1	9.9±5.3	17.0±8.0	15.0±5.4	42.4±11.0*	31.2±2.1	49.5±8.7
(ng/ml)	2	11.2±6.5	9.2±3.9	8.3±2.6	9.3±6.2	13.4±1.4	15.7±9.1
2.3-DHBA	1	3.9±3.9	8.6±4.4	6.9±3.3	33.5±7.1*	27.7±2.5	41.4±9.1
(ng/ml)	2	0.6±0.6	8.5±3.7*	6.7±2.7	10.9±1.9	15.1±1.7	26.3±9.8
Cathechol+	1	5.0±4.8	11.3±5.7	8.0±3.9	34.6±7.8*	27.7±2.7	47.1±10.0
2,3-DHBA	2	0.6±1.1	11.0±4.9*	7.6±4.1	13.1±3.5	16.6±2.6	27.7±10.6
Total=Cat+	1	14.9±10.1	28.3±13.7	23.0±9.4	77.0±18.8*	58.9±4.8	96.6±18.7
DHBA	2	11.8±7.6	20.2±8.8	15.9±5.7	22.4±9.7	30.0±4.0	43.4±19.7

Earlier findings showing that increasing ischemic duration results in an analogous increase in the total *and* the 'free' fraction of iron were substantiated here. The pool of 'free' cytosolic iron, in mammalian cells, is controlled predominantly by ferritin (Ft). This multimeric protein incorporates and stores excessive 'free' iron, functioning as an iron scavenger (41-43). Ft can also release its iron causing an increase of the cellular 'free' iron pool (36, 37, 44). These indicate that Ft may be responsible for modulations of the amounts of 'free' iron in the heart. Therefore, Ft contents in these hearts have become of interest.

The levels of iron (and Cu) in the CFF, following the PC episodes, were small, but significant. Table V shows the concentrations of iron and copper that were mobilized from the heart *(i)* during the ischemic-PC phase alone, *(ii)* following prolonged ischemia of 35min (no PC, group III), and *(iii)* after PC *and* 35min ischemia (group I). It is clear that the amounts mobilized following prolonged ischemia (without PC) are markedly higher (> 10-fold) than the small levels associated with the PC phase alone.

Table 5: Mobilization of iron and copper from the heart tissue to the first coronary flow fractions, following prolonged ischemia, and under the following conditions:

Group	**Iron mobilization ng/ml**
Prolonged Ischemia and Reperfusion	**108**
PC followed by Ischemia and Reperfusion	**26**
Preconditioning only	**2-4**

Ft contents were determined in heart tissue extracts by ELISA using polyclonal antibodies against rat heart Ft (Table 4). Subjecting hearts to PC prior to the prolonged ischemic insult (35min) yielded substantially higher levels of Ft in the cardiac tissue (0.90 *versus* 0.54-0.64μg/mg protein, for all other groups; p<0.05).

The result of Ft contents in heart tissue was found to be in accord with the data concerning the degree of saturation of Ft with iron. In group I, heart Ft-saturation was 0.22μg Fe/μg Ft, a value lower than those for the groups II & III, which were 0.31-0.32μg Fe/μg Ft. These data indicate that an increase in heart Ft content took place *only* in the PC group (group I), and not in the continuously perfused hearts (group II), nor in those that were subjected to prolonged ischemia without prior PC (group III).

Table 6: Ferritin levels in hearts and in coronary flow of following ischemia and reperfusion with or without CPC. * = $p \leq 0.05$.

	Ferritin/Protein mg/mg	**Fe in Ferritin** mg/mg	**Total ferritin in Coronary flow** (mg)
Group I: PC+Ischemia (80 min)	**0.90 ± 0.13‡**	**0.22 ± 0.04**	**0.73 ± 0.11*,‡**
Group II: Normal perfusion (80')	**0.64 ± 0.10**	**0.32 ± 0.04**	**0.19 ± 0.05‡**
Group III: Ischemia without PC (80')	**0.54 ± 0.07**	**0.31 ± 0.04**	**1.30 ± 0.14***

*** denotes p<0.05 of groups I or III *versus* group II;.**
‡ denotes p<0.05 of groups I or II *versus* group III.

PC yields a marked decrease of the levels of cellular re-distribution and extra-cellular mobilization of iron (and copper), following prolonged ischemia. PC is further associated with an accumulation of intracellular ferritin, and a concomitant decrease in ferritin-iron saturation. It is suggested that the low but significant and reproducible levels of mobilization of intracellular iron, following each cycle of PC, have led to the relief of the inhibitory control of ferritin synthesis, by virtue of converting the iron responsive proteins, notably IRP-1, to cytoplasmic aconitase.

The ability of ferritin to incorporate *and* release iron renders this protein a major active regulator of and passive responder to cellular 'free' iron pool, playing dual roles in oxidative stress. On one hand, scavenging of catalytic iron from the cytosol inhibiting the formation of reactive oxygen species (ROS), thus producing a protective effect (45, 46). On the other hand, releasing iron and increasing its availability for Fenton chemistry, thus producing a pro-oxidant effect (36, 37, 41, 42). Therefore, it is expected that the balance between its protection and pro-oxidant activity will determine the net effect of ferritin. An increase in ferritin synthesis led to a concomitant increase in iron incorporation (42, 43, 47-49), while degradation of ferritin allowed the release of iron (35-38, 50). The changes in ferritin levels reflected the balance between synthesis and degradation, and indicate the resultant direction of cellular-iron distribution.

The resultss showed that ferritin levels (protein content) correlated with the levels of iron mobilization from cardiac tissue to the coronary flow: only following PC, when the level of mobilization was small, a marked increase in tissue ferritin was observed. No change in ferritin level was demonstrated without ischemia, when no mobilization of iron took place. Analogously, no change was noticed following prolonged ischemia (without PC), when a relatively high level of iron mobilization was recorded.

Enhanced protein catabolism by virtue of intracellular proteolysis occurs in an ischemic organ (51-54). Ferritin degradation during prolonged ischemia, together with acidosis and reducing environment of the ischemic cell lead to the release of iron (55). Each iron-loaded ferritin molecule (containing ~1500-2500 Fe atoms), releases many redox active iron ions that catalyze the formation of free radicals, during the reperfusion phase, and yields tissue injury. The prominent protective effect following PC is explained by *de novo* synthesis of ferritin in the preconditioned hearts, culminating in the preparation of the heart to scavenge excessive 'free' iron that had been recently released (56-61).

The typical function of IRP-1 is to inhibit the synthesis of apo-ferritin, while maintaining an adequate level of inhibitory control of translation of the mRNA. Upon small influx of iron the inhibition is relieved, ferritin synthesis is activated, protecting the cell against iron-mediated injury. Ischemic PC leads to re-distribution of small amounts of iron within the cell and its mobilization out of the cell. The intracellular newly released iron, serve as the trigger for the relief of the inhibitory control of translation of the ferritin message through the conversion of IRP-1 to the cytoplasmic aconitase. The result is the production of a marked reservoir of apo-ferritin, which is ready to scavenge 'free' iron, to be released only following the prolonged ischemia.

Further support to this pproposed novel mechanism can be found in the followinf data:

(i) - Chelators of iron have been shown to protect against reperfusion injury of the ischemic heart. Desferrioxamine (DFO) at mM concentration was proven protective. Here, we used very low levels of DFO, or its building block (hydroxamic acid derivatives such as acetyl hydroxamic acid), or the zinc complex of DFO that has already been shown to infiltrate into cells. When ~1μM of these compounds was included in the perfusate the protection of the heart by PC was abolished.

(ii) - Using very low levels of an hydrophobic complex of iron, such as ferric-1,10-phenanthroline-penta-chlorophenol complex, a PC-like effect was demonstrated. This protection was interpreted by the infiltration of iron (from the complex) into the myocytes, and its reaction with the IRPs converting them to a non-functional form, and thus relieving their inhibitory control in ferritin synthesis.

Acknowledgements:

M.C. is the incumbent of the Dr. William Ganz Chair of Heart Studies, at the Hebrew University of Jerusalem. This study was supported by the 'Pepka and Dr. Moshe Bergman Memorial Fund' and by a research grant from the Israel Science Foundation (Research Grant 585/02).

References

[1] Kitagawa K, Matsumoto M, Oda T, Niinobe M, Hata R, Handa N, et al. Free radical generation during brief period of cerebral ischemia may trigger delayed neuronal death. Neuroscience 1990;35(3):551-8.

[2] Kitagawa K, Matsumoto M, Kuwabara K, Tagaya M, Ohtsuki T, Hata R, et al. 'Ischemic tolerance' phenomenon detected in various brain regions. Brain Res 1991;561(2):203-11.

[3] Emerson MR, Samson FE, Pazdernik TL. Effects of hypoxia preconditioning on expression of metallothionein-1,2 and heme oxygenase-1 before and after kainic acid-induced seizures. Cell Mol Biol (Noisy-le-grand) 2000;46(3):619-26.

[4] Emerson MR, Nelson SR, Samson FE, Pazdernik TL. A global hypoxia preconditioning model: neuroprotection against seizure-induced specific gravity changes (edema) and brain damage in rats. Brain Res Brain Res Protoc 1999;4(3):360-6.

[5] Emerson MR, Nelson SR, Samson FE, Pazdernik TL. Hypoxia preconditioning attenuates brain edema associated with kainic acid-induced status epilepticus in rats. Brain Res 1999;825(1-2):189-93.

[6] Olsson T, Hansson O, Nylandsted J, Jaattela M, Smith ML, Wieloch T. Lack of neuroprotection by heat shock protein 70 overexpression in a mouse model of global cerebral ischemia. Exp Brain Res 2003.

[7] Fujiki M, Kobayashi H, Abe T, Ishii K. Astroglial activation accompanies heat shock protein upregulation in rat brain following single oral dose of geranylgeranylacetone. Brain Res 2003;991(1-2):254-7.

[8] Kirino T. Ischemic tolerance. J Cereb Blood Flow Metab 2002;22(11):1283-96.

[9] Emerson MR, Samson FE, Pazdernik TL. Effects of hypoxia preconditioning on expression of metallothionein-1,2 and heme oxygenase-1 before and after kainic acid-induced seizures. Cell Mol Biol (Noisy-le-grand) 2000;46(3):619-626.

[10] Rajdev S, Hara K, Kokubo Y, Mestril R, Dillmann W, Weinstein PR, et al. Mice overexpressing rat heat shock protein 70 are protected against cerebral infarction. Ann Neurol 2000;47(6):782-91.

[11] Andoh T, Chock PB, Chiueh CC. Preconditioning-mediated neuroprotection: role of nitric oxide, cGMP, and new protein expression. Ann N Y Acad Sci 2002;962:1-7.

[12] Fiscus RR, Yuen JP, Chan SL, Kwong JH, Chew SB. Nitric oxide and cyclic GMP as pro- and anti-

apoptotic agents. J Card Surg 2002;17(4):336-9.
[13] Fiscus RR. Involvement of cyclic GMP and protein kinase G in the regulation of apoptosis and survival in neural cells. Neurosignals 2002;11(4):175-90.
[14] Guarente L. Mutant mice live longer. Nature 1999;402(6759):243, 245.
[15] Andoh T, Chock PB, Chiueh CC. The roles of thioredoxin in protection against oxidative stress-induced apoptosis in SH-SY5Y cells. J Biol Chem 2002;277(12):9655-60.
[16] Skaper SD, Facci L, Strijbos PJ. Neuronal protein kinase signaling cascades and excitotoxic cell death. Ann N Y Acad Sci 2001;939:11-22.
[17] Murray B, Alessandrini A, Cole AJ, Yee AG, Furshpan EJ. Inhibition of the p44/42 MAP kinase pathway protects hippocampal neurons in a cell-culture model of seizure activity. Proc Natl Acad Sci U S A 1998;95(20):11975-80.
[18] Tomai F, Crea F, Chiariello L, Gioffre PA. Ischemic preconditioning in humans: models, mediators, and clinical relevance. Circulation 1999;100(5):559-563.
[19] Das DK, Engelman RM, Maulik N. Oxygen free radical signaling in ischemic preconditioning. Ann. N. Y. Acad. Sci. 1999;30(874):49-65.
[20] Przyklenk K, Simkhovich BZ, Bauer B, Hata K, Zhao L, Elliott GT, et al. Cellular mechanisms of infarct size reduction with ischemic preconditioning. Role of calcium? Ann. N. Y. Acad. Sci. 1999;30(874):192-210.
[21] Das DK, Engelman RM, Kimura Y. Molecular adaptation of cellular defences following preconditioning of the heart by repeated ischaemia. Cardiovasc. Res. 1993;27(4):578-584.
[22] Yue Y, Krenz M, Cohen MV, Downey JM, Critz SD. Menadione mimics the infarct-limiting effect of preconditioning in isolated rat hearts. Am. J. Physiol. Heart Circ. Physiol. 2001;281(2):H590-595.
[23] Zeltcer G, Berenshtein E, Samuni A, Chevion M. Nitroxide radicals prevent metal-aggravated reperfusion injury in isolated rat heart. Free Radic. Res. 1997;27(6):627-635.
[24] Chevion M, Jiang Y, Har-El R, Berenshtein E, Uretzky G, Kitrossky N. Copper and iron are mobilized following myocardial ischemia: possible predictive criteria for tissue injury. Proc. Natl. Acad. Sci. U. S. A. 1993;90(3):1102-1106.
[25] Berenshtein E, Mayer B, Goldberg C, Kitrossky N, Chevion M. Patterns of mobilization of copper and iron following myocardial ischemia: possible predictive criteria for tissue injury. *J. Mol. Cell.* Cardiol. 1997;29(11):3025-3034.
[26] Eaton S, Pourfarzam M, Bartlett *K*. The effect of respiratory chain impairment of beta-oxidation in rat heart mitochondria. Biochem. J. 1996;319(Pt 2):633-640.
[27] White K, Munro HN. Induction of ferritin subunit synthesis by iron is regulated at both the transcriptional and translational levels. J. Biol. Chem. 1988;263(18):8938-8942.
[28] Van der Kraaij AM, Van Eijk HG, Koster JF. Prevention of postischemic cardiac injury by the orally active iron chelator 1,2-dimethyl-3-hydroxy-4-pyridone (L1) and the antioxidant (+)-cyanidanol-3. Circulation 1989;80(1):158-164.
[29] Van Jaarsveld H, Kuyl JM, De Wet EH, Alberts DW, Van der Westhuizen *FD*. Effect of various mixtures of diethylether, halothane, nitrous oxide and oxygen on low molecular weight iron content and mitochondrial function of the rat myocardium. Free Radic. Res. Commun. 1991;15(3):151-157.
[30] Halliwell B, Gutteridge JM, Cross CE. Free radicals, antioxidants, and human disease: where are we now? J. Lab. Clin. Med. 1992;119(6):598-620.
[31] Allen DR, Wallis GL, McCay PB. Catechol adrenergic agents enhance hydroxyl radical generation in xanthine oxidase systems containing ferritin: implications for ischemia/reperfusion. Arch. Biochem. Biophys. 1994;315(2):235-243.
[32] Lesnefsky EJ, Ye J. Exogenous intracellular, but not extracellular, iron augments myocardial reperfusion injury. Am. J. Physiol. 1994;266(2 Pt 2):H384-392.
[33] P, Swaak AJ, van Eijk HG, Koster *JF*. Superoxide dependent iron release from ferritin in inflammatory diseases. Free Radic. Biol. Med. 1988;4(3):185-198.
[34] Bando Y, Aki K. Superoxide-mediated release of iron from ferritin by some flavoenzymes. *Biochem. Biophys. Res. Com*mun. 1990;168(2):389-395.
[35] Vaisman B, Fibach E, Konijn AM. Utilization of intracellular ferritin iron for hemoglobin synthesis in developing human erythroid precursors. *B*lood 1997;90(2):831-838.
[36] Sakaida I, Kyle ME, Farber JL. Autophagic degradation of protein generates a pool of ferric iron required for the killing of cultured hepatocytes by an oxidative stress. Mol. Pharmacol. 1990;37(3):435-442.
[37] Rothman RJ, Serroni A, Farber JL. Cellular pool of transient ferric iron, chelatable by deferoxamine and distinct from ferritin, that is involved in oxidative cell injury. Mol. Pharmacol. 1992;42(4):703-710.
[38] Roberts S, Bomford A. Ferritin iron kinetics and protein turnover in K562 cells. *J. Biol. C*hem. 1988;263(35):19181-19187.

[39] Udassin R, Ariel I, Haskel Y, Kitrossky N, Chevion M. Salicylate as an in vivo free radical trap: studies on ischemic insult to the rat intestine. Free Radic. Biol. Med. 1991;10(1):1-6.
[40] Halliwell B, Grootveld M, Gutteridge JM. Methods for the measurement of hydroxyl radicals in biomedical systems: deoxyribose degradation and aromatic hydroxylation. Methods Biochem. Anal. 1988;33:59-90.
[41] Harrison PM, Arosio P. The ferritins: molecular properties, iron storage function and cellular regulation. *Biochim. Biophys. Acta.* 1996;1275(3):161-203.
[42] Picard V, Renaudie F, Porcher C, Hentze MW, Grandchamp B, Beaumont C. Overexpression of the ferritin H subunit in cultured erythroid cells changes the intracellular iron distribution. Blood 1996;87(5):2057-2064.
[43] Picard V, Epsztejn S, Santambrogio P, Cabantchik ZI, Beaumont C. Role of ferritin in the control of the labile iron pool in murine erythroleukemia cells. *J. Biol.* Chem. 1998;273(25):15382-15386.
[44] Konijn AM, Glickstein H, Vaisman B, Meyron-Holtz EG, Slotki IN, Cabantchik ZI. The cellular labile iron pool and intracellular ferritin in K562 cells. Blood 1999;94(6):2128-2134.
[45] Balla G, Jacob HS, Balla J, Rosenberg M, Nath K, Apple F, et al. Ferritin: a cytoprotective antioxidant strategem of endothelium. *J.* Biol. Chem. 1992;267(25):18148-18153.
[46] Cermak J, Balla J, Jacob HS, Balla G, Enright H, Nath K, et al. Tumor cell heme uptake induces ferritin synthesis resulting in altered oxidant sensitivity: possible role in chemotherapy efficacy. *Cancer* Res. 1993;53(21):5308-5313.
[47] Theil EC. Iron regulatory elements (IREs): a family of mRNA non-coding sequences. *Biochem.* J. 1994;304(Pt 1):1-11.
[48] Klausner RD, Rouault TA, Harford JB. Regulating the fate of mRNA: the control of cellular iron metabolism. Cell 1993;72(1):19-28.
[49] Hentze MW, Kuhn LC. Molecular control of vertebrate iron metabolism: mRNA-based regulatory circuits operated by iron, nitric oxide, and oxidative stress. Proc. Natl. Acad. Sci. U. S. A. 1996;93(16):8175-8182.
[50] Roberts S, Bomford A. Chelation of transferrin iron by desferrioxamine in K562 cells. The partition of iron between ferrioxamine and ferritin. Biochem. J. 1988;254(3):869-875.
[51] Shibata T, Yamamoto F, Suehiro S, Kinoshita H. Effects of protease inhibitors on postischemic recovery of the heart. *Cardiovasc. Drugs* Ther. 1997;11(4):547-556.
[52] Matsumura Y, Kusuoka H, Inoue M, Hori M, Kamada T. Protective effect of the protease inhibitor leupeptin against myocardial stunning. *J. Cardiovasc. Pharmacol.* 1993;22(1):135-142.
[53] Ivanova TN, Poliakova ED, Ivanov AI. [Activity of lysosomal enzymes in isolated perfused rat heart in reversible ischemia and post-ischemic reperfusion with administration of dibutyryl-cAMP and isoproterenol]. *Vopr. Med.* Khim. 1990;36(6):28-32.
[54] Karapetian RG, , Oganesian SS, , Akopian TN, , Dzhanpoladian EG. [Activity of proteolytic enzymes and their inhibitors in experimental myocardial ischemia]. Vopr. Med. Khim. 1993;39(1):29-31.
[55] Cottin Y, Doise JM, Maupoil V, Tanniere-Zeller M, Dalloz F, Maynadie M, et al. Plasma iron status and lipid peroxidation following thrombolytic therapy for acute myocardial infarction. Fundam. Clin. Pharmacol. 1998;12:236-241.
[56] Chevion M. A site-specific mechanism for free radical induced biological damage: the essential role of redox-active transition metals. Free Radic Biol Med 1988;5(1):27-37
[57] Gelvan D, Saltman P, Powell SR. Cardiac reperfusion damage prevented by a nitroxide free radical. Proc. Natl. Acad. Sci. U. S. A. 1991;88(11):4680-4684.
[58] Gelvan D, Konijn AM. The perils of free radicals in ferritin iron depletion. In: 11-th International Conference on Iron and Iron Proteins.; 1993, May 2-7,: Jerusalem, Israel,; 1993, May 2-7,. p. p 44.
[59] Ambrosio G, Flaherty JT, Duilio C, Tritto I, Santoro G, Elia PP, et al. Oxygen radicals generated at reflow induce peroxidation of membrane lipids in reperfused hearts. J. Clin. Invest. 1991;87(6):2056-2066.
[60] Caraceni P, De Maria N, Ryu HS, Colantoni A, Roberts L, Maidt ML, et al. Proteins but not nucleic acids are molecular targets for the free radical attack during reoxygenation of rat hepatocytes. Free Radic. Biol. Med. 1997;23(3):339-344.
[61] Karwatowska-Prokopczuk E, Czarnowska E, Beresewicz A. Iron availability and free radical induced injury in the isolated ischaemic/reperfused rat heart. Cardiovasc. Res. 1992;26(1):58-66.

Frontiers in Neurodegenerative Disorders and Aging:
Fundamental Aspects, Clinical Perspectives and New Insights
T. Özben and M. Chevion (Eds.)
IOS Press, 2004

Cardiovascular Aging and Cardiovascular Diseases in Elderly Patients

Beste Özben, Ahmet Kaya Bilge, Nevres Koylan
Department of Cardiology, Istanbul Faculty of Medicine, Istanbul University, İstanbul, Turkey

Abstract: Elderly population is increasing year by year as a result of the improvements in civilization, medicine and living conditions. This fact leads to huge increases in certain clinical conditions such as coronary artery disease, heart failure, hypertension, and diabetes among elderly people. For this result, understanding age-associated changes in healthy people is a necessity. Aging causes arterial stiffening with decreased elasticity and compliance of the aorta and great arteries leading to higher systolic arterial pressures and increased resistance to left ventricular ejection. Subsequent mild left ventricular hypertrophy and interstitial fibrosis leading to a decrease in myocardial relaxation follows this fact increasing the importance of atrial contraction in diastolic filling of left ventricle. With aging, connective tissue increases in all parts of the heart including the conduction system which may lead to a partial or complete separation of the sinus node from the atrial musculature causing to the loss of sinoatrial pacemaker cells up to 50- 75 % resulting in a decrease of sinus rate with altered autonomic modulation. Calcification of the aortic and mitral annuli, with central fibrous body and upper part of the interventricular septum occurs with aging affecting the neighboring parts of conduction system as atrioventricular node, AV bundle and proximal bundle branches. Aging decreases the sensitivity of the heart to adrenergic stimulation and diminishes chemoreceptor and baroreceptor reactivity. Although myocardial contractility does not change primarily with aging, but age associated diseases like hypertension and coronary artery disease may lead to the deterioration of ventricular performance. On the other hand, age related decreases in heart rate and left ventricular filling causes a reduction in cardiac output. A decrease in maximum capacity for physical work with aging is due to both diminished cardiac and peripheral factors. Physical conditioning might improve or at least delay some of the age related cardiovascular deficits. Due to all of these age associated cardiovascular changes, elderly people are more likely to develop cardiovascular disease or the preexisting cardiovascular diseases may worsen rapidly in the elderly.

1. Epidemilogical Aspects of Aging

Both number and proportion of elderly people in population is in an increase as a result of technological and medical improvements and social and environmental welfare. There are 35 million people in the US which consists almost 15 % of population; and this number is expected to reach 25 % in 2030. Life expectancy in Turkey is 68,5 years in 2002 with an increase of 2,2 years in the last 10 years. As result of this increase, an increased attention to age related problems is needed. Aging is associated with a gradual loss of function in many organs without any pathological conditions and frequently comorbid diseases complicate aging related changes. Cardiovascular diseases and conditions, such as coronary atherosclerosis, hypertension, stroke, congestive heart failure and atrial fibrillation reach epidemic proportions among elderly people and their course and prognosis worsen with increasing age [1] (**Figure 1**).

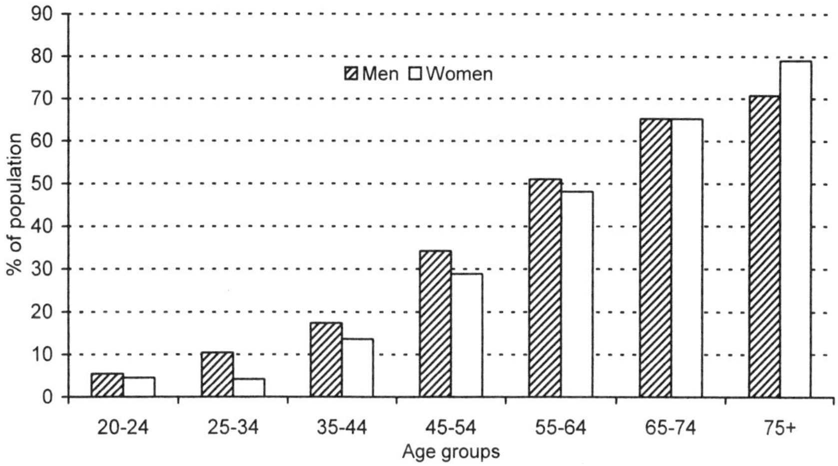

Figure 1- Estimated Prevalence of Cardiovascular Diseases among United States Population Aged 20 and Older by Age and Sex through 1988- 1994 (Adapted from American Heart Association. *2001 Heart and Stroke Statistical Update*. Dallas, Texas: American Heart Association, 200).

Although it may start at any age, hypertension is one of the greatest health problems in the elderly. More than half of the people over the age of 60 and almost two thirds of people over 70 years are hypertensives [2]. Hypertension is not only a disease state in the elderly, but also one of the most important risk factors for coronary heart disease, stroke, heart failure, and even atrial fibrillation.

The incidence of coronary heart disease increases rapidly with advancing age. The prevalence of coronary heart disease is almost 18% in men over 65 years of age and more than 13 % in women in the same age group. Although this prevalence remains the same in men after the age 75, the prevalence in women over 75 exceeds 16 %. On the other hand, the number of men having diagnosed heart attack doubles after the age 65. The increase in the number of heart attacks in women is more prominent, showing almost five fold increase [1]. Not only does clinically overt coronary disease increase dramatically with aging, but also do subclinical or occult diseases, such as silent coronary atherosclerosis. A substantial percentage of older, community-dwelling, otherwise healthy volunteers have evidence of inducible ischemia during combined thallium/ECG treadmill stress testing, and their prognosis is found to be poor compared with their counterparts without subclinical coronary disease[3]. On the other hand, total cholesterol levels and body mass index often decline in the elderly [4-7] despite the increase in the prevalence of hypertension and diabetes population. These age-related trends suggest a changing role for total cholesterol and body mass index in the development of CHD in older individuals and an increased role for hypertension and diabetes.

Stroke is the most frequent cause of disability in the elderly. There is a three fold increase of cerebrovascular events after the age of 65, reaching to 0,5- 0,6 % per year, and this incidence doubles again after the age 75[8]. According to the NHLBI's Framingham Heart Study, only 28 % of the people who suffer a stroke in a given year are under age 65. For people over age 55, the incidence of stroke more than doubles in each successive decade and the chance of having a stroke before age 70 is 1 in 20 for both sexes. The estimated prevalence of stroke shows a 50% increase in men after the age 65. In women, the increase in stroke prevalence is more than double. These rates double again after the age of 75 in both sexes [1].

The prevalence of heart failure show huge increases with advancing age. The decrease of premature morbidity and mortality from heart disease causes this increase of heart failure in the aged population as the common result of most heart disease. It has been increasingly appreciated that the development of heart failure with apparently preserved systolic function, as evidenced by a "normal" ejection fraction, occurs in about one-third to one-half of older patients with heart failure[9-12]. In a patient with heart failure, a diagnosis of diastolic heart failure can be inferred, largely by exclusion, when other comorbidities that masquerade as heart failure are ruled out and left ventricular ejection fraction is intact[13].

Atrial fibrillation (AF) is detected in approximately 3% to 4% of healthy volunteers over age 60 years who are rigorously screened to exclude clinical coronary artery disease; this is a rate 10-fold higher than in the general adult population [15]. The proportion of AF cases that occur in the absence of an identifiable cause differs between studies due to changes in study populations and methodologies. A history of atrial fibrillation without identifiable cause (so-called "lone" atrial fibrillation) was present 16.8% of men and 6.0% of women with AF at a mean age of about 70 years in Framingham population [15]. During long-term follow-up, individuals with lone AF suffered over 4 times as many strokes as control subjects, although their rates of coronary events or congestive heart failure were similar to those of controls.

Left ventricular hypertrophy is well known to be strongly associated with increased risk for coronary heart disease, sudden death, stroke, and overall cardiovascular disease[16, 17]. Left ventricular wall thickness, measured via M-mode echocardiography, increases progressively with age in both sexes; not only in people with hypertension or apparent cardiac disease, but also in healthy subjects[18-20]. On the other hand, cardiac myocyte enlargement was observed at autopsy, along with a decrease in the estimated myocyte number in older hospitalized patients without apparent cardiovascular disease, in whom overall LV mass was not increased [21].

There is strong evidence supporting the hypothesis that age-associated changes in cardiovascular structure/function are implicated in the markedly increased risk for cardiovascular disease in older persons. Thus, therapies to prevent or delay cardiovascular changes that accompany aging may reduce the risk for age-associated cardiovascular diseases. Understanding the nature and effectiveness of such therapies, however, requires an understanding of heart and arterial aging at the cellular and molecular levels. Fortunately, many of the age-associated changes in cardiac and arterial structure or function that have been observed in humans also occur across a wide range of other species and data obtained from cellular and molecular studies in these animal models may hold clues that will assist in directing future efforts toward developing novel therapies for age-associated arterial and cardiac structural and functional remodeling in humans.

2. The Effect of Aging on Cardiovascular Structure

2.1 Vascular Aging

2.1.1 Aging Associated Changes in Vascular Structure and Function

Age-associated changes at the walls of large arteries include luminal dilation, intimal and medial thickening, vascular smooth muscle hypertrophy, vascular stiffening, fragmentation of the internal elastic membrane and an increase in the amount of collagen and collagen crosslinking in arterial walls as well as the acompanying endothelial dysfunction [22-29]. The thickened intima in the elderly mainly consists of matrix molecules including collagen, fibronectin, and proteoglycans, as well as vascular smooth muscle cells (SMC). On the other hand, a decrease in the elastin content occurs due to increased elastase activity with aging. Increased levels for transforming growth factor-beta (TGF-β), interstitial cell adhesion molecule (ICAM-1), the zinc-dependent endopeptidase type-2 metalloproteinase (MMP-2), and its activator, membrane type metalloproteinase-1 can be detected through intima. Aortic MMP-2 is active in situ and accumulates in areas surrounding SMCs that are located near breaks in the internal elastic lamina, suggesting that it may play a role in the observed fragmentation of the elastic lamina [23]. Asummary of age associated cellular changes is given in **Table 1** [30].

Table 1- A summary of age associated changes in the vasculature (Adapted from [30] with changes)

↑ Diameter	**Matrix**
↑ Wall stiffness	↑ Collagen content
↑ Wall thickness	↑ Collagen cross-linking (nonenzymatic glycation)
Intima	↑ Fibronectin
↑ Thickness: SMC and matrix	↓ Elastin: calcification and fragmentation
↑ TGF-_, but ↓ antiproliferative effects	↑ Glycosaminoglycans
↑ MMP-II levels and activity	**Vasoreactivity**
↑ Expression of adhesion molecules	↓ Free NO, ↑ superoxide, ↑ peroxynitrite
↑ Nitrite and nitrate	↑ Expression of adhesion molecules
↑ Activity of ACE	↑ Permeability
Media	↓ Angiogenesis, ↓ VEGF*
↑ Thickness	**Endothelial dysfunction**
SMC: ↑ size, ↓ number	

Aging associated arterial remodeling consists of luminal dilation, and intimal and medial thickening. The thickening of intima is composed of matrix molecules such as collagen, proteoglycan and vascular smooth muscle cells and and contains high levels of matrix metalloproteinases [23] which play a very crucial role on intimal breakdown and remodeling in the elderly. High levels of transforming growth factor β (TGF- β) suppresses protease activity by activating tissue inhibitors of matrix metalloproteinase[31] and is a potent factor for synthesis of extracellular matrix proteins[32] These facts may account for the concomitant increase in fibronectin with aging[33].

Aging is associated with enhanced expression of adhesion molecules in aorta [23] and increased adherence of monocytes to the endothelium[34]. Thus, the serum levels of these adhesion molecules may be used as the indicators of age-associated alterations in endothelial function[35]. Aging is also associated with glycosaminoglycan induced increase in arterial permeability [34, 36].

Angiogenesis is found to be impaired with advancing age[37]. As endothelial cells play a pivotal role in angiogenesis, the migration and proliferation of endothelial cells in response to cytokines is significantly impaired in the elderly [38-40]. Thus, the age-associated impairment in angiogenesis is due, in part, to changes in the levels of extracellular enzymes, matrix proteins, and growth factors, which affect endothelial cell proliferation and migration.

The same metabolic, enzymatic, cellular, and endothelial alterations are increasingly recognized as playing a critical role in the genesis and promotion of atherosclerosis, vascular inflammation, vascular remodeling, and oxidant stress. In other words, many of the same factors that underlie the age-associated structural and functional intimal and medial alterations are also implicated in the pathogenesis of clinical cardiovascular diseases. The age-associated intimal-medial thickening that is observed in humans is often ascribed to "subclinical" atherosclerosis[41, 42]. In other words, early phases of atherosclerosis may be regarded as premature aging of the vessel. On the other hand, aging associated vascular remodeling makes it sensitive to risk factors[43].

Aging associated endothelial changes also resembles, in some ways, the changes observed after vascular injury induced by arterial catheter balloon inflation [44, 45] or after aortocoronary saphenous vein graft implantation [46], except the absence of atherosclerotic plaques and inflammatory cells. Enhancement of neointimal growth in response to injury in aging is due to factors intrinsic to the vessel wall [47, 48].

After balloon injury to arteries, medial smooth muscle cells are activated, begin to proliferate, and subsequently migrate to the intimal layer. Invasion of the complex extracellular matrix of the vessel wall leads to discontinuities in the internal elastic lamina. Recent evidence suggests that hematopoietic stem cells also contribute to the neointimal proliferation after arterial injury by migrating to subendothelium from the vascular lumen and differentiating into vascular smooth muscle cells [49] as a result of the action of elastases and gelatinases (such as MMP-2) secreted by the activated SMC [50]. Thus, the exaggerated response of old vessels to experimental injury in vivo [47, 48] may be attributable, in part, to enhanced SMC chemotaxis or proliferation in response to growth factors such as PDGF and TGF-β [51, 52]. TGF-β suppresses the activity of proteases, activates tissue inhibitors of matrix metalloproteinases, and is a potent factor for the synthesis of extracellular matrix proteins while its antiproliferative actions decrease with age [53].

Although nitric oxide-dependent mechanical and agonist mediated endothelial vasodilation decreases with age [54], vasoconstrictor response to angiotensin II is also attenuated in the elderly which is normalized by the reduction of nitric oxide synthesis[55]. The decrease in the nitric oxide content of aged endothelium may be a result of either age associated decrease of endothelial nitric oxide synthase (eNOS) activity, or the increase of oxygen free radicals which leads to the increased degradation of nitric oxide[56].Fibronectin and TGF-β expression are both regulated by angiotensin II [57]. Aortic angiotensin converting enzyme (ACE) activity increases with age [58, 59] and many of the age-associated intimal and matrix changes can be prevented by chronic administration of ACE inhibitors or angiotensin II receptor blockers, suggesting that age associated changes in the local vascular angiotensin system may play a central role in age-associated vascular remodeling [22].

2.1.2 Vascular Aging in Clinical Setting

Age associated subclinical changes in arterial structure and function is a strong predictor of forthcoming vascular disease. It has been observed that, wall thickening and dilatation are the main structural changes that occur within large elastic arteries during aging [109]. Age associated aortic wall thickening that occurs with aging consists mainly of intimal thickening and is widespread even in populations with a low incidence of atherosclerosis[60]. Although carotid wall intima- media thickness increases 2- to 3 fold with aging, huge differences may be observed among individuals of the same age group and there is not enough data regarding the causes of this variability.

Age-associated endothelial dysfunction, arterial stiffening, and arterial pulse pressure widening can also be considered similarly. Combinations of these processes in varying degrees determine the overall vascular aging profile of a given individual. In an average individual, additional risk factors, including hypertension, smoking, dyslipidemia, diabetes, diet, and unidentified genetic factors interact with vascular aging to activate an atherosclerotic plaque. According to this view, atherosclerosis, which increases with aging, is not a specific disease but rather an interaction of atherosclerotic plaque with intrinsic features related to vascular aging modulated by atherosclerotic risk factors [61]. Hence, it is possible that atherosclerosis occurring at younger ages may be regarded not only as a result of traditional risk factors, but also as a result of accelerated vascular aging; which may, in fact, implicate that the traditional risk factors may themselves accelerate aging of the vasculature. This fact is demonstrated in various population studies with the application of pharmacological and lifestyle interventions [62-66].

On the other hand, increased intima- media thickness is a strong predictor of atherosclerotic events. As it is accepted as an early manifestation of atherosclerosis, its presence is accepted as an evidence for subclinical coronary artery disease, and thus, future ckinical cardiovascular events. Indeed, the potency of intima- media thickness as a risk factor equals or exceeds those of conventional risk factors [67].

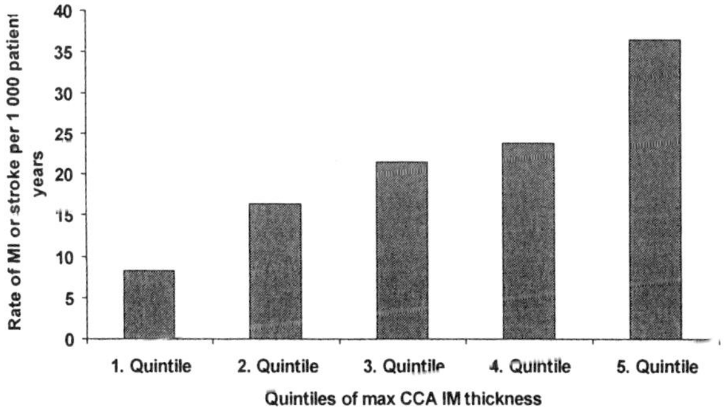

Figure 2- The relation of carotid intima- media thickness with future cardiovascular events (CCA: Common carotid artery, IM thickness: Intima- media thickness, MI: myocardial infarction) (From ref. [67], with changes)

Age-associated intima media thickening is accompanied by both luminal dilatation and a reduction in compliance or distensibility, with an increase in vessel stiffness [68]. These changes are due to structural alterations in the vascular media, including increased collagen, reduced elastin content, elastin fractures, and calcification. These structural changes may develop in the elderly with little or no atherosclerosis as well as in the young with atherosclerosis and/or diabetes [69, 70], which gives the impression that stiffness is determined not only by the structural changes within the matrix, as noted above, but also by endothelial regulation of vascular smooth muscle tone and of other aspects of vascular wall.

As the walls of large arteries become stiffer, systolic pressure increases and diastolic pressure decreases, which causes increased pulse pressure. Pulse pressure elevations are associated with progression of intima media thickening [71]. Elevated pulse pressure is a very strong predictor of future cardiovascular events [72-76]. Thus, altered structure/ function due to the stiffening of the vessel wall, in addition to the associated increase in systolic and pulse pressures, act as a risk factor for future vascular events. In addition to this, it has been demonstrated that increased vascular stiffness precedes the development of hypertension [77]. Such observations give rise to the notion that hypertension is in part a disease of the arterial wall.

2.1.3 The Clinical Manifestations of Vascular Aging

2.1.3.1 Hypertension

As a result of increased vascular stiffness, systolic pressure increases progressively with age while diastolic pressure remains the same or decreases. This leads to high pulse pressures which is linked to increased risk of major cardiovascular events and heart failure. Evidence shows that the lower the blood pressure (and pulse pressure), the lower the risk of cardiovascular events; even among the elderly. Thus, antihypertensive therapy should be given to every hypertensive elderly, even the mildly hypertensive ones. Recent data indicates that systolic blood pressure must be kept below 140 mmHg in hypertensive ones; and, must be further reduced to levels below 130 mmHg in people with diabetes or renal dysfunction. As coincident diseases, and associated clinical conditions are high in the elderly, the selection of drug therapy must be made individually. Combination drug therapy for hypertension generally increases treatment success with less side effects. In addition, nonpharmacologic therapy including salt restriction, limited alcohol intake, weight loss and regular exercise is also important in management of hypertension [78-82].

On the other hand; orthostatic hypotension (drop of more than 20 mmHg in blood pressure on going from supine or sitting position to a standing position) due to noncompliant vessels and hypovolemia and postprandial hypotension (drop of more than 20 mmHg in blood pressure occurring 30 to 120 minutes after a meal) due to vasodilation associated with excessive insulin response to a glucose load are more common in elderly people.

2.1.3.2 Carotid disease

Stroke remains a major public health problem and carotid artery disease is the most leading cause of all strokes. The patients with carotid stenosis have either occult or symptomatic coronary artery disease. Presence and severity of carotid atherosclerosis correlates with the presence and severity of coronary atherosclerosis and peripheral vascular disease [83]. The risk factors for coronary atherosclerosis are also associated with carotid atherosclerosis. Smoking, hypertension, diabetes, male gender, elevated systolic blood pressure and hypercholesterolemia are the important risk factors. The incidence of severe carotid disease increases with age both in men and in women. One-half of men over 75 years are found to have some degree of carotid atherosclerosis by ultrasonography [84]. Management of carotid disease includes the same medical approaches and risk modifications as in systemic atherosclerosis.

2.1.3.3 Peripheral Arterial Diseases

The term peripheral arterial disease (PAD) generally refers to atherosclerosis when it obstructs the blood supply to the lower or upper extremities. PAD is a strong marker of risk for major cardiovascular events since it is frequently associated with coronary and cerebral atherosclerosis. In a free-living population participating in a lipid research clinic protocol, PAD was detected in less than 3 percent of those younger than 60 but in more than 20 percent of those 75 years and olderand was 27 percent more prevalent in men than women [85], however in another study the prevalence was found similar or greater in women [86]. The very well-known risk factors associated with coronary atherosclerosis are also associated with peripheral arterial disease. Cigarette smoking, diabetes mellitus, hyperlipidemia, hypertension, hyperhomocysteinemia increase the risk of PAD. An increase in fibrinogen or elevated levels of C-reactive protein are also associated with an increased risk of PAD. As aging increase the risk of development of atherosclerosis, it is not surprising that the incidence of PAD increases with age. Intermittent claudication (pain, ache, a sense of fatigue occurring during exercise and resolving with rest in the affected extremity) is typical in the affected patients although one third of the patients do not suffer from claudication. The prevalence and incidence of claudication increase with age [85]. Segmental pressure measurement, Doppler ultrasound imaging may be used as diagnostic tests. Risk factor modification (lipid lowering therapy, smoking cessation, strict glucose control in diabetic patients and fine regulation of blood pressure) and antiplatelet therapy are given as treatment modality. In addition, supervised exercise rehabilitation programs improve symptoms of claudication in patients with PAD.

2.1.3.4 Aortic Aneurysms and Aortic Dissection

Aortic aneurysm is the pathological dilatation of the normal aortic lumen (having a diameter at least 1.5 times that of the expected normal diameter of that segment) involving one or several segments. Abdominal aortic aneurysms are much more common than thoracic aortic aneurysms. Age is an important factor as the incidence rapidly increases after 55 years of age in men and 70 years of age in women [87]. The prevalence of abdominal aortic aneurysms in the population 50 years of age and older is at least 3 percent [88]. Classically, atherosclerosis has been considered the common underlying etiology; however genetic and cellular factors play important roles as well. Aterosclerotic disease causes thickening of the intima and may thereby compromise the diffusion of oxygen and nutrients to the medial layer. Exacerbated by increases in aortic wall stress from hypertension, as tissue hypoxia may injure the media and initiate degeneration of the media and its elastic elements leading to the weakening of the aortic wall which results in the formation of either fusiform or saccular dilatation of the aorta. The majority of aortic aneurysms are asymptomatic whereas symptomatic patients mostly suffer from pain. Physical examination, computed tomography, aortography or magnetic resonance angiography are used for diagnosis. The paramount concern in managing aortic aneurysms is their tendency to rupture. Mortality from rupture is quite high; sixty percent of patients die before receiving medical attention [89] and the operative mortality for those reaching the hospital is approximately 50 percent [90] for an overall mortality from rupture of 80 percent. Surgical repair remains the therapy of choice for aneurysms considered to be at risk of rupture. Risk factor modification such as careful control of hyperlipidemia and hypertension or cessation of smoking is fundamental in the medical management of aortic aneurysms. Beta blockers are shown to reduce the risk of aneurysm expansion and rupture.

Acute aortic dissection is an uncommon but potentially catastrophic illness with an early mortality rate as high as 1 percent per hour if untreated. Thus prompt clinical recognition and definitive diagnostic testing are essential in the management of patients with aortic dissection. Medial degeneration is considered to be the main predisposing factor in most nontraumatic cases of aortic dissection. Advanced age and hypertension appear to be two of the most important risk factors. The peak incidence of aortic dissection is in the sixth and seventh decades of the life. Men are affected twice as often as women and a coexisting history of hypertension is found in 72 to 80 percent of cases [91]. Aortic dissection has also been reported to occur in association with hereditary defects of connective tissue such as Marfan and Ehlers-Danlos syndromes, certain congenital cardiovascular abnormalities such as Noonan and Turner syndromes and sometimes direct trauma to the aorta may also cause aortic dissection, particularly in the young ones.

2.2 The Aging Heart

2.2.1 Aging associated cardiac changes

Aging associated myocardial changes include an increase in LV mass due to an enlargement of myocyte size despite the reduction of the number of myocytes as a result of necrosis and apoptosis, and focal matrix proliferation caused by the altered cardiac fibroblast number or function [92, 93]. Stimuli for aging associated myocardial enlargement include an age-associated increase in vascular load due to arterial stiffening and stretching of cells caused by the loss of neighboring myocytes [94]. Growth factor signaling (eg, angiotensin II/TGF-β) induced by the stretching of myocardial cells, which, in addition to modulating cell growth and matrix production, also leads to apoptosis [95]. The production of atrial natriuretic and opioid peptides is also increased in the aged heart resembling their response to chronic stress [96, 97].

Aging associated changes in the cardiac cell excitation-contraction coupling process result in a prolonged action potential (AP), a prolonged cytosolic calcium (Ca_i) transient after excitation, and a prolonged contraction [98, 99] (Table 2). Both the number and the activity of individual cardiac L-type Ca channels increase with age while they inactivate more slowly, and this, as well as reductions in outwardly directed K^+ currents, could account, in part, for the prolonged AP [100, 101]. The age-associated prolonged Ca^{2+} transience and contraction may impair myocardial relaxation during early diastole which results in a reduced early diastolic filling rate that accompanies aging. It has been shown that gene therapy or exercise conditioning may improve impaired relaxation and Ca^{2+} sequestration [102, 103]. This altered pattern of Ca^{2+} regulation and resulting myosin protein expression allows the myocardium of older hearts to generate force and active stiffness for a longer time after excitation [104]. The prolonged isovolumic relaxation period in the aged heart may be in part a result of prolonged contractile protein Ca^{2+} activation, enabling the continued ejection of blood during late systole, a beneficial adaptation with respect to enhanced central arterial stiffness and early reflected pulse waves [105].

Acute myocardial Ca^{2+} due to neurotransmitters, postischemic reperfusion, or oxidative stress loading leads to dysregulation of Ca^{2+} homeostasis, impaired diastolic and systolic function, arrhythmias, and cell death [106]. Interestingly, this fact not only occuse in the aged, but also in the young subjects chronically exposed to pressure overload. The main causes of reduced Ca^{2+} tolerance of the aged heart are changes in the amounts of Ca^{2+} regulating proteins, increase in the stress associated generation of intracellular reactive oxygen species and age associated alterations in the composition of cellular membranes [107, 108].

Another manifestation of cardiac aging is the alterations in the β- adrenergic receptor signaling cascade [109]. These mainly include the reduction of myocardial contractial response to β- adrenergic stimulation due to the decreased responsiveness of L- type Ca^{2+} channels [110, 111], and multiple changes in the molecular and biochemical steps that couple the receptor to postreceptor effectors, as well as an adaptive process to limit the risk of Ca_{2} overload and cell death in these cells.

Interestingly, many of the molecular and cellular changes observed in senescent hearts also occur in the young with chronic pressure or volume overload [112]. On the other hand, hypertension or mechanical factors causing pressure or volume overload induce myocardial hypertrophy in a lesser extent in the elderly when compared with the young [113], as well as the myocardial response to acute ischemia.

2.2.2 The Clinical Aspects of Cardiac Aging

Left ventricular wall thickness increases progressively with age mostly due to an increase in average myocyte size in both sexes [94]. Olivetti et al [114] reported that an increase in cardiac myocyte volume was prevalent in the autopsies of older hospitalized patients with no known cardiovascular disease, with age cardiac myocyte enlarged and the number of myocyte decreased (decrease in number was found higher in frequency in older male than female patients) and autopsy overall left ventricle mass was found decreased. Aging increases the magnitude of the L-type calcium current in parallel with enlargement of cardiac myocytes; but this increase is balanced by the enlarged cell size in aged myocytes and the overall density becomes normalized. Aging also changes the amount and physical properties of collagen within the myocardium while the cardiac myocyte-to-collagen ratio in the older heart either remains constant or increases. With aging elastic and collagenous tissue increase in all parts of the heart as well as the conduction system. Fat accumulations around the sinoatrial node may lead to a partial or complete separation of the node from the atrial musculature. There may be a 50 to 75 percent loss of pacemaker cells in the sinoatrial node beginning at the age of 60 accompanied by a decrease in intrinsic and maximum sinus rate [115] Calcification of the aortic and mitral annuli, the central fibrous body and the summit of the interventricular septum occurs with aging affecting the atrioventricular node, AV bundle and proximal left and right bundle branches because of their proximity to these structures [115] and may cause certain degrees of heart block or bundle branch blocks.

In many studies performed either by echocardiography [116], radionuclide angiography [117] or Doppler ultrasonography [118] it has been observed that there is a reduction in the early diastolic filling rate progressively after the age of 20 which is compensated by increased atrial contraction [117] often accompanied by atrial enlargement. This is clinically detected as the fourth heart sound (atrial gallop). In the Baltimore Longitudinal Study on Aging (BLSA) [119], it was observed that aging caused no differences in left ventricle end-diastolic volumes in elderly patients when compared with the young. However, there was a remarkable age-associated reduction in end-systolic volumes which resulted in the preservation of left ventricular ejection fraction. The stroke volumes were found to be preserved in older persons over a wide range of performance. However, older people failed to reduce end-systolic volumes failed to augment the stroke volumes during progressive exercise. The loss of acute cardiac reserve in the exhaustive exercise in elderly patients was found to be nearly 30% of the cardiac reserve of healthy young men. This reduction was shown entirely due to reduction in heart rate reserve as systolic volume index at max exercise was found preserved.

Although the reduction of the heart rate in healthy men was not found to be age related in the BLSA study, reduction in the spontaneous and respiratory variations in resting heart rate is observed in many other populations due to the altered autonomic modulation due to aging. Heart rate increases slightly less in elderly people and this age related reduction increases progressively with exercise leading to about one-third of maximum acute dynamic reserve range of the young ones.

Resting cardiac output seems to be preserved rest. However, its exercise induced increases are reduced in the elderly people both due to the age-associated decrease of exercise induced heart rate incrementations and oxygen consumption. Impaired left ventricle ejection reserve is the most dramatic age related change in cardiac function in healthy people. This impairment is due to reduced heart rate reserve, left ventricular end-diastolic dilation and an altered diastolic filling pattern [119]. On the other hand, age associated decline in the aerobic capacity may reach to 50% of the young at peak exercise mainly because of age associated reduction in cardiac function and reductions in oxygen consumption during maximum exercise such as age related reduction in muscle mass [119].

There is no decrease in myocardial contractility, solely, as a result of aging. However, a decrease in the maximal intrinsic contractility of older people might be expected due to the reduced maximum heart rate since the heart rate is a determinant of the myocardial contractile state. In the presence of β-adrenergic blockade, left ventricle of the elderly dilates at end diastole in response to a given increase in afterload [119, 120].

Cardiac afterload increases with age as a result of increases at both left ventricular volume and vascular load. Vascular load on the heart has four components: conduit artery compliance characteristics, reflected pulse waves, inertance and resistance. The age related structural changes in the conduit arteries lead to the increase of vascular load as well as the increase of resting systolic pressure. Diastolic blood pressure tend to decrease with aging due to the reduced conduit artery compliance and early reflected pulse waves occurring centrally in late systole rather than in diastole [115]. On the other hand, total systemic vascular resistance increases modestly or does not appreciably change at rest with aging in otherwise healthy persons [119]. These age associated changes in arterial structure and cardiac function lead to an increase in the left ventricular wall thickness principally due to the increased systolic pressure rather than aging itself [121].

The abovementioned age associated changes in cardiovascular structure and function imply that there are some age associated changes in sympathetic system modulation. Plasma norepinephrine and epinephrine levels was shown to be increased with age due to increased spillover and reduced clearance. The efficiency of postsynaptic β-adrenergic signaling was also shown to decrease with aging [122]. Aging also decreases sensitivity of the heart to β-adrenergic agonists [123-127].

2.2.3 Age associated cardiac disorders

2.2.3.1 Coronary Heart Disease

In general, aging, solely, is known as one of the major risk factors in the development of atherosclerosis and thereby coronary heart disease as well as the age associated increases in the incidence of some other classical risk factors like hypertension and diabetes. The prognoses of all clinical manifestations of coronary heart disease is poorer in the elderly as well as the difficulties of the application of diagnostic and therapeutic interventions.

2.2.3.1.1 Acute Coronary Syndromes

In certain studies [128-130] it was reported that older patients were more likely to be female, have a preexisting history of angina, present with a typical symptoms of acute myocardial ischemia and infarction such as confusion, syncope or shortness of breath and experience a non-Q wave myocardial infarction. On the other hand, nearly one-half of myocardial infarctions in the elderly were misdiagnosed clinically [131]. But in all of these studies age was shown as a powerful independent predictor of short and long term mortality of patients having acute myocardial infarction. Despite the appropriate treatment with aspirin, thrombolytic agents, β-blocking agents and angiotensin converting enzyme inhibitors, age increases short-term mortality and morbidity following acute myocardial infarction [132, 133]. This increased risk of complications might be due to age related changes in diastolic filling patterns of left ventricle, aortic compliance, decreased catecholamine sensitivity that lead to decrease in cardiac reserve. Long term mortality and morbidity after an acute coronary event is also higher in the elderly.

As the mortality and morbidity are higher in the elderly with acute coronary syndromes, aggressive treatment modalities are necessary. Many studies showed that the patients with high risks, especially the elderly patients were the ones who benefited most from the optimal medical intervention such as aspirin, nitrates, β-blockers, calcium-channel blockers, ACE inhibitors, thrombolytics and anticoagulants such as heparin and warfarin [134, 135]. On the other hand, large registry data in the United States indicate that thrombolytic-eligible patients older than 75 are significantly less likely to receive thrombolytic therapy than patients younger than 65 [136]. This low rate of thrombolytic usage in the elderly patients might be due to the increased risk of intracranial hemorrhage with age.

Primary angioplasty is another treatment approach in the elderly patients with acute coronary syndromes. Data from meta-analyses show a decrease in short-term mortality and nonfatal reinfarction in patients with ST segment elevation myocardial infarction treated with primary angioplasty compared with thrombolytic treatment, with a particular benefit in the elderly [137]. Overall stroke and intracranial hemorrhage risks are lower in direct angioplasty compared with thrombolytic treatment. In addition, angioplasty is helpful in relieving ischemia in elderly patients with postinfarction angina and unstable angina [138, 139].

2.2.3.1.2 Chronic Coronary Artery Disease

All patients with chronic coronary artery disease should get an optimal medical therapy including aspirin, β-blocker, angiotensin converting enzyme inhibitor and lipid lowering drug as long as they can tolerate. β-blockers are the antiischemic drugs of choice in the elderly with stable angina. β-blocking agents decrease the incidence of ventricular arrhythmia, sudden cardiac death and early morning acute myocardial infarction. β-blockers and angiotensin converting enzyme inhibitors are shown to decrease the mortality and morbidity in many studies [140, 141]. ACE inhibitors prevent left ventricular remodeling and the onset of congestive heart failure after a large myocardial infarction. Aspirin plays an important role as an antiplatelet drug and all patients must be informed to take 325 mg aspirin a day. Cholesterol lowering is also beneficial for elderly patients with chronic coronary artery disease [142].

The number of the elderly patients with chronic coronary disease who had undergone either percutaneous transluminal coronary angioplasty or coronary artery bypass surgery is significantly increasing while the mortality and morbidity risk are decreasing with technical advances. Coronary artery bypass surgery enables significant relief in angina and improvement in quality of life in many elderly patients [143]. Nevertheless, decision for bypass surgery should be taken carefully assessing both the risks and benefits. The morbidity and mortality rates are higher in the elderly patients as age increases the severity of coronary artery disease and the risk of neurological events and wound infections. Morbidity and mortality depend on the presence of comorbidity, the ejection fraction and the diffuseness of the coronary artery disease. Angioplasty outcomes have improved with the usage of new techniques and stents, especially the coated stents. Elderly patients with high-risk coronary artery disease or angina unresponsive to medical therapy are underwent percutaneous interventions. Angioplasty is a less invasive procedure and has less complication risk than bypass surgery especially in the elderly patients. The number of the vessels with critical coronary artery disease, the extent and the site of stenosis and the physical status and the coexisting diseases of the patients are important factors in the decision between angioplasty and bypass surgery.

Participation in cardiac rehabilitation programs is important especially in the elderly patients with ischemic heart diseases. Exercise training may be helpful in patients' daily activities and education may be given to come over the psychological problems.

2.2.3.2 Congestive Heart Failure

Congestive heart failure is a highly lethal condition with high mortality and morbidity. The prevalence of heart failure increases with age due to both the increase of coronary artery disease and hypertension with aging, and, aging associated myocardial and vascular changes [144].

In the management of heart failure, the goals of treatment consist of improving survival and increasing quality of life. Appropriate medical treatment, full compliance to lifestyle changes, intensive patient education and close monitoring of the patient are essential to reach these goals. It has been demonstrated that angiotensin converting enzyme inhibitors [145], β-blockers (carvedilol [146] and metoprolol [147]) and aldosterone inhibition [148] improve survival even in the elderly. Diuretics, and digitalis improve symptomatology without affecting overall survival [149]. Multisite pacing, mechanical assist devices and surgical treatment including heart transplantation are other treatment modalities in people with refractory heart failure.

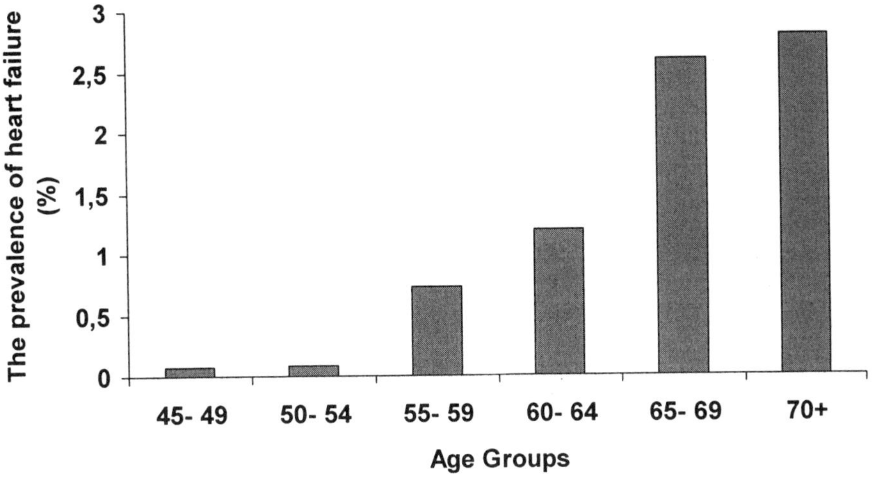

Figure 3- The age associated prevalence of heart failure according to the Framingham Study

2.2.3.3 Arrhythmia

The frequency of supraventricular and ventricular arrhythmias increase with aging [150] due to age related disturbances in impulse generation and conduction, and increased incidence of coronary and hypertensive heart disease. Hyperthyroidism, anemia, hypoxia, electrolyte imbalance, infections, hypotension and hypertension are the other less frequent causes of arrhythmias in the elderly. Longterm ambulatory electrocardiographic monitoring during patients' daily activities enable the detection of the nature, severity and duration of the arrhythmia noninvasively. As an invasive method, electrophysiologic studies are used both for diagnosis of the arrhythmia and determination of its mechanism and therapeutic approaches. Older individuals are more likely to develop hemodynamic and ischemic deterioration during an arrhytmic episode, thus more attention should be given to old individuals with arrhythmias.

Atrial fibrilation is the most common supraventricular arrhythmia in the elderly and is associated with increasing age, heart failure, valvular heart disease, coronary artery disease, diabetes and hypertension. Both anticoagulation and antiarrhythmic (rhythm control/rate control) therapies should be applied properly for both to decrease stroke risk and improve cardiac performance. The most frequently used treatment modalities for rhythm control are electrical or pharmacological cardioversion, In addition AV node ablation with pacemaker insertion, electrophysiologic ablation procedures like pulmonary vein isolation and surgical treatment are other therapeutic procedures which can be used when necessary.

Ventricular arrhythmias are frequent in the elderly, especially in the presence of ischemia, left ventricular dysfunction, and electrolyte disturbances. As most of the ventricular arrhythmias except simple ectopic beats are life threatening, aggressive drug management, implantable cardioverter defibrilators and electrophysiologic approaches may be used.

Conduction defects are more common in the elderly. Due to the age associated changes in cardiac pacemakers and conduction system, as well as the decreased sensitivity to adrenergic stimulus lead to conduction disturbances like sick sinus syndrome and AV and bundle branch blocks. Pacemaker implantation is the treatment of choice in most cases, especially in those with or having the risk of syncope or presyncope.

2.2.3.4 Valvular Heart Disease

Any valve lesion may be seen in the elderly people. The most frequently clinically seen valvular heart disease in the elderly people is calcific aortic stenosis and mitral regurgitation due to myxomatous mitral valve.

Aortic valve sclerosis may result from stiffening and calcification of the aortic annulus and base of the semilunar cusps and may or may not be associated with other manifestations of atherosclerosis, especially the coronary artery disease [151]. The development of clinically significant aortic stenosis may be very rapid in the elderly people leading to congestive heart failure rather than angina and syncope, which that are more common in the younger ones. Doppler echocardiography is useful in the diagnosis. Aortic valve replacement often improves symptoms as well as left ventricular function and survival [152, 153]. Chronic aortic regurgitation may be seen in elderly people secondary to aortic root dilation. Rarely, infective endocarditis may also cause aortic regurgitation and must be kept in mind as the clinical manifestations of endocarditis may be frust in the elderly. Angina and congestive heart failure may accompany aortic regurgitation. Vasodilation may improve survival and time to surgery, but surgery is the treatment of choice in the patients with left ventricular dilatation.

The most common causes of mitral stenosis in the elderly are rheumatic disease and mitral annular calcification. Doppler echocardiography is useful in the diagnosis.. Surgery or balloon mitral valvuloplasty should be performed. Mitral regurgitation in the elderly is often associated with coronary heart disease (either acute ischemia or previous myocardial infarction) and myxomatous degeneration of mitral valve, as well as the calcification of the mitral annulus, ruptured chordae, endocarditis and trauma. Mitral valve repair or mitral valve replacement are surgical approaches for these facts. Atrial fibrillation commonly accompanies and causes functional deterioration in older individuals with mitral valve disease.

2.2.3.5 Cardiomyopathy

Both dilated and hypertrophic cardiomyopathies may be seen in the elderly people. Dilated cardiomyopathies may be of idiopathic or may be a result of coronary artery disease, diabetes, arrhythmias, infections, valvular diseases or amyloid depositions. Hypertrophic cardiomyopathy is increasing in the elderly and β-blockers and calcium channel blockers are the first line drugsa. Surgical septal myomectomy and alcohol-induced transcoronary ablation of septal hypertrophy might be used when medical therapy is not adequate to reduce subvalvular pressure gradient.

References

[1] American Heart Association. 2001 Heart and Stroke Statistical Update. Dallas, Texas: American Heart Association, 2000.

[2] Burt VL, Whelton P, Roccella EJ, et al. Prevalence of hypertension in the US adult population: results from the Third National Health and Nutrition Examination Survey, 1988-1991. Hypertension. 1995 Mar;25(3):305–313.

[3] Fleg JL, Gerstenblith G, Zonderman AB, et al. Prevalence and prognostic significance of exercise-induced silent myocardial ischemia detected by thallium scintigraphy and electrocardiography in asymptomatic volunteers Circulation 1990 Feb;81(2):428-436.
[4] Cornoni-Huntley JC, Harris TB, Everett DF, et al. An overview of body weight of older persons, including the impact on mortality. The National Health and Nutrition Examination Survey I: Epidemiologic Follow-up Study. J Clin Epidemiol. 1991;44(8):743–753.
[5] Ferrara A, Barrett-Connor E, Shan J. Total, LDL, and HDL cholesterol decrease with age in older men and women: The Rancho Bernardo Study 1984–1994. Circulation. 1997 Jul 1;96(1):37–43.
[6] Wilson PW, Anderson KM, Harris T, Kannel WB, Castelli WP. Determinants of change in total cholesterol and HDL-C with age: The Framingham Study. J Gerontol. 1994 Nov;49(6):M252–M257.
[7] Weijenberg MP, Feskens EJ, Kromhout D. Age-related changes in total and high-density-lipoprotein cholesterol in elderly Dutch men. Am J Public Health. 1996 Jun;86(6):798–803.
[8] Kannel WB, Wolf PA, Garrison RJ, eds. Framingham Study: An Epidemiological Investigation of Cardiovascular Disease. Section 34. NIH Publication No.87–2703. Bethesda, Md: National Heart, Lung and Blood Institute; 1987.
[9] Vasan RS, Larson MG, Benjamin EJ, Evans JC, Reiss CK, Levy D. Congestive heart failure in subjects with normal versus reduced left ventricular ejection fraction: prevalence and mortality in a population-based cohort. J Am Coll Cardiol. 1999 Jun;33(7):1948–1955.
[10] Mosterd A, Hoes AW, de Bruyne MC, et al. Prevalence of heart failure and left ventricular dysfunction in the general population: the Rotterdam Study. Eur Heart J. 1999 Mar;20(6):447–455.
[11] Senni M, Tribouilloy CM, Rodeheffer RJ, et al. Congestive heart failure in the community: a study of all incident cases in Olmsted County, Minnesota, in 1991. Circulation. 1998 Nov 24;98(21):2282–2289.
[12] Kitzman DW, Gardin JM, Gottdiener JS, et al. Importance of heart failure with preserved systolic function in patients > or = 65 years of age: CHS Research Group. Cardiovascular Health Study. Am J Cardiol. 2001 Feb 15;87(4):413–419.
[13] Vasan RS, Levy D. Defining diastolic heart failure: a call for standardized diagnostic criteria. Circulation. 2000 May 2;101(17):2118–2121.
[14] Manolio TA, Furberg CD, Rautaharju PM, et al. Cardiac arrhythmias on 24-hour ambulatory electrocardiography in older women and men: the Cardiovascular Health Study. J Am Coll Cardiol. 1994 Mar 15;23(4):916–925.
[15] Brand FN, Abbott RD, Kannel WB, Wolf PA. Characteristics and prognosis of lone atrial fibrillation: 30-year follow-up in the Framingham Study. JAMA. 1985 Dec 27;254(24):3449–3453.
[16] Haider AW, Larson MG, Benjamin EJ, Levy D. Increased left ventricular mass and hypertrophy are associated with increased risk for sudden death. J Am Coll Cardiol. 1998 Nov;32(5):1454–1459.
[17] Levy D, Garrison RJ, Savage DD, Kannel WB, Castelli WP. Prognostic implications of echocardiographically determined left ventricular mass in the Framingham Heart Study. N Engl J Med. 1990 May 31;322(22):1561–1566.
[18] Lauer MS, Anderson KM, Levy D. Influence of contemporary versus 30-year blood pressure levels on left ventricular mass and geometry: the Framingham Heart Study. J Am Coll Cardiol. 1991 Nov 1;18(5):1287–1294.
[19] Lauer MS, Anderson KM, Levy D. Separate and joint influences of obesity and mild hypertension on left ventricular mass and geometry: the Framingham Heart Study. J Am Coll Cardiol. 1992 Jan;19(1):130–134.
[20] Levy D, Anderson KM, Savage DD, Kannel WB, Christiansen JC, Castelli WP. Echocardiographically detected left ventricular hypertrophy: prevalence and risk factors: The Framingham Heart Study. Ann Intern Med. 1988 Jan;108(1):7–13.
[21] Olivetti G, Giordano G, Corradi D, et al. Gender differences and aging: effects on the human heart. J Am Coll Cardiol. 1995 Oct;26(4):1068–1079.
[22] Michel JB, Heudes D, Michel O, et al. Effect of chronic ANG I-converting enzyme inhibition on aging processes: II: large arteries. Am J Physiol. 1994 Jul;267(1 Pt 2):R124–R135.
[23] Li Z, Froehlich J, Galis ZS, Lakatta EG. Increased expression of matrix metalloproteinase-2 in the thickened intima of aged rats. Hypertension. 1999 Jan;33(1):116–123.
[24] Haudenschild CC, Prescott MF, Chobanian AV. Aortic endothelial and subendothelial cells in experimental hypertension and aging. Hypertension. 1981 May-Jun;3(3 Pt 2):I148–I153.
[25] Asai K, Kudej RK, Shen YT, et al. Peripheral vascular endothelial dysfunction and apoptosis in old monkeys. Arterioscler Thromb Vasc Biol. 2000 Jun;20(6):1493–1499.
[26] Wang M, Lakatta EG. Altered regulation of matrix metalloproteinase-2 in aortic remodelling during aging. Hypertension. 2002 Apr;39(4):865–873.

[27] Michel JB, Heudes D, Michel O, Poitevin P, Philippe M, Scalbert E, Corman B, Levy BI. Effect of chronic ANG-I-converting enzyme inhibition on aging processes: II. Large arteries. Am J Physiol. 1994 Jul;267(1 pt 2): R124-135.
[28] Fornieri C, Quaglino D Jr, Mori G. Role of the extracellular matrix in age-related modifications of the rat aorta. Ultrastructural, morphometric, and enzymatic evaluations. Arterioscler Thromb. 1992 Sep;12(9):1008-1016.
[29] Guyton JR, Lindsay KL, Dao DT. Comparison of aortic intima and inner media in young adult versus aging rats. Stereology in a polarized system. Am J Pathol. 1983 May;111(2):234-246.
[30] Lakatta EG: Arterial and Cardiac Aging: Major Shareholders in Cardiovascular Disease Enterprises. Part III: Cellular and Molecular Clues to Heart and Arterial Aging. Circulation. 2003 Jan 28;107(3):490-497.
[31] Border WA, Ruoslahti E. Transforming growth factor-beta in disease: The dark side of tissue repair. J Clin Invest. 1992 Jul;90(1):1-7 (Rewiev).
[32] Majesky MW, Lindner V, Twardzik DR, Schwartz SM, Reidy MA. Production of transforming growth factor beta 1 during repair of arterial injury. J Clin Invest. 1991 Sep;88(3):904-910.
[33] Takasaki I, Chobanian AV, Sarzani R, Brecher P. Effect of hypertension on fibronectin expression in the rat aorta. J Biol Chem. 1990 Dec 15;265(35):21935-21939.
[34] Orlandi A, Marcellini M, Spagnoli LG. Aging influences development and progression of early aortic atherosclerotic lesions in cholesterol-fed rabbits. Arterioscler Thromb Vasc Biol. 2000 Apr;20(4):1123–1136.
[35] Morisaki N, Saito I, Tamura K, et al. New indices of ischemic heart disease and aging: studies on the serum levels of soluble intercellular adhesion molecule-1 (ICAM-1) and soluble vascular cell adhesion molecule-1 (VCAM-1) in patients with hypercholesterolemia and ischemic heart disease. Atherosclerosis. 1997 May;131(1):43–48.
[36] Belmin J, Corman B, Merval R, et al. Age-related changes in endothelial permeability and distribution volume of albumin in rat aorta. Am J Physiol. 1993 Mar;264(3 Pt 2):H679–H685.
[37] Rivard A, Fabre JE, Silver M, et al. Age-dependent impairment of angiogenesis. Circulation. 1999 Jan 5-12;99(1):111–120.
[38] Reed MJ, Corsa AC, Kudravi SA, McCormick RS, Arthur WT. A deficit in collagenase activity contributes to impaired migration of aged microvascular endothelial cells. J Cell Biochem. 2000 Feb;77(1):116–126.
[39] Reed MJ, Corsa A, Pendergrass W, Penn P, Sage EH, Abrass IB. Neovascularization in aged mice: delayed angiogenesis is coincident with decreased levels of transforming growth factor beta1 and type I collagen. Am J Pathol. 1998 Jan;152(1):113–123.
[40] Rivard A, Berthou-Soulie L, Principe N, et al. Age-dependent defect in vascular endothelial growth factor expression is associated with reduced hypoxia-inducible factor 1 activity. J Biol Chem. 2000 Sep 22;275(38):29643–29647.
[41] Salonen R, Nyssonen K, Porkkala-Sarataho E, Salonen JT. The Kuopio Atherosclerosis Prevention Study (KAPS): effect of pravastatin treatment on lipids, oxidation resistance of lipoproteins, and atherosclerotic progression. Am J Cardiol. 1995 Sep 28;76(9):34C–39C.
[42] Woo KS, Chook P, Raitakari OT, McQuillan B, Feng JZ, Celermajer DS. Westernization of Chinese adults and increased subclinical atherosclerosis. Arterioscler Thromb Vasc Biol. 1999 Oct;19(10):2487–2493.
[43] Homma S, Hirose N, Ishida H, Ishii T, Araki G. Carotid plaque and intima-media thickness assessed by b-mode ultrasonography in subjects ranging from young adults to centenarians. Stroke. 2001 Apr;32(4):830–835.
[44] Jenkins GM, Crow MT, Bilato C, et al. Increased expression of membrane-type matrix metalloproteinase and preferential localization of matrix metalloproteinase-2 to the neointima of balloon-injured rat carotid arteries. Circulation. 1998 Jan 6-13;97(1):82–90.
[45] Galis ZS, Sukhova GK, Libby P. Microscopic localization of active proteases by in situ zymography: detection of matrix metalloproteinase activity in vascular tissue. FASEB J. 1995 Jul;9(10):974–980.
[46] Motwani JG, Topol EJ. Aortocoronary saphenous vein graft disease: pathogenesis, predisposition, and prevention. Circulation. 1998 Mar 10;97(9):916–931.
[47] Stemerman MB, Weinstein R, Rowe JW, et al. Vascular smooth muscle cell growth kinetics in vivo in aged rats. Proc Natl Acad Sci U S A. 1982 Jun;79(12):3863–3866.
[48] Hariri RJ, Alonso DR, Hajjar DP, Coletti D, Weksler ME. Aging and arteriosclerosis: I: development of myointimal hyperplasia after endothelial injury. J Exp Med. 1986 Oct 1;164(4):1171–1178.
[49] Sata M, Saiura A, Kunisato A, et al. Hematopoietic stem cells differentiate into vascular cells that participate in the pathogenesis of atherosclerosis. Nat Med. 2002 Apr;8(4):403–409.

[50] Cheng L, Mantile G, Pauly R, et al. Adenovirus-mediated gene transfer of the human tissue inhibitor of metalloproteinase-2 blocks vascular smooth muscle cell invasiveness in vitro and modulates neointimal development in vivo. Circulation. 1998 Nov 17;98(20):2195–2201.
[51] Pauly RR, Passaniti A, Crow M, et al. Experimental models that mimic the differentiation and dedifferentiation of vascular cells. Circulation. 1992 Dec;86(6 suppl):III68–III73.
[52] McCaffrey TA, Nicholson AC, Szabo PE, Weksler ME, Weksler BB. Aging and arteriosclerosis: The increased proliferation of arterial smooth muscle cells isolated from old rats is associated with increased platelet-derived growth factor-like activity. J Exp Med. 1988 Jan 1;167(1):163–174.
[53] McCaffrey TA, Falcone DJ. Evidence for an age-related dysfunction in the antiproliferative response to transforming growth factor-beta in vascular smooth muscle cells. Mol Biol Cell. 1993;4:315–322.
[54] Hongo K, Nakagomi T, Kassell NF, et al. Effects of aging and hypertension on endothelium-dependent vascular relaxation in rat carotid artery. Stroke. 1988 Jul;19(7):892–897.
[55] Cernadas MR, Sanchez de Miguel L, Garcia-Duran M, et al. Expression of constitutive and inducible nitric oxide synthases in the vascular wall of young and aging rats. Circ Res. 1998 Aug 10;83(3):279–286.
[56] Van der Loo B, Labugger R, Skepper JN, et. al. Enhanced peroxynitrite formation is associated with vascular aging. J Exp Med. 2000 Dec 18;192(12):1731–1744.
[57] Crawford DC, Chobanian AV, Brecher P. Angiotensin II induces fibronectin expression associated with cardiac fibrosis in the rat. Circ Res. 1994 Apr;74(4):727–739.
[58] Challah M, Nadaud S, Philippe M, et al. Circulating and cellular markers of endothelial dysfunction with aging in rats. Am J Physiol. 1997 Oct;273(4 Pt 2):H1941–H1948.
[59] Wang M, Takagi G, Asai K, et al. Aging increases aortic MMP-2 activity and angiotensin II in nonhuman primates. Hypertension. 2003 Jun;41(6):1308-16.
[60] Virmani R, Avolio AP, Mergner WJ, et al. Effect of aging on aortic morphology in populations with high and low prevalence of hypertension and atherosclerosis: comparison between occidental and Chinese communities. Am J Pathol. 1991 Nov;139(5):1119–1129.
[61] Spagnoli LG, Orlandi A, Mauriello A, et al. Aging and atherosclerosis in the rabbit: distribution, prevalence, and morphology of atherosclerotic lesions. Atherosclerosis. 1991 Jul;89(1):11–24.
[62] Hodis HN, Mack WJ, LaBree L, et al. Reduction in carotid arterial wall thickness using lovastatin and dietary therapy: a randomized, controlled clinical trial. Ann Intern Med. 1996 Mar 15;124(6):548–556.
[63] Hedblad B, Wikstrand J, Janzon L, Wedel H, Berglund G. Low-dose metoprolol CR/XL and fluvastatin slow progression of carotid intima-media thickness: main results from the Beta-Blocker Cholesterol-Lowering Asymptomatic Plaque Study (BCAPS). Circulation. 2001 Apr 3;103(13):1721–1726.
[64] Furberg CD, Adams HP, Applegate WB, et al. Effect of lovastatin on early carotid atherosclerosis and cardiovascular events. Asymptomatic Carotid Artery Progression Study (ACAPS) Research Group. Circulation. 1994 Oct;90(4):1679–1687.
[65] Lonn EM, Yusuf S, Dzavik V, et al. Effects of ramipril and vitamin E on atherosclerosis: the study to evaluate carotid ultrasound changes in patients treated with ramipril and vitamin E (SECURE). Circulation. 2001 Feb 20;103(7):919–925.
[66] de Groot E, Jukema JW, Montauban van Swijndregt AD, et al. B-mode ultrasound assessment of pravastatin treatment effect on carotid and femoral artery walls and its correlations with coronary arteriographic findings: a report of the Regression Growth Evaluation Statin Study (REGRESS). J Am Coll Cardiol. 1998 Jun;31(7):1561–1567.
[67] O'Leary DH, Polak JF, Kronmal RA, Manolio TA, Burke GL, Wolfson SK Jr. Carotid-Artery Intima And Media Thickness As A Risk Factor For Myocardial Infarction And Stroke In Older Adults. Cardiovascular Health Study Collaborative Research Group. N Engl J Med. 1999 Jan 7;340(1):14-22.
[68] Vaitkevicius PV, Fleg JL, Engel JH, et al. Effects of age and aerobic capacity on arterial stiffness in healthy adults. Circulation 1993 Oct;88(4 Pt 1):1456-1462.
[69] Avolio A. Genetic and environmental factors in the function and structure of the arterial wall. Hypertension. 1995 Jul;26(1):34–37. Review.
[70] Blacher J, Asmar R, Djane S, London GM, Safar ME. Aortic pulse wave velocity as a marker of cardiovascular risk in hypertensive patients. Hypertension. 1999 May;33(5):1111–1117.
[71] Zureik M, Touboul PJ, Bonithon-Kopp C, et al. Cross-sectional and 4-year longitudinal associations between brachial pulse pressure and common carotid intima-media thickness in a general population: the EVA Study. Stroke. 1999 Mar;30(3):550–555.
[72] Franklin SS, Larson MG, Khan SA, et al. Does the relation of blood pressure to coronary heart disease risk change with aging? The Framingham Heart Study. Circulation. 2001 Mar 6;103(9):1245–1249.

[73] Sesso HD, Stampfer MJ, Rosner B, et al. Systolic and diastolic blood pressure, pulse pressure, and mean arterial pressure as predictors of cardiovascular disease risk in men. Hypertension. 2000 Nov;36(5):801–807.

[74] Franklin SS, Khan SA, Wong ND, Larson MG, Levy D. Is pulse pressure useful in predicting risk for coronary heart disease? The Framingham Heart Study. Circulation. 1999 Jul 27;100(4):354–360.

[75] Blacher J, Staessen JA, Girerd X, et al. Pulse pressure not mean pressure determines cardiovascular risk in older hypertensive patients. Arch Intern Med. 2000 Apr 24;160(8):1085–1089.

[76] Glynn RJ, Chae CU, Guralnik JM, Taylor JO, Hennekens CH. Pulse pressure and mortality in older people. Arch Intern Med. 2000 Oct 9;160(18):2765–2772.

[77] Liao D, Arnett DK, Tyroler HA, et al. Arterial stiffness and the development of hypertension: the ARIC Study. Hypertension 1999 Aug;34(2):201–206.

[78] Himmelmann A, Kjeldsen SE, Hedner T. Recent hypertension guidelines: JNC-7 and 2003 ESH/ESC. Blood Press. 2003;12(4):196–197.

[79] Verdecchia P, Angeli F. The Seventh Report of the Joint National Committee on the Prevention, Detection, Evaluation and Treatment of High Blood Pressure: the weapons are ready. Rev Esp Cardiol. 2003 Sep;56(9):843–847.

[80] Sica DA. JNC 7: has the definition of hypertension changed? Heart Dis. 2003 Sep-Oct;5(5):305–307.

[81] Phillips B. The JNC 7 hypertension guidelines. JAMA. 2003 Sep 10;290(10):1314

[82] National Cholesterol Education Program. Second Report of the Expert Panel on Detection, Evaluation, and Treatment of High Blood Cholesterol in Adults (Adult Treatment Panel II).Circulation. 1994 Mar;89(3):1333–1445.

[83] Von Kemp K, van den Brande P, Peterson T, et al. Screening for concomitant diseases in peripheral vascular patients. Results of a systematic approach. Intern Angiol. 1997. Jun;16(2):114–122.

[84] Colgan MP, Strode GR, Sommer JD, Gibbs JL, Sumner DS. Prevalence of asymptomatic carotid disease: Results of duplex scanning in 348 unselected volunteers. J Vasc Surg. 1988 Dec;8(6):674–678.

[85] Criqui MH, Fronek A, Barrett-Connor E, Klauber MR, Gabriel S, Goodman D. The prevalence of peripheral arterial disease in a defined population. Circulation 1985 Mar;71(3):510–515.

[86] Gofin R, Kark JD, Friedlander Y, et al. Peripheral vascular disease in a middle-aged population sample. The Jerusalem Lipid Research Clinic Prevalence Study. Isr J Med Sci 1987 Mar;23(3):157–167.

[87] Bengtsson H, Bergqvist D, Sternby NH. Increasing prevalence of abdominal aortic aneurysms: A necropsy study. Eur J Surg 1992 Jan;158(1):19–23.

[88] Anidjar S, Kieffer E. Pathogenesis of acquired aneurysms of the abdominal aorta. Ann Vasc Surg 1992 May;6(3):298–305.

[89] Ingoldby CJ, Wujanto R, Mitchell JE. Impact of vascular surgery on community mortality from ruptured aortic aneurysm. Br J Surg 1986 Jul;73(7):551–553.

[90] Hollier LH, Taylor LM, Ochsner J. Recommended indications for operative treatment of abdominal aortic aneurysms. Report of a subcommittee of the Joint Council of the Society for Vascular Surgery and the North American Chapter of the International Society for Cardiovascular Surgery. J Vasc Surg. 1992 Jun;15(6):1046–1056. Review.

[91] Hagan PG, Nienaber CA, Isselbacher EM, et al. The International Registry of Acute Aortic Dissection (IRAD)—new insights into an old disease. JAMA. 2000 Feb 16;283(7):897–903.

[92] Fraticelli A, Josephson R, Danziger R, Lakatta E, Spurgeon H. Morphological and contractile characteristics of rat cardiac myocytes from maturation to senescence. Am J Physiol. 1989 Jul;257(1 Pt 2):H259–H265.

[93] Anversa P, Palackal T, Sonnenblick EH, Olivetti G, Meggs LG, Capasso JM. Myocyte cell loss and myocyte cellular hyperplasia in the hypertrophied aging rat heart. Circ Res. 1990 Oct;67(4):871–885.

[94] Lakatta EG. Cardiovascular aging research: the next horizons. J Am Geriatr Soc. 1999 May;47(5):613–625.

[95] Cigola E, Kajstura J, Li B, Meggs LG, Anversa P. Angiotensin II activates programmed myocyte cell death in vitro. Exp Cell Res. 1997 Mar 15;231(2):363–371.

[96] Younes A, Boluyt MO, O'Neill L, Meredith AL, Crow MT, Lakatta EG. Age-associated increase in rat ventricular ANP gene expression correlates with cardiac hypertrophy. Am J Physiol. 1995 Sep;269(3 Pt 2):H1003–H1008.

[97] Caffrey JL, Boluyt MO, Younes A, et al. Aging, cardiac proenkephalin mRNA and enkephalin peptides in the Fisher 344 rat. J Mol Cell Cardiol. 1994 Jun;26(6):701–711.

[98] Wei JY, Spurgeon HA, Lakatta EG. Excitation-contraction in rat myocardium: alterations with adult aging. Am J Physiol. 1984 Jun;246(6 Pt 2):H784–H791.

[99] Orchard CH, Lakatta EG. Intracellular calcium transients and developed tensions in rat heart muscle: a mechanism for the negative interval-strength relationship. J Gen Physiol. 1985 Nov;86(5):637–651.
[100] Josephson IR, Guia A, Stern MD, Lakatta EG. Alterations in properties of L-type Ca channels in aging rat heart. J Mol Cell Cardiol. 2002 Mar;34(3):297–308.
[101] Walker KE, Lakatta EG, Houser SR. Age associated changes in membrane currents in rat ventricular myocytes. Cardiovasc Res. 1993 Nov;27(11):1968–1977.
[102] Brenner DA, Apstein CS, Saupe KW. Exercise training attenuates age-associated diastolic dysfunction in rats. Circulation. 2001 Jul 10;104(2):221–226.
[103] Schmidt U, del Monte F, Miyamoto MI, et al. Restoration of diastolic function in senescent rat hearts through adenoviral gene transfer of sarcoplasmic reticulum Ca(2+)-ATPase. Circulation. 2000 Feb 22;101(7):790–796.
[104] Spurgeon HA, Thorne PR, Yin FC, Shock NW, Weisfeldt ML. Increased dynamic stiffness of trabeculae carneae from senescent rats. Am J Physiol. 1977 Apr;232(4):H373–H380.
[105] Lakatta EG, Levy D. Arterial and cardiac aging: major shareholders in cardiovascular disease Enterprises: part II: the aging heart in health: links to heart disease. Circulation. 2003 Jan 21;107(2):346–354.
[106] Hano O, Bogdanov KY, Sakai M, Danziger RG, Spurgeon HA, Lakatta EG. Reduced threshold for myocardial cell calcium intolerance in the rat heart with aging. Am J Physiol. 1995 Nov;269(5 Pt 2):H1607–H1612.
[107] Pepe S, Tsuchiya N, Lakatta EG, Hansford RG. PUFA and aging modulate cardiac mitochondrial membrane lipid composition and Ca2+ activation of PDH. Am J Physiol. 1999 Jan;276(1 Pt 2):H149–H158.
[108] Lucas DT, Szweda LI. Cardiac reperfusion injury: aging, lipid peroxidation, and mitochondrial dysfunction. Proc Natl Acad Sci U S A. 1998 Jan 20;95(2):510–514.
[109] Lakatta EG. Cardiovascular regulatory mechanisms in advanced age. Physiol Rev. 1993 Apr;73(2):413–467.
[110] Sakai M, Danziger RS, Staddon JM, Lakatta EG, Hansford RG. Decrease with senescence in the norepinephrine-induced phosphorylation of myofilament proteins in isolated rat cardiac myocytes. J Mol Cell Cardiol. 1989 Dec;21(12):1327–1336.
[111] Xiao RP, Spurgeon HA, O'Connor F, Lakatta EG. Age-associated changes in beta-adrenergic modulation on rat cardiac excitation-contraction coupling. J Clin Invest. 1994 Nov;94(5):2051–2059.
[112] Yin FC, Spurgeon HA, Weisfeldt ML, Lakatta EG. Mechanical properties of myocardium from hypertrophied rat hearts. A comparison between hypertrophy induced by senescence and by aortic banding. Circ Res. 1980 Feb;46(2):292–300.
[113] Nitta Y, Abe K, Aoki M, Ohno I, Isoyama S. Diminished heat shock protein 70 mRNA induction in aged rat hearts after ischemia. Am Physiol Soc. 1994 Nov;267(5 Pt 2):H1795–H1803.
[114] Olivetti G, Melissari M, Capasso JM, Anversa P. Cardiomyopathy of the aging human heart. Myocyte loss and reactive cellular hypertrophy. Circ Res. 1991 Jun;68(6):1560–1568.
[115] Braunwald E, Zipes DP, Libby P. Heart Disease. A textbook of cardiovascular medicine. 6th edition. W.B. Saunders Company. Philadelphia. 2001.
[116] Gerstenblith G, Frederiksen J, Yin FC, Fortuin NJ, Lakatta EG, Weisfeldt ML. Echocardiographic assessment of a normal adult aging population. Circulation 1977 Aug;56(2):273–278.
[117] Swinne CJ, Shapiro EP, Lima SD, Fleg JL. Age-associated changes in left ventricular diastolic performance during isometric exercise in normal subjects. Am J Cardiol. 1992 Mar 15;69(8):823–826.
[118] Fleg JL, Schulman SP, Gerstenblith G, Becker LC, O'Connor FC, Lakatta EG. Additive effects of age and silent myocardial ischemia on the left ventricular response to upright cycle exercise. J Appl Physiol. 1993 Aug;75(2):499–504.
[119] Fleg JL, O'Connor FC, Gerstenblith G, Becker LC, Clulow J, Schulman SP, Lakatta EG. Impact of age on the cardiovascular response to dynamic upright exercise in healthy men and women. Baltimore Longitudinal Study on Aging. J Appl Physiol. 1995 Mar;78(3):890–900.
[120] Yin FC, Raizes GS, Guarnieri T, Spurgeon HA, Lakatta EG, Fortuin NJ, Weisfeldt ML. Age-associated decrease in ventricular response to haemodynamic stress during beta-adrenergic blockade. Br Heart J. 1978 Dec;40(12):1349–1355.
[121] Chen CH, Ting CT, Lin SJ, et al. Which arterial and cardiac parameters best predict left ventricular mass? Circulation. 1998 Aug 4;98(5):422–428.
[122] Lakatta EG. Deficient neuroendocrine regulation of the cardiovascular system with advancing age in healthy humans. Circulation. 1993 Feb;87(2):631–636.

[123] Davies CH, Ferrara N, Harding SE. Beta-adrenoceptor function changes with age of subject in myocytes from non-failing human ventricle. Cardiovasc Res. 1996 Jan;31(1):152–156.
[124] Fleg JL, Schulman S, O'Connor F, Becker LC, Gerstenblith G, Clulow JF, Renlund DG, Lakatta EG. Effects of acute beta-adrenergic receptor blockade on age-associated changes in cardiovascular performance during dynamic exercise. Circulation. 1994 Nov;90(5):2333–2341.
[125] Lakatta EG. Cardiovascular regulatory mechanisms in advanced age. Physiol Rev. 1993 Apr;73(2):413–467.
[126] Stratton JR, Cerqueira MD, Schwartz RS, et al. Differences in cardiovascular responses to isoproterenol in relation to age and exercise training in healthy men. Circulation. 1992 Aug;86(2):504–512.
[127] White M, Roden R, Minobe W, et al. Age-related changes in beta-adrenergic neuroeffector systems in the human heart. Circulation. 1994 Sep;90(3):1225–1238.
[128] Nicod P, Gilpin E, Dittrich H, et al. Short- and long-term clinical outcome after Q wave and non-Q wave myocardial infarction in a large patient population. Circulation. 1989 Mar;79(3):528–536.
[129] Goldberg RJ, Gore JM, Gurwitz JH, et al. The impact of age on the incidence and prognosis of initial acute myocardial infarction: The Worcester Heart Attack Study. Am Heart J. 1989 Mar;117(3):543–549.
[130] Nadelmann J, Frishman WH, Ooi WL, et al. Prevalence, incidence and prognosis of recognized and unrecognized myocardial infarction in persons aged 75 years or older: The Bronx Aging Study. Am J Cardiol. 1990 Sep 1;66(5):533–537.
[131] Maggioni AP, Maseri A, Fresco C, et al. Age-related increase in mortality among patients with first myocardial infarctions treated with thrombolysis. The Investigators of the Gruppo Italiano Per lo Studio della Sopravvivenza nell'Infarto Miocardico (GISSI-2). N Engl J Med. 1993 Nov 11;329(20):1442–1448.
[132] An international randomized trial comparing four thrombolytic strategies for acute myocardial infarction. The GUSTO Investigators. N Engl J Med. 1993 Sep 2;329(10):673–682.
[133] White HD, Barbash GI, Califf RM, et al. Age and outcome with contemporary thrombolytic therapy. Results from the GUSTO-I trial. Global Utilization of Streptokinase and TPA for Occluded coronary arteries trial. Circulation. 1996 Oct 15;94(8):1826–1833.
[134] Smith SC Jr. Drug treatment after acute myocardial infarction: Is treatment the same for the elderly as in the young patient? Am J Geriatr Cardiol. 1998 Jan;7(1):60–64.
[135] Indications for fibrinolytic therapy in suspected acute myocardial infarction: Collaborative overview of early mortality and major morbidity results from all randomized trials of more than 1000 patients. Fibrinolytic Therapy Trialists' (FTT) Collaborative Group. Lancet. 1994 Feb 5;343(8893):311–322.
[136] Barron HV, Bowlby LJ, Breen T, et al. Use of reperfusion therapy for acute myocardial infarction in the United States: Data from the National Registry of Myocardial Infarction 2. Circulation. 1998 Mar 31;97(12):1150–1156.
[137] Weaver WD, Simes RJ, Betriu A, et al. Comparison of primary coronary angioplasty and intravenous thrombolytic therapy for acute myocardial infarction. A quantitative review. JAMA. 1997 Dec 17;278(23):2093–2098.
[138] Iniguez A, Macaya C, Hernandez R, et al. Long-term outcome of coronary angioplasty in elderly patients with post-infarction angina. Eur Heart J. 1994 Apr;15(4):489–494.
[139] Effects of tissue plasminogen activator and a comparison of early invasive and conservative strategies in unstable angina and non-Q wave myocardial infarction: Results of the TIMI IIIB Trial. Thrombolysis in Myocardial Ischemia. TIMI IIIB Investigators. Circulation. 1994;89:1545–1556.
[140] Krumholz HM, Radford MJ, Wang Y, Chen J, Heiat A, Marciniak TA. National use and effectiveness of beta-blockers for the treatment of elderly patients after acute myocardial infarction: National Cooperative Cardiovascular Project. JAMA. 1998 Aug 19;280(7):623–629.
[141] Schroeder AP, Sorensen K, Nielsen JC, et al. Clinical assessment of indication for ACE-inhibitor treatment early after acute myocardial infarction. Scand Cardiovasc J. 1999;33(3):137–142.
[142] Miettinen TA, Pyorala K, Olsson AG, et al. Cholesterol-lowering therapy in women and elderly patients with myocardial infarction or angina pectoris: findings from the Scandinavian Simvastatin Survival Study (4S), for the Scandinavian Simvastatin Study Group. Circulation. 1997 Dec 16;96(12):4211–4218.
[143] Glower DD, Christopher TD, Milano CA, et al. Performance status and outcome after coronary artery bypass grafting in persons aged 80 to 93 years. Am J Cardiol. 1992 Sep 1;70(6):567–571.
[144] Love MP, McMurray JV. The public health problem in heart failure in Managing heart failure in primary care (eds HJ Dargie, JJV Mc Murray, PA Poole-Wilson), Blackwell, London 1996, s:23-35
[145] Effects of enalapril on mortality in severe congestive heart failure. Results of the Cooperative North Scandinavian Enalapril Survival Study (CONSENSUS). The CONSENSUS Trial Study Group. N Engl J Med. 1987 Jun 4;316(23):1429–1435.

[146] Packer M, Bristow MR, Cohn JN, et al. The effect of carvedilol on morbidity and mortality in patients with chronic heart failure. U.S. Carvedilol Heart Failure Study Group. N Engl J Med. 1996 May 23;334(21):1349–1355.
[147] Effect of metoprolol CR/XL in chronic heart failure: Metoprolol CR/XL randomized intervention trial in congestive heart failure (MERIT-HF). MERIT-HF Study Group. Lancet. 1999 Jun 12;353(9169):2001–2007.
[148] Pitt B, Zannad F, Remme WJ, et al. The effect of spironolactone on morbidity and mortality in patients with severe heart failure. Randomized Aldactone Evaluation Study Investigators. N Engl J Med. 1999 Sep 2;341(10):709–717.
[149] The effect of digoxin on mortality and morbidity in patients with heart failure. The Digitalis Investigation Group. N Engl J Med. 1997 Feb 20;336(8):525–533.
[150] Fleg JL, Kennedy HL. Cardiac arrhythmias in a healthy elderly population: detection by 24-hour ambulatory electrocardiography. Chest. 1982 Mar;81(3):302–307.
[151] Otto CM, Lind BK, Kitzman DW, Gersh BJ, Siscovick DS. Association of aortic-valve sclerosis with cardiovascular mortality and morbidity in the elderly. N Engl J Med. 1999 Jul 15;341(3):142–147.
[152] Lindblom D, Lindblom U, Qvist J, Lundstrom H. Long-term relative survival rates after heart valve replacement. J Am Coll Cardiol. 1990 Mar 1;15(3):566–573.
[153] Bernard Y, Etievent J, Mourand JL, et al. Long-term results of percutaneous aortic valvuloplasty compared with aortic valve replacement in patients more than 75 years old. J Am Coll Cardiol. 1992 Oct;20(4):796–801.

Frontiers in Neurodegenerative Disorders and Aging: Fundamental Aspects, Clinical Perspectives and New Insights
T. Özben and M. Chevion (Eds.)
IOS Press, 2004

Dipeptidyl Peptidase IV (DP IV/CD26) as a Regulator of T Cell Functions and Target of Immunotherapy

Stefan Brocke[1], Aliza Biton[1], Maya Ratner[1], Sabine Wrenger[2], Klaus Neubert[3], Siegfried Ansorge[4], and Dirk Reinhold[2]

[1]Department of Pathology, Hebrew University Faculty of Medicine, P. O. Box 12272, 91120 Jerusalem, Israel; [2]Institute of Immunology, Otto-von-Guericke University Magdeburg, Leipziger Str. 44, 39120 Magdeburg, Germany; [3]Institute of Biochemistry, Department of Biochemistry and Biotechnology, Martin-Luther University Halle-Wittenberg, 61120 Halle, Germany [4]Institute of Experimental Internal Medicine, Otto-von-Guericke University Magdeburg, Leipziger Str. 44, 39120 Magdeburg, Germany

Abstract. Activated T lymphocytes express high levels of ectopeptidases, including dipeptidyl peptidase IV (DP IV, CD26). Among a multitude of functions, ectopeptidases play an important role in the regulation of T cell activation, growth, differentiation and effector functions. This article provides a short overview of DP IV/CD26 expression and functions on immune cells *in vitro* and *in vivo*. A major focus of this review are clinical aspects of the role of CD26 on hematopoietic cells and the potential use of synthetic DP IV inhibitors as therapeutics in inflammatory disorders.

1. Introduction

The ectoenzyme dipeptidyl peptidase IV (DP IV, E.C. 3.4.14.5) was first described by Hopsu-Havu and Glenner [1] 36 years ago. DP IV is an exopeptidase catalyzing the release of N-terminal dipeptides from oligo- and polypeptides preferentially with proline, hydroxyproline and, with less efficiency, alanine in the penultimate position. The post proline cleaving substrate specificity makes DP IV relatively unique among other proteases. Among the rare group of proline-specific proteases, DP IV was originally believed to be the only membrane-bound enzyme specific for proline as the penultimate residue at the amino-terminus of the polypeptide chain. However, recent studies have identified a number of additional molecules bearing DP IV-like enzymatic activity [2].

The cDNA encoding human DP IV predicts a protein of 766 amino acids with 9 potential glycosylation sites. In the plasma membrane, DP IV occurs as a homodimer with a total molecular mass of 220–240 Kd [3]. The human DP IV gene is localized on chromosome 2q24.3 and is composed of 26 small exons.

Distribution and function of DP IV are only partially known and complex. DP IV is ubiquitously distributed with exceptional high expression in intestine, kidney and liver [3]. In 1977, Lojda [4] demonstrated for the first time DP IV activity on human peripheral blood lymphocytes. 11 years later, it was discovered that DP IV is identical with the leukocyte surface antigen CD26. Subsequently at the 4th Workshop on Leukocytes Differentiation Antigens a number of monoclonal antibodies recognizing DP IV were subsumed under the term CD26 [3].

The physiological functions of DP IV greatly differ depending on the type of tissue where it is expressed. For example, within the gastrointestinal system the main function of DP IV is probably the delivery of proline-containing dipeptides for reutilization by final digestion of nutrients. Pauly [5] expanded this function by reporting DP IV-mediated processing of gastrointestinal hormones such as glucagon-like peptide-1(7-36) and glucose-dependent insulinotropic polypeptide.

Within the hematopoietic system, DP IV is expressed on the surface of resting and activated T, B, and NK cells. In general, CD26 expression is upregulated following stimulation of T cells with mitogen, antigen, anti-CD3 antibodies or IL-2, B cell stimulation with staphylococcal proteins and IL-2 stimulation of NK cells. Thus, activated antigen-specific $CD4^+$ T cell clones express high levels of DP IV/CD26 [for review see ref 6]. Albeit extensively studied, the role of CD26 in T cell biology has not yet been clarified. The wide range of DP IV/CD26 activity within the hematopoietic system is related to soluble mediators and cellular functions. DP IV exopeptidase activity has been shown to play a role in the activation or inactivation of biological peptides [7]. DP IV/CD26 has attracted great interest due to its ability to process and either inactivate or alter the specificity of many chemokines, including CXCL10 (IFN-inducible protein 10 kDa; IP-10) and CXCL12 (stromal cell-derived factor-1; SDF-1) [8], and has been described to be preferentially expressed by T helper-1 (Th-1) [9] and T regulatory-1 (Tr-1) cells [10]. Thus, processing of CXCL10 and CXCL11 (IFN-inducible T cell α-chemoattractant; I-TAC) by DP IV/CD26 results in reduced CXCR3-binding and more than 10-fold reduced chemotactic potency [11]. On the other hand, DP IV/CD26 differentially regulates the chemotaxis of T cells and monocytes toward the chemokine CCL5 (regulated on activation, normal T expressed and secreted; RANTES), enhancing directed T cell migration by a factor of two [12]. Of note, anergic T cells have been reported to exert antigen-independent inhibition of cell-cell interactions via chemokine metabolism. Instrumental to this effect may be the increased cell surface expression and enzymatic activity of CD26, which may act by metabolizing chemoattractants bound to the endothelial/epithelial cell surface [13]. Apart from processing polypeptides, DP IV/CD26 can interact either as a receptor or ligand with various proteins playing a role in immune responses. The enzyme has been described as a collagen receptor [14] and adenosine deaminase (ADA) binding protein [15]. Furthermore, it appears to be associated with CD45 [16]. Previous studies have shown that CD26 directly binds to the cytoplasmic domain of CD45 [17]. According to this report, CD26 localizes into lipid rafts while aggregation of CD26 by anti-CD26 mAb crosslinking causes coaggregation of CD45 into rafts. Finally, several groups have shown a key role of DP IV in the regulation of differentiation and growth of T lymphocytes [16, 18-19].

2. The role of DP IV/CD26 in lymphocyte activation

The development of specific synthetic DP IV inhibitors facilitated the study of the cellular functions of this enzyme on the surface of immune cells. In 1985 Schön and coworkers [20] showed for the first time that N-Ala-Pro-O-(nitrobenzoyl-)hydroxylamine, which irreversibly inhibits DP IV, is capable of suppressing the proliferation of human peripheral blood mononuclear cells (PBMC) stimulated with mitogens. This was the first evidence that

DP IV plays a critical role in the regulation of DNA synthesis of immune cells and that the enzymatic activity of DP IV is involved in this process.

In the meantime, a multitude of biochemically distinct synthetic inhibitors of DP IV have been studied under different stimulation conditions using a variety of target cells. The most potent reversible inhibitors produced and tested in our laboratories were Lys[Z(NO_2)]-thiazolidide, -piperidide, and -pyrrolidide which cause a 50 % inhibition of DP IV in the range of 2 - 3 μM.

The inhibitory effects of DP IV-specific inhibitors on leukocyte proliferation and cytokine production was confirmed in different T cell models. Previously, we reported the dose-dependent suppression of DNA synthesis of pokeweed mitogen (PWM)- and phytohemagglutinin (PHA)-stimulated human PBMC and purified T cells [21]. The same holds true for myelin basic protein (MBP)-stimulated T cell clones derived from patients with multiple sclerosis (MS) [22]. These cells also express high levels of DP IV/CD26 on their surface.

Likewise, mouse splenocytes and thymocytes express high levels of DP IV/CD26 [23]. We could show that Lys[Z(NO_2)]-thiazolidide and Lys[Z(NO_2)]-pyrrolidide inhibit the enzymatic activity of freshly isolated murine splenocytes and thymocytes as well as the DNA synthesis of activated mouse spleno- and thymocytes [24]. In addition, the antigen-specific proliferation of murine lymph node cells, T cell lines and clones can be suppressed by these inhibitors [25-26].

Besides their influence on DNA synthesis, DP IV inhibitors also exhibit strong suppressive effects on the production of various cytokines. It was shown that Lys[Z(NO_2)]-thiazolidide, -piperidide, and -pyrrolidide inhibit the production of IL-2, IL-10, IL-12, and IFN-γ of PWM-stimulated PBMC and purified T cells [21] as well as the production of IL-2, IL-6 and IL-10 of PHA-stimulated mouse splenocytes and Con A-stimulated mouse thymocytes [24]. These inhibitors also reduce in a dose-dependent manner IFN-γ, IL-4, and TNF-α production of myelin basic protein (MBP)-stimulated T cell clones from MS patients [22]. As shown by competitive RT-PCR, also the levels of IL-2 and IFN-γ mRNA in mitogen-stimulated T cells were found to be decreased after exposure of cells to Lys[Z(NO_2)]-thiazolidide [27].

Interestingly, DP IV inhibitors elicit the enhanced production and secretion of latent transforming growth factor-ß1 (TGF-ß1). To determine whether this "immunoinhibitory" cytokine is involved in the suppression of DNA synthesis and cytokine production induced by DP IV inhibitors, the concentrations of latent TGF-ß1 in supernatants of PWM-stimulated PBMC and T cells were assayed in the presence or absence of DP IV inhibitors. Interestingly, these inhibitors induce a three to fourfold increased secretion of latent TGF-ß1, as measured with a specific TGF-ß1 enzyme-linked immunosorbent assay (ELISA) and in the Mv1Lu bioassay [21]. Levels of TGF-ß1 mRNA were found 2- to 3-fold increased in PHA-stimulated T cells in presence of Lys[Z(NO_2)]-thiazolidide [6]. Previously, it had been demonstrated that TGF-ß1 exhibits the same inhibitory effects as DP IV inhibitors on DNA synthesis and cytokine production [28-29]. A neutralising chicken anti-TGF-ß1 antibody was capable of abolishing the DP IV inhibitor-induced suppression of DNA synthesis of PWM-stimulated PBMC and T cells, suggesting that TGF-ß1 might have key functions in the molecular action of DP IV/CD26 concerning the regulation of DNA synthesis and cytokine production. Moreover, TGF-ß1 as well as DP IV inhibitors have been demonstrated to downregulate the mRNA expression of DP IV/CD26 itself [27].

3. Naturally occurring inhibitors of DP IV/CD26

If DP IV inhibitor-mediated modulation of T cell activity is a pathway with physiological importance, endogenous as well as exogenous molecules with an inhibitory function on DP IV may play a role in regulating immune responses *in vivo*. Interestingly, inhibition of the enzymatic activity of porcine kidney DP IV was observed with a number of non-substrate oligopeptides containing a N-terminal Xaa-Xaa-Pro- sequence, e. g. HIV-1 Tat(1-86) and Met-IL-2(1-6) [30-31]. The short N-terminal nonapeptide of HIV-1 Tat, Tat(1-9), also inhibiting human DP IV, interferes with the proliferation of tetanus-toxoid-stimulated peripheral blood mononuclear cells [31]. The exchange of aspartic acid at position two in Tat(1-9) by tryptophan results in a peptide which strongly enhanced DP IV inhibition and suppression of DNA synthesis. The inhibitory effect of W^2-Tat(1-9) is in the range of those of the inhibitors TMC-2A and TSL-225, (K_i values of 5.3 μM and 3.6 μM, respectively, compared to 2.12 μM for W^2-Tat(1-9)) [32]. Thus, the N-terminal motif XWP turned out to be important for DP IV inhibition.

By database searches for the N-terminal XWP motif, the thromboxane A2 receptor (TXA2-R) sequence was identified. TXA2-R is a broadly distributed G protein-coupled receptor with seven putative transmembrane helices locating the MWP-bearing N-terminus (29 amino acids) at the outer site of the plasma membrane. The N-terminal nonapeptide of TXA2-R, TXA2-R(1-9), exerts comparable inhibitory effects as W^2-Tat(1-9) on DP IV activity and on DNA synthesis of activated PBMC [33]. Interestingly, TXA2 receptors have been identified on peripheral blood monocytes. Monocytes participate in the activation of T lymphocytes by presenting antigens via the major histocompatibility complex II (MHC II) to the T cell receptor (TCR). At the same time multiple molecular interactions between ligand-receptor pairs of antigen presenting cells and T cells occur (e. g. CD2-CD58, CD28-CD80), requiring a close contact between both cells. Therefore it is highly probable that the N-terminal part of TXA2-R expressed on monocytes is able to interact with T cell-expressed DP IV during antigenic T cell activation. We speculate that TXA2-R might be an endogenous ligand of DP IV, contributing to the aforementioned complex molecular interplay modulating T cell activation. A hypothetical mechanism of the modulation of T cell activation by inhibition of DP IV via synthetic inhibitors or inhibitory ligands such as the TXA2-R is shown in Figure 1.

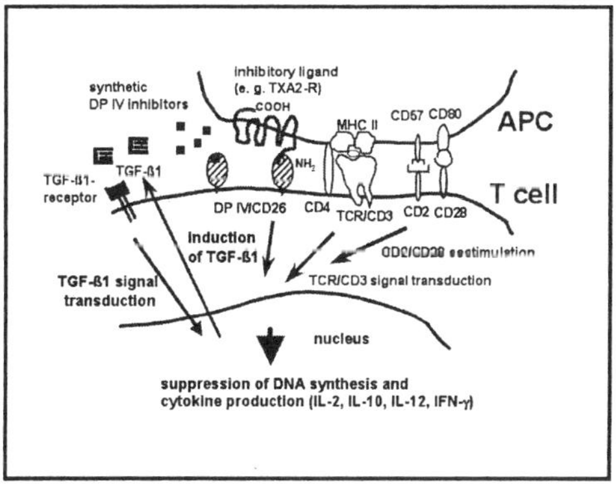

Figure 1: Model of the TGF-ß1-mediated modulation of T cell activation following inhibition of DP IV/CD26 by synthetic inhibitors or inhibitory ligands such as the thromboxane A2 receptor.

4. Targeting DP IV *in vivo*

Due to their blocking effects on T cell activation, it is conceivable to assume that DP IV inhibitors could be used for immunosuppressive therapy *in vivo*. The role of DP IV/CD26 and the effect of synthetic DP IV inhibitors were thus examined in several animal models of human diseases *in vivo* (Table 1). In these studies, various mechanisms have been suggested to account for the therapeutic effects of DP IV/CD26 inhibitors *in vivo*.

Table 1: *In vivo* studies examining DP IV inhibitors

Model	**References**
Rat cardiac transplantation	[34-36]
Collagen- and alkyldiamine-induced arthritis	[32, 37]
Experimental autoimmune encephalomyelitis	[25, 26]

Korom and coworkers analyzed the influence of the inhibitor pro-pro-diphenyl-phosphonate (prodipine) on the immune cascade triggered by organ transplantation. The treatment abrogated acute rejection, resulting in prolonged allograft survival in a rat cardiac transplantation model [34-36]. The inhibition of DP IV was associated with severely impaired host cytotoxic T cell responses.

Other studies demonstrated that different synthetic DP IV inhibitors like Ala-boro-Pro, Lys[Z(NO_2)]-thiazolidide, Ala-Pro-nitrobenzoyl-hydroxyl-amine, TMC-2A and TSL-225 suppressed collagen- or alkyldiamine-induced arthritis in a dose-dependent fashion [32, 37]. Based on these results, the authors conclude that DP IV inhibitors had antiarthritic effects, although the precise mechanisms of their therapeutic effects remain to be elucidated.

DP IV/CD26 has attracted interest as a potential target in developing anti-inflammatory therapy for MS. As with other T cells, CD26 is expressed on myelin-reactive T cell lines from patients with MS. In addition, patients with MS have an increased median percentage of $CD26^+$ cells among $CD4^+$ T cells in the peripheral blood. CD26 expression decreases somewhat in peripheral blood and cerebrospinal fluid after oral high-dose methylprednisolone treatment [38-40]. Others found correlations between changes in the CD26-expressing T cells and lesion activity on magnetic resonance imaging in MS patients with relapsing-remitting and chronic progressive disease, consistent with the presumed function of CD26 in T cell activation [41]. For these reasons, we addressed the role of CD26/DP IV in murine experimental autoimmune encephalomyelitis (EAE), a well characterized $CD4^+$ T-cell mediated autoimmune disease leading to CNS inflammation and demyelination in susceptible strains of rodents [25-26]. We demonstrated that the clinical signs of EAE can be suppressed by DP IV inhibition *in vivo* both in a preventive and therapeutic fashion. CNS inflammation associated with acute EAE was reduced. We could show that the protective effect of DP IV inhibition is caused by a modulation of T cell effector function. DP IV activity was detected on the cell surface of all autoreactive T cell clones examined. The DP IV inhibitors Lys[Z(NO_2)]-thiazolidide and -pyrrolidide had strong antiproliferative effects *in vitro* on the T cell clones examined, on both an encephalitogenic Th1 clone and a nonencephalitogenic Th2 clone. Lys[Z(NO_2)]-thiazolidide and -pyrrolidide also suppressed the proliferation of lymphe node cells and, importantly, their secretion of TNF-α and, to a lesser extent, IFN-γ. It is widely accepted that EAE can be mediated by Th1 $CD4^+$ T cells typically secreting IFN-γ, TNF-α, and lymphotoxin. We therefore suggest that the inhibition of T cell proliferation and effector functions including proinflammatory cytokine secretion may in part be responsible for the *in vivo* effect. More importantly, we found an up-regulation of latent TGF-ß1 production *in vivo* both in spinal cord tissues and in plasma from Lys[Z(NO_2)]-pyrrolidide-treated mice as compared to mice treated with PBS or Lys[Z(NO_2)]-OH. We demonstrated furthermore that Lys[Z(NO_2)]-pyrrolidide increases the secretion of latent TGF-ß1 by antigen-stimulated lymphe node cell populations. We extended these findings, demonstrating for the first time that anti-TGF-ß1 can also block the effect of DP IV inhibition on antigen-specific T cell proliferation. Our *in vitro* data suggested that the cell types induced to secrete latent TGF-ß1 by Lys[Z(NO_2)]-pyrrolidide treatment include T cells. One can assume that TGF-ß1 secretion is increased both by the encephalitogenic T cells initiating the infiltrate and by T cells that are attracted and activated during the later stages of lesion formation in a bystander fashion. Not surprisingly, macrophages and microglia, in addition to a majority of T cells, appear to produce TGF-ß1 in acute EAE lesions. Whether those or other cell types are susceptible to regulation of DP IV remains to be investigated. Taken together, our data suggest that this therapeutic effect may be mediated at least in part by upregulation of the immunosuppressive cytokine TGF-ß1 *in situ* and the inhibition of T cell effector functions.

In conclusion, these findings from *in vitro* and *in vivo* studies demonstrate that DP IV activity associated with CD26 plays an important role in the activation of autoreactive T cells. Inhibition of DP IV activity and possibly other ectopeptidases *in vivo* provides a new approach to downmodulate tissue-specific autoimmunity. These results may have important implications for the treatment of human diseases with a putative autoimmune pathogenesis. At present, major research efforts are directed at the investigation of DP IV as a potentially powerful and safe pharmacological target.

Acknowledgements

This work was supported by the Deutsche Forschungsgemeinschaft (SFB 387) and the BMBF (01770110), by grant no. 5063 from the Chief Scientist's Office, Ministry of Health, Israel and by grant no. 1809 from the MOS and BMBF, Israel and Germany.

References

[1] Hopsu-Havu, K.V., and Glenner, G.G. (1966) A new dipeptide naphthylamidase hydrolyzing glycyl-prolyl-beta-naphthylamide. Histochemie *7*, 197-201.

[2] Sedo, A., Malik, R. (2001) Dipeptidyl peptidase IV-like molecules: homologous proteins or homologous activities? Bioch. Biophys. Acta *1550*, 107-116.

[3] Fleischer, B. (1994) CD26: a surface protease involved in T-cell activation. Immunol. Today *15*, 180-184.

[4] Lojda, Z. (1977) Studies on glycyl-proline naphthylamidase. I. Lymphocytes. Histochemistry *54*, 299-309.

[5] Pauly, R.P., Rosche, F., Wermann, M., McIntosh, C.H.S., Pederson, R.A., and Demuth, H.U. (1996) Investigation of glucose-dependent insulinotropic polypeptide-(1-42) and glucagon-like peptide-1-(7-36) degradation *in vitro* by dipeptidyl peptidase IV using matrix-assisted laser desorption/ionization time of flight mass spectrometry - A novel kinetic approach. J. Biol. Chem. *271*, 23222-23229.

[6] Kähne, T., Lendeckel, U., Wrenger, S., Neubert, K., Ansorge, S., and Reinhold, D. (1999) Dipeptidyl peptidase IV: A cell surface peptidase involved in regulating T cell growth. (Review) Int. J. Mol. Med. *4*, 3-15.

[7] De Meester, I., Korom, S., Van Damme, J., and Scharpe´, S. (1999) CD26, let it cut or cut it down. Immunol. Today *20*, 367-375.

[8] Lambeir, A.M., Proost, P., Durinx, C., Bal, G., Senten, K., Augustyns, K., Scharpe, S., Van Damme, J., and De Meester, I. (2001) Kinetic investigation of chemokine truncation by CD26/Dipeptidyl peptidase IV reveals a striking selectivity within the chemokine family. J. Biol. Chem. *276*, 29839-29845.

[9] Rogge, L., Bianchi, E., Biffi, M., Bono, E., Chang, S.Y., Alexander, H., Santini, C., Ferrari, G., Sinigaglia, L., Seiler, M., Neeb, M., Mous, J., Sinigaglia, F., and Certa, U. (2000) Transcript imaging of the development of human T helper cells using oligonucleotide arrays. Nat. Genet. *25*, 96-101.

[10] Cavani, A., Nasorri, F., Prezzi, C., Sebastiani, S., Albanesi, C., and Girolomoni, G. (2000) Human CD4+ T lymphocytes with remarkable regulatory functions on dendritic cells and nickel-specific Th1 immune responses. J. Invest. Dermatol. *114*, 295-302.

[11] Proost, P., Schutyser, E., Menten, P., Struyf, S., Wuyts, A., Opdenakker, G., Detheux, M., Parmentier, M., Durinx, C., Lambeir, A.M., Neyts, J., Liekens, S., Maudal, P.C., Billiau, A., and Van Damme, J. (2001) Amino-terminal truncation of CXCR3 agonists impairs receptor signaling and lymphocyte chemotaxis, while preserving antiangiogenic properties. Blood *13*, 3554-3561.

[12] Iwata, S., Yamaguchi, N., Munakata, Y., Ikushima, H., Lee, J.F., Hosono, O., Schlossman, S:F., and Morimoto, C. (1999) CD26/dipeptidyl peptidase IV differentially regulates the chemotaxis of T cells and monocytes toward RANTES: possible mechanism for the switch from innate to acquired immune response. Int. Immunol. *11*, 417-426.

[13] James, M.J., Belaramani, L., Prodromidou, K., Datta, A., Nourshargh, S., Lombardi, G., Dyson, J., Scott, D., Simpson, E., Cardozo, L., Warrens, A., Szydlo, R.M., Lechler, R.I., and Marelli-Berg, F.M. (2003) Anergic T cells exert antigen-independent inhibition of cell-cell interactions via chemokine metabolism. Blood. *102*, 2173-2179.

[14] Hanski, C., Huhle, T., and Reutter, W. (1985) Involvement of plasma membrane dipeptidyl peptidase IV in fibronectin-mediated adhesion of cells on collagen. Biol. Chem. Hoppe-Seyler *366*, 1169-1176.

[15] Kameoka, J., Tanaka, T., Nojima, Y., Schlossman, S.F., and Morimoto, C. (1993) Direct association of adenosine deaminase with a T cell activation antigen, CD26. Science *261*, 466-469.

[16] Torimoto, Y., Dang, N.H., Vivier, E., Tanaka, T., Schlossman, S.F., and Morimoto, C. (1991) Coassociation of CD26 (dipeptidyl peptidase IV) with CD45 on the surface of human T lymphocytes. J. Immunol. *147*, 2514-2517.

[17] Ishii, T., Ohnuma, K., Murakami, A., Takasawa, N., Kobayashi, S., Dang, N.H., Schlossman, S.F., and Morimoto, C. (2001) CD26-mediated signaling for T cell activation occurs in lipid rafts through its association with CD45RO. Proc. Natl. Acad. Sci. USA *98*, 12138-12143.

[18] Ansorge, S., Schön, E., and Kunz, D. (1991) Membrane-bound peptidases of lymphocytes: Functional implications. Biomed. Biochem. Acta *50*, 799-807.

[19] Dang, N.H., Torimoto, Y., Deusch, K., Schlossman, S.F., and Morimoto, C. (1990) Comitogenic effect of solid-phase immobilized anti-1F7 on human CD4 T cell activation via CD3 and CD2 pathways. J. Immunol. *144*, 4092-4100.

[20] Schön, E., Mansfeld, H.W., Demuth, H.U., Barth, A., and Ansorge, S. (1985) The dipeptidyl peptidase IV, a membrane enzyme involved in the proliferation of T lymphocytes. Biomed. Biochem. Acta *44*, K9-K15.

[21] Reinhold, D., Bank, U., Bühling, F., Lendeckel, U., Faust, J., Neubert, K., and Ansorge, S. (1997) Inhibitors of dipeptidyl peptidase IV induce secretion of transforming growth factor-β_1 in PWM-stimulated PBMC and T cells. Immunology *91*, 354-360.

[22] Reinhold, D., Hemmer, B., Gran, B., Born, I., Faust, J., Neubert, K., McFarland, H.F., Martin, R., and Ansorge, S. (1998) Inhibitors of dipeptidyl peptidase IV/CD26 suppress activation of human MBP-specific CD4+ T cell clones. J. Neuroimmunol. *87*, 203-209.

[23] Vivier, I., Marguet, D., Naquet, P., Bonicel, J., Black, D., Xiao-Yan, Li C., Bernard, A.M., Gorvel, J.P., and Pierres, M. (1991) Evidence that thymocyte-activating molecule is mouse CD26 (dipeptidyl peptidase IV). J. Immunol. *147*, 447-454.

[24] Reinhold, D., Bank, U., Bühling, F., Täger, M., Born, I., Faust, J., Neubert, K., and Ansorge, S. (1997) Inhibitors of dipeptidyl peptidase IV (DP IV, CD26) induces secretion of transforming growth factor-ß1 (TGF-ß1) in stimulated mouse splenocytes and thymocytes. Immunol. Lett. *58*, 29-35.

[25] Steinbrecher, A., Reinhold, D., Quigley, L., Gado, A., Tresser, N., Izikson, L., Born, I., Faust, J., Neubert, K., Martin, R., Ansorge, S., and Brocke, S. (2000) Dipeptidyl peptidase IV in inflammatory CNS disease. Adv. Exp. Med. Biol. *477*, 145-153.

[26] Steinbrecher, A., Reinhold, D., Quigley, L., Gado, A., Tresser, N., Izikson, L., Born, I., Faust, J., Neubert, K., Martin, R., Ansorge, S., and Brocke, S. (2001) Targeting dipeptidyl peptidase IV (CD26) suppresses autoimmune encephalomyelitis and upregulates TGF-ß1 secretion in vivo. J. Immunol. *166*, 2041-2048.

[27] Arndt, M., Lendeckel, U., Spiess, A., Faust, J., Neubert, K., Reinhold, D., and Ansorge, S. (2000) Dipeptidyl peptidase IV (DP IV/CD26) mRNA expression in PWM-stimulated T-cells is suppressed by specific DP IV inhibition, an effect mediated by TGF-ß1. Biochem. Biophys. Res. Comm. *274*, 410-414.

[28] Reinhold, D., Bank, U., Bühling, F., Lendeckel, U., Ulmer, A.J., Flad, H., and Ansorge, S. (1994) Transforming growth factor-ß1 (TGF-ß1) inhibits DNA synthesis of PWM stimulated PBMC via suppression of IL-2 and IL-6 production. Cytokines *6*, 382-388.

[29] Reinhold, D., Bank, U., Bühling, F., Lendeckel, U., and Ansorge, S. (1995) Transforming Growth Factor beta1 inhibits Interleukin-10 mRNA expression and production in pokeweed mitogen-stimulated peripheral blood mononuclear cells and T cells. J. Interferon Cytokine Res. *15*, 685-690.

[30] Hoffmann, T., Reinhold, D., Kähne, T., Faust, J., Neubert, K., Frank, R., and Ansorge, S. (1995) Inhibition of dipeptidyl peptidase IV by anti-DP IV antibodies and non-substrate X-X-Pro-oligopeptides ascertained by capillary electrophoresis. J. Chromatogr.*716*, 355-362.

[31] Wrenger, S., Hoffmann, T., Faust, J., Mrestani-Klaus, C., Brandt, W., Neubert, K., Kraft, M., Olek, S., Frank, R., Ansorge, S., and Reinhold, D. (1997) The N-terminal structure of HIV-1 Tat is required for suppression of CD26-dependent T cell growth. J. Biol. Chem. *272*, 30283-30288.

[32] Tanaka, S., Murakami, T., Nonaka, N., Ohnuki, T., Yamada, M., and Sugita, T. (1998) Anti-arthritic effects of the novel dipeptidyl peptidase IV inhibitors TMC-2A and TSL-225. Immunopharmacol. *40*, 21-26.

[33] Wrenger, S., Faust, J., Mrestani-Klaus, C., Fengler, A., Stöckel-Maschek, A., Lorey, S., Kähne, T., Brandt, W., Neubert, K., Ansorge, S., and Reinhold, D. (2000) Down-regulation of T cell activation following inhibition of dipeptidyl peptidase IV/CD26 by the N-terminal part of the thromboxane A2 receptor. J. Biol. Chem. *275*, 22180-22186.

[34] Korom, S., De Meester, I., Onodera, K., Stadlbauer, T.H.W., Borloo, M., Lambeir, A.M., and Kupiec-Weglinski, J.W. (1997) The efffects of CD26/DPP IV-targeted therapy on acute allograft rejection. Transplant. Proc. *29*, 1274-1275.

[35] Korom, S., De Meester, I., Stadlbauer, T.H.W., Chandraker, A., Schaub, M., Sayagh, M.H., Belyaev, A., Haemers, H., Scharpe', S., and Kupiec-Weglinski, J.W. (1997) Inhibition of CD26/Dipeptidyl peptidase IV activity in vivo prolongs cardiac allograft survival in rat recipients. Transplantation *63*, 1495-1500.

[36] Korom, S., De Meester, I., Coito, A.J., Graser, E., Pratschke, J., König, S., Grimm, H., Volk, H.D., Scharpe', S., and Kupiec-Weglinski, J.W. (1999) CD26/DPP IV-mediated modulation of acute rejection. Transplant. Proc. *31*, 873.

[37] Tanaka, S., Murakami, T., Horikawa, H., Sugiura, M., Kawashima, K., and Sugita, T. (1997) Suppression of arthritis by the inhibitors of dipeptidyl peptidase IV. Int. J. Immunopharmacol. *19*, 15-24.

[38] Hafler, D.A., Fox, D.A., Manning, M.E., Schlossman, S.F., Reinherz, E.L., and Weiner, H.L. (1985) In vivo activated T lymphocytes in the peripheral blood and cerebrospinal fluid of patients with multiple sclerosis. N Engl. J. Med. *312*, 1405-1411.

[39] Sellebjerg, F., Madsen, H.O., Jensen, C.V., Jensen, J., and Garred, P. (2000) CCR5 delta32, matrix metalloproteinase-9 and disease activity in multiple sclerosis. J. Neuroimmunol. *102*, 98-106.

[40] Sellebjerg, F., Christiansen, M., Jensen, J., and Frederiksen, J.L. (2000) Immunological effects of oral high-dose methylprednisolone in acute optic neuritis and multiple sclerosis. Eur. J. Neurol. *7*, 281-289.

[41] Khoury, S.J., Guttmann, C.R., Orav, E.J., Kikinis, R., Jolesz, F.A., and Weiner, H.L. (2000) Changes in activated T cells in the blood correlate with disease activity in multiple sclerosis. Arch. Neurol. *57*, 1183 1189.

Frontiers in Neurodegenerative Disorders and Aging: Fundamental Aspects, Clinical Perspectives and New Insights
T. Özben and M. Chevion (Eds.)
IOS Press, 2004

Oxidative Stress in Neurodegenerative Diseases

Mutay Aslan and Tomris Özben
Department of Biochemistry, Akdeniz University Medical School, 07059 Antalya, Turkey.

Abstract: Neurodegenerative disorders, which are chronic and progressive, are characterized by selective and symmetric loss of neurons in motor, sensory, or cognitive systems. The most important risk factors for neurodegenerative diseases are old age and a positive family history. In addition to the possible involvement of aging, oxidative damage may also play an important role in the slowly progressive neuronal death that is characteristic of several neurodegenerative disorders including Alzheimer's disease (AD), Parkinson's disease (PD), amyotrophic lateral sclerosis (ALS) and Huntington's disease. These diseases of the brain are thought to involve oxidative processes either as a primary cause or as a consequence of disease progression. This review discusses the role of reactive oxygen species in the pathogenesis of neurodegenerative diseases and examines the relevance of antioxidant therapy in preventing neurodegeneration.

1. Reactive Oxygen Species

Reactive oxygen and nitrogen species are formed in vivo via oxidation-reduction reactions, they are highly reactive and thus very short lived. Superoxide ($O_2^{\cdot-}$) is the primary free radical formed within the cell by the reduction of molecular oxygen. The spontaneous or enzyme catalyzed dismutation of $O_2^{\cdot-}$ generates hydrogen peroxide (H_2O_2) which can undergo further reactions yielding hydroxyl radical ($OH^{\cdot}$). In an iron catalyzed Haber-Weiss reaction, $O_2^{\cdot-}$, ascorbate, thiols and other reductants can reduce Fe(III) to Fe(II), which in turn reduces H_2O_2 to hydroxyl radical [1].

As confirmed by many recent studies, not only oxygen centered but also nitrogen centered free radicals play an important role in physiological and pathological processes. Nitric oxide ($^{\cdot}NO$), a freely diffusible radical, is produced by a variety of mammalian cells including vascular endothelium, neurons, smooth muscle cells, macrophages, neutrophils, platelets and pulmonary epithelium [2]. $^{\cdot}NO$ is synthesized by a family of three NOS enzymes that have a C-terminal reductase and an N-terminal oxygenase domain [3]. The generation of $^{\cdot}NO$ occurs by the oxidative deamination of L-arginine to L-citrulline in the presence of the cofactors

NADPH, flavin adenine dinucleotide (FAD), flavin mononucleotide (FMN), iron protoporphyrin IX and tetrahydrobiopterin (H_4 biopterin) [3]. Superoxide accelerates the destruction of $^{\cdot}NO$ via the facile radical reaction of these species to form the potent oxidant peroxynitrite ($ONOO^-$) and its conjugate acid peroxynitrous acid (ONOOH, pKa=6.8) [4]. The rate constant for this reaction (2×10^{10} $M^{-1}sec^{-1}$) is faster than the SOD-catalyzed enzymatic dismutation of superoxide [4]. Peroxynitrite is a potent oxidant with a half-life of about 1.6 sec at neutral pH. Peroxynitrous acid reacts by two pathways, with the first pathway yielding nitrate (NO_3^-) without forming strong oxidant intermediates [4]. The second pathway forms hydroxyl radical and nitrogen dioxide ($NO_2^{\cdot}$), a potent oxidant that can initiate fatty acid oxidation and nitration of aromatic amino acids [5]. $ONOO^-$ reactivity is also influenced by CO_2, with the formation of a reactive nitrosoperoxocarbonate ($ONOOCO_2^-$) intermediate. Consequently, CO_2 stimulates both $ONOO^-$ decay and enhances $ONOO^-$-mediated nitration of molecules by nearly 2-fold [6].

2. Defense Mechanisms Against Oxidative Stress

The enzymatic antioxidant system that protects aerobic organisms from free radical damage includes cytoplasmic, mitochondrial and extracellular superoxide dismutases (SODs), glutathione peroxidase (GPx) and catalase. SOD is a metalloprotein that dismutates $O_2^{\cdot -}$ to yield H_2O_2 and oxygen. At pH 7.4, the rate constant for this enzyme-catalyzed reaction is $\sim 2 \times 10^9$ M^{-1} sec^{-1} which is approximately 10^4 times faster than the spontaneous dismutation of $O_2^{\cdot -}$ [7]. The H_2O_2 that is formed from this reaction and following divalent reduction of oxygen is removed by the heme-containing enzyme catalase, by GPx or by thioredoxin-dependent peroxidases [8]. Catalase catalyzes the dismutation of H_2O_2 to water and oxygen or in the presence of alcohols, catalyzes the peroxidatic scavenging of H_2O_2 [8]. GPx catalyzes the reduction of H_2O_2 by reduced glutathione (GSH). The resulting glutathione disulfide is reduced by NADPH derived in large part from the pentose phosphate pathway [8].

There are also a variety of low molecular weight antioxidants that are important in the cellular defenses against oxidative stress. α-Tocopherol and β-carotene (vitamin A) are lipophilic molecules that scavenge free radicals and thus inhibit lipid peroxidation [1]. α-Tocopherol and ascorbate can also serve as reducing agents and, during pathological conditions, induce heme release or reduce metals and act as prooxidants. In such cases, the amount of vitamin E that is present and availability of redox-active metal centers determines its prooxidant or antioxidant effect [9, 10]. The intracellular thiol reductant that directly scavenges reactive species and serves as a GPx cofactor, GSH, contributes to the reduction of H_2O_2, lipid peroxides and other oxidizing species [1].

3. Oxidative Stress in Brain

Isolated mitochondria from the brain and other organs show that 2-5% of the total oxygen consumed in mitochondrial respiration yields reactive oxygen species (ROS) mostly as hydrogen peroxide (H_2O_2) [11, 12]. Since the major portion of total reactive species production during aerobic metabolism comes from byproducts of the electron transport chain, the brain is particularly vulnerable to oxidative damage due to utilizing glucose as an energy source and consuming high levels of oxygen during the metabolic process [13]. Indeed, brain ischemia initiates a complex cascade of metabolic events, several of which involve the generation of nitrogen and oxygen free radicals. These free radicals and related reactive chemical species mediate much of the damage that occurs after transient brain ischemia [14-20]. It has also been shown that enzymatic antioxidants, such as catalase, are found in lower concentrations in the brain as compared to other tissues [11, 21].

Another risk factor for increased oxidative damage in the brain is the high content of easily oxidizable unsaturated fatty acids [22]. The oxidation of unsaturated membrane lipids can result in bilayer fluidity changes, increased ion permeability, covalent crosslinking of protein and lipid membrane constituents, inactivation of membrane enzymes and receptors, polypeptide strand scission, DNA damage and mutagenesis [22]. Malondialdehyde and hydroxynonenal, products of lipid peroxidation, can additionally react with proteins, nucleic acids and lipids to further exert toxic effects [22].

It is important to note that the brain has areas enriched in Fe and ascorbate which can also contribute to increased oxidative damage [11, 23]. As stated previously, Fe(III) can initiate lipid peroxidation reactions when a reducing agent like ascorbate is present. Ascorbate is known to serve as a pro-oxidant during pathological conditions by reducing metal ions [1].

4. Neurodegenerative Diseases and Oxidative Stress

4.1. Alzheimer's Disease

Alzheimer's disease is clinically characterized by loss of memory, reasoning and speech [24]. The most important risk factors for AD are old age and a positive family history [25]. The frequency of the disease reaches to 20-40 % in the population over the age of 85 [26]. Autopsy findings have indicated that the most severe pathology in AD occurs in the hippocampus, temporal cortex and the basal nucleus [27]. There is a reduction in the volume of the hippocampus in patients with AD compared with that of age-matched controls [27]. The most important microscopic findings are senile plaques and neurofibrillary tangels. These two lesions can be seen in small numbers during normal aging of the brain but occur in large amounts during AD [28].

Neurofibrillary tangels (NFTs) associated with AD, can be observed as paired helical filaments in neuronal cytoplasm via silver staining [29]. NFTs represent abnormally phosphorylated tau protein which is associated with microtubules [29]. It is suggested that increased phosphorylation of tau may disturb the function of the protein that may be involved in the assembly and stabilization of microtubules [30]. Several mutations have also been reported in tau that are associated with NFTs and dementia [24].

Senile plaques observed in AD, are composed of a central core consisting of β-amyloid, proteoglycans, Apo E, α_1 antichymotrypsin, presenilin 1 and 2 [24]. Amyloid staining in senile plaques and in small blood vessels of the cerebral cortex provided the basis for cloning the β-amyloid gene. This gene encodes a large protein, amyloid precursor protein (APP), which contains the 40-42 amino acid β-amyloid fragment [25]. APP is a membrane-spanning protein that is processed into smaller units including the β-amyloid protein [24]. Seven different mutations have been found in the gene for the amyloid precursor, all of which increase the production of β-amyloid leading to fibrillar aggregation toxic to neurons [25]. However, it is important to note that these mutations account for less that 1% of all early-onset Alzheimer's disease [24].

Investigation of families with familial AD led to the discovery of two additional genes called the presenilins (PS-I and II) [31]. Mutations in these genes are transmitted in an autosomal fashion and account for early-onset AD [31]. The functions of APP and presenilins are unknown but presenilins may be involved in signal transduction [24].

The Apo E gene that encodes apolipoprotein E has also been implicated in the pathogenesis of AD [32]. No mutations have been reported for Apo E which is involved in cholesterol transport. Among the three genetic variants of Apo E (ϵ2, ϵ3 and ϵ4), ϵ4 shows a strong association with late-onset familial and sporadic forms of AD [32]. However, it is reported that although Apo E4 is an important risk factor for AD, it is neither essential nor specific for the development of the disease [24].

4.1.1. Alzheimer's Disease and Oxidative Stress

The mechanism of β-amyloid-induced neurotoxicity is unknown but several lines of evidence suggest that increased formation of ROS may play an important role. Cell-free incubation of β-amyloid 1–40 peptide generated free radicals in oxygenated buffer systems as observed by EPR spectroscopy [33]. Similarly, it was demonstrated that β-amyloid induces increased intracellular H_2O_2 accumulation in hippocampal neurons which causes lipid peroxidation in cell membranes, probably via hydroxyl radical generation [34]. Peroxidation of polyunsaturated fatty acids results in the formation of multiple aldehydes including 4-HNE, which is capable of inducing apoptosis in neuronal cells [35]. Consistent with these findings, exposure of cultured hippocampal neurons to β-amyloid significantly increased 4-hydroxy-2-*trans*-nonenal (4-HNE) formation suggesting that oxidized lipids may mediate oxidative stress-induced apoptosis observed in AD [36]. Indeed, it was shown that 4-HNE, like β-amyloid was able to inhibit ion motive ATPases and induce neuronal apoptosis [37].

The findings that radical scavengers like vitamin E, the spin-trap compound PBN (α-phenyl-*tert*-butyl nitrone) and lazoroids attenuate β-amyloid aggregation further support the concept of oxidant-induced neurodegeneration in AD [38, 39].

Identification of oxidatively altered proteins in AD is important for understanding the relationship between protein oxidation, protein aggregation and neurodegeneration. Reactive carbonyl groups on proteins can be used as a marker for ROS-mediated protein damage [40]. Carbonyl derivatives, formed following ROS-mediated oxidation of sugar and membrane lipids, are able to form adducts commonly known as CO-proteins (proteins bearing carbonyl groups) with structural proteins, lipoproteins, enzymes and with DNA, causing alterations in their biological activity [41]. Reactive carbonyl groups on proteins can also be formed by direct oxidation of protein side-chains. ROS may oxidize amino acid residue side-chains into ketone or aldehyde derivatives [42]. Histidine, arginine, and lysine are the most susceptible amino acids for the ROS-mediated carbonyl formation [42]. Measurement of carbonyl groups is thought to be a good estimation for the extent of oxidative damage of proteins associated with various conditions of oxidative stress, aging, physiological disorders, and disease [43].

Most methods detecting protein-bound carbonyls are based on the covalent reaction of the carbonylated protein side chain with 2,4-dinitrophenylhydrazine (DNPH) and detection of 2,4-dinitrophenylhydrazone groups with a specific anti-dinitrophenyl (DNP) antibody [41]. A histofluorescence method for protein carbonyl measurement showed that β-amyloid added to cultured hippocampal neuronal or astrocytic cells led to the formation of oxidized proteins [44, 45].

EPR spin labeling technique using the protein specific spin label, 2,2,6,6-tetramethyl-4-maleimido-piperidine-1-oxyl (MAL-6) has also been used to investigate protein oxidation in AD [46]. MAL-6 forms covalent bonds with cysteine SH groups and forms a typical EPR spectrum that can be used to assess structural information [47]. The EPR spectrum reflects at least two sites of MAL-6 binding to membrane proteins, characterized as strongly (S) and weakly (W)-immobilized reaction sites. Conformational alterations in proteins or increased protein-protein interactions lead to decreased W/S ratio [47]. Hydroxyl radical modifications of membrane proteins via fenton reactions also show a decreased W/S ratio of MAL-6 [46], suggesting the presence of motional resistance that may be due to steric hindrance resulting form increased protein-protein interactions. As predicted, β-amyloid also causes a decreased W/S ratio of MAL-6 in cortical synaptosomal membranes [48].

In agreement with data obtained from cell culture studies, markers of oxidative stress were also found to be increased in transgenic mouse models and humans with AD [49-52]. Clinical findings show that oxidative stress occurs in AD as indicated by data showing higher than normal levels of lipid, protein and DNA oxidations [53]. Isolated synaptosomal membranes from hippocampal and inferior parietal regions of AD brain rich in β-amyloid containing senile plaques showed decreased W/S ratio [48] and increased levels of protein carbonyls [44]. Similarly, lipid peroxidation measured as thiobarbituric acid reactive substances were also found to be increased in various brain regions of AD patients [54, 55].

With reference to preclinical and clinical data supporting the presence of oxidative stress in AD, a clinical trial was performed to test the effect of D,L-α-tocopherol in patients with AD. Patients with moderately severe functional impairment showed some beneficial effects with respect to rate of deterioration of cognitive function [56].

4.2. Parkinson's Disease

Parkinson's disease (PD) is a syndrome consisting of rest tremor, rigidity, bradykinesia and a characteristic disturbance of gait and posture [57]. Although the cause of the disease is unknown, symptoms are caused by a loss of dopaminergic neurons from the substantia nigra, globus pallidus and putamen [58]. The disease occurs in all ethnic groups and has an equal sex distribution [59]. It is the second most common neurodegenerative disorder after AD, with a prevalence of 2% among people over the age of 65 [60]. Although idiopathic PD is usually sporadic, approximately 5-10% of PD patients have a familial form of parkinsonism with an autosomal-dominant form of inheritance [60]. Large intracytoplasmic inclusions called Lewy bodies are the pathological hallmark of the disease, occurring mainly in the melanin-containing neurons of the sustantia nigra [61]. Lewy bodies are intraneuronal hyaline inclusions that are immunoreactive with antibodies to α-synuclein [62]. In patients with both inherited and sporadic PD, the Lewy bodies contain α-synuclein and ubiquitin [61, 62]. Mutations in the genes encoding these proteins are thought to lead to protein aggregations as Lewy bodies [63].

4.2.1 Parkinson's Disease and Oxidative Stress

The cause of Parkinson's disease is unknown but accumulating evidence suggests that endogenous dopamine may act as a neurotoxin and thereby participate in the pathophysiology of the disease [64]. Dopamine is inactivated by the enzyme monoamine oxidase (MAO), a reaction that yields significant amounts of hydrogen peroxide [65]. It is hypothesized that increased dopamine turnover in early stages of PD may generate excess hydrogen peroxide and subsequent formation of hydroxyl radical leading to dopaminergic cell death [65]. It is important to note that MAO activity increases with age, thus, exposing cells to oxidative stress-mediated injury [66]. Dopamine also has a potential to decompose by auto-oxidation generating quinones and semiquinones, which themselves are toxic and may lead to the generation of ROS [67]. Indeed, quinone addition to reduced sulfhydryls produces covalently linked protein adducts that can inactivate or alter protein function [68, 69].

The concept that oxidative processes are the link between dopamine toxicity and neuronal degeneration is based on studies showing that oxidants and nitrating agents generated by dopamine promote α-synuclein aggregation [70]. Dopamine adducts with α-synuclein inhibit formation of α-synuclein fibrils by promoting protofibril formation, which have been shown to be toxic [71]. Furthermore, a reduction in dopamine levels have been shown to inhibit α- synuclein induced apoptosis [72].

A potential role of oxidative stress in PD is also supported by the findings of mitochondrial defects in complex I activity of the electron transport chain [73]. The reported alterations in the oxidant status observed in PD is also accompanied by changes in antioxidant defense mechanisms. Increased total iron and decreased GSH levels in the substantia nigra have been reported in post-mortem tissue from individuals with PD [74-76]. Since GSH is involved in the detoxification of H_2O_2, a reduction in GSH levels could result in increased concentrations of H_2O_2, which in the presence of metals could lead to the formation of $^{\cdot}OH$.

In 1987, the DATATOP (Deprenyl and Tocopherol Antioxidant Therapy of Parkinsonism) clinical trial was initiated to examine the benefits of deprenyl (selegiline) and alpha-tocopherol in slowing the progression of PD [77]. Alpha-tocopherol produced no benefits while deprenyl 10 mg/day was found to significantly delay the time until enough disability developed to warrant the initiation of levodopa therapy. However, being a MAO-B inhibitor, this drug has symptomatic effects of its own, which has confounded interpretation of the results [77]. Advances in understanding the pathogenesis of PD hold promise in the coming decade for developing and achieving neuroprotective therapies for PD.

4.3. Amyotrophic Lateral Sclerosis

Amyotrophic lateral sclerosis (ALS) is characterized by a selective and progressive degeneration of the lower motor neurons in the spinal cord and the upper motor neurons in the cerebral cortex [78]. It is the most common motor-neuron disorder which usually begins in the fifth and sixth decades of life [79]. ALS is usually sporadic, but in 1 to 10 percent of patients it is familial, being inherited as an autosomal dominant trait [79]. Lower motor neuron dysfunction and early denervation observed in ALS presents itself with insidiously developing asymmetric weakness, usually evident distally in one of the limbs [78]. Weakness caused by denervation is associated with progressive wasting and atrophy of muscles. If the initial denervation involves bulbar rather than limb muscles, the problem at onset is difficulty with chewing, swallowing and movements of the face and tongues [78]. Early involvement of the muscles of respiration may lead to death before the disease is far advanced elsewhere [79]. Neuropathological studies show that the effected motor neurons undergo shrinkage often with accumulation of the pigmented lipid (Lipofuscin) that normally develops in these cells with advancing age [80]. Observed neuronal cell death is preceded by the formation of webs of ubiquitin-positive threads and axonal swellings that stain for ubiquitin and α-synuclein [81].

4.3.1. Amyotrophic Lateral Sclerosis and Oxidative Stress

The cause of motor-neuron loss in ALS remains unknown, but about 15-20% of patients with familial ALS carry mutations in the gene encoding for the free radical scavenging enzyme SOD-1 [82]. Over 50 different SOD-1 mutations have been documented in familial ALS patients [83]. Transgenic mice have been generated that express mutant forms of SOD-1 found in familial ALS cases, which develop motor neuron disease and death within 4-6 months if the mutant enzyme is expressed at sufficient levels [84]. The observed Cu/Zn-SOD mutations appear to be a cause for oxidative stress in ALS. Indeed, lipid peroxidation and nitrotyrosine can be found in both transgenic mice and human patients [85].

It was reported that the mutant Cu/Zn-SODs that cause the most rapid forms of ALS can form perfectly functional proteins with normal SOD activity [86]. However it was shown that the mutant proteins were less stable and more susceptible to losing their zinc and copper atoms [87]. Because zinc is held less tightly than copper, the mutations favor the accumulation of zinc-deficient SOD [88]. It was shown that zinc-deficient SOD rapidly oxidizes many intracellular oxidants, while the copper transfers these electrons to oxygen producing $O_2^{\cdot-}$ [86]. In the presence of low concentration of $NO^{\cdot}$, zinc-deficient SOD generates $ONOO^-$ and depletes cellular antioxidant defenses [87]. Delivering zinc-deficient SOD to motor neurons was shown to cause motor neuron cell death probably via a peroxynitrite-dependent mechanism [87].

Reducing oxidative stress via various drugs has been used as a potential therapeutic strategy in transgenic mice expressing the mutated human SOD-1 enzyme [89]. Polyamine- or putrescine-modified catalase has been shown to increase the survival of SOD mutant transgenic mice [90]. The copper chelators, Vitamine E and N-acetylcysteine have also been reported to increase the survival time and delay the onset of the disease in this mouse model [90]. However, no beneficial effect of α-tocopherol, selegiline, N-acetylcysteine or an antioxidant cocktail has been obtained in humans [91].

4.4. Huntington's Disease

Huntington's disease (HD) is an autosomal dominant degenerative brain disorder. HD involves the extrapyramidal motor system and is characterized by chorea, a dementia which is progressive, and other psychiatric symptoms [92]. It has a population frequency of about 10/100,000 with an onset usually in the fourth or fifth decade [93]. Neuropathologically, there is a progressive, massive loss of neurons, particularly in the striatum [94]. Microscopically, there are no dramatic changes such as the plaques and tangles seen in AD. However there is gliosis and neuronal loss, especially of medium sized spiny neurons in the caudate and putamen [95]. Neurochemically there is a marked decrease of gamma-aminobutyric acid (GABA) and its synthetic enzyme glutamic acid decarboxylase throughout the basal ganglia [96]. The levels of other neurotransmitters, including substance P and enkephalins, are also reduced [97].

Huntington's disease was initially linked to a gene defect on chromosome 4 [98]. The HD gene was found to contain an unstable CAG repeat region at the 5`-end [99]. Normal subjects have a median of 19 CAG repeats with a range of 11 to 34, whereas nearly all patients with HD have more than 40 [100]. The increased number of CAG repeats in the HD gene are expressed as an elongated huntingtin protein with 40-150 glutamine residues [101]. The function of huntingtin is not known but it is found in many cells in both neural and nonneural tissues [101]. It is reported that the expression of an expanded polyglutamine tract in huntingtin causes protein aggregates in neuronal nuclei and dystrophic neuritis in HD brains [101].

4.4.1. Huntington's Disease and Oxidative Stress

One potential cause of cell death in HD that has received much interest is oxidative stress. However, a detailed investigation of oxidative stress indices in the caudate nucleus, putamen, and frontal cortex of HD brains revealed no alterations in concentrations of thiobarbituric acid–malondialdehyde adducts and lipid peroxides or of oxidative DNA and protein damage [102]. These data strongly suggest that oxidative stress is not a major contributor to neurodegeneration in HD. However, evidence indicates that an alternative marker of oxidation, isoprostane concentration is increased [103]. It was reported that F2-isoprostane concentration was moderately but significantly higher in HD patients than in the control group (35% of increase). However, the overlap of levels between the two groups suggested that the oxidative damage to the brain may not occur uniformly in the early phase of the disease. As in the case of AD, there was no correlation between F2-isoprostanes and age or disease duration, and no difference was observed between men and women.

5. Conclusions

There is sufficient evidence that oxidative and nitrative processes play an important role in the pathogenesis of neuronal loss and neurodegeneration. However, despite all documentation of experimental data there is still limited evidence for a neuroprotective effect of antioxidants in the treatment of neurodegenerative disorders in humans. Probably, an effective mode of protective therapy in neurodegenerative disorders would be to start the therapeutic interventions at an early stage of the disease and target specific sites of reactive species generation. It is desirable that future studies and clinical trails will eventually advance our understanding on neurodegenerative diseases and help in the design of more effective therapies.

References

[1] Freeman BA, Crapo JD. Biology of disease: free radicals and tissue injury. *Lab Invest* 47:412-426, 1982.

[2] Moncada S. Nitric oxide. *J Hypertens Suppl* 12:S35-39, 1994.

[3] Mayer B, Hemmens B. Biosynthesis and action of nitric oxide in mammalian cells. *Trends Biochem Sci* 22:477-481, 1997.

[4] Beckman JS, Beckman TW, Chen J, Marshall PA, Freeman BA. Apparent hydroxyl radical production by peroxynitrite: implications for endothelial injury from nitric oxide and superoxide. *Proc Natl Acad Sci USA* 87:1620-1624, 1990.

[5] Rubbo H, Darley-Usmar V, Freeman BA. Nitric oxide regulation of tissue free radical injury. *Chem Res Toxicol* 9:809-820, 1996.

[6] Radi R, Denicola A, Freeman BA. Peroxynitrite reactions with carbon dioxide-bicarbonate. *Methods Enzymol* 301:353-67, 1999.

[7] Fridovich I. Superoxide dismutases. *Annu Rev Biochem* 44:147-59, 1975.

[8] Mates JM, Sanchez-Jimenez F. Antioxidant enzymes and their implications in pathophysiologic processes. *Front Biosci* 4:D339-45, 1999.

[9] Frei B, England L, Ames BN. Ascorbate is an outstanding antioxidant in human blood plasma. *Proc Natl Acad Sci USA* 86:6377-81, 1989.

[10] Yamamoto K, Niki E. Interaction of alpha-tocopherol with iron: antioxidant and prooxidant effects of alpha-tocopherol in the oxidation of lipids in aqueous dispersions in the presence of iron. *Biochim Biophys Acta* 958:19-23, 1988.

[11] Floyd RA. Antioxidants, oxidative stress, and degenerative neurological disorders. *Proc Soc Exp Biol Med* 222:236-45, 1999.

[12] Papa S, Skulachev VP. Reactive oxygen species, mitochondria, apoptosis and aging. *Mol Cell Biochem* 174:305-19, 1997.

[13] Floyd RA, Hensley K. Oxidative stress in brain aging. Implications for therapeutics of neurodegenerative diseases. *Neurobiol Aging* 23:795-807, 2002.

[14] Serteser M, Ozben T, Gumuslu S, Balkan S, Balkan E. The effects of NMDA receptor antagonist MK-801 on lipid peroxidation during focal cerebral ischemia in rats. *Prog Neuropsychopharmacol Biol Psychiatry* 26:871-7, 2002.

[15] Serteser M, Ozben T, Gumuslu S, Balkan S, Balkan E. Lipid peroxidation in rat brain during focal cerebral ischemia: prevention of malondialdehyde and lipid conjugated diene production by a novel antiepileptic, lamotrigine. *Neurotoxicology* 23:111-9, 2002.

[16] Serteser M, Visvikis S, Ozben T, Herbeth T, Balkan S, Siest G. Lipid profile and apolipoprotein E genotyping in stroke: A case-control study. *Neuroscience-net* 3:10015, 2001.

[17] Serteser M, Ozben T, Gumuslu S, Balkan S, Balkan E. Biochemical evidence of crossed cerebellar diaschisis in terms of nitric oxide indicators and lipid peroxidation products in rats during focal cerebral ischemia. *Acta Neurol Scand* 103:43-8, 2001.

[18] Gumuslu S, Serteser M, Ozben T, Balkan S, Balkan E. Inhibitory role of N omega-nitro-L-arginine methyl ester (L-NAME), a potent nitric oxide synthase inhibitor, on brain malondialdehyde and conjugated diene levels during focal cerebral ischemia in rats. *Clin Chim Acta* 267:213-23, 1997.

[19] Balkan S, Ozben T, Balkan E, Oguz N, Serteser M, Gumuslu S. Effects of Lamotrigine on brain nitrite and cGMP levels during focal cerebral ischemia in rats. Acta Neurol Scand 95:140-6, 1997.

[20] Balkan E, Balkan S, Ozben T, Serteser M, Gumuslu S, Oguz N. The effects of nitric oxide synthase inhibitor, L-NAME on NO production during focal cerebral ischemia in rats: could L-NAME be the future treatment of sudden deafness? *Int J Neurosci* 89:61-77, 1997.

[21] Marklund SL, Westman NG, Lundgren E, Roos G. Copper- and zinc-containing superoxide dismutase, manganese-containing superoxide dismutase, catalase, and glutathione peroxidase in normal and neoplastic human cell lines and normal human tissues. *Cancer Res* 42:1955-61, 1982.

[22] Floyd RA, Carney JM. Free radical damage to protein and DNA: mechanisms involved and relevant observations on brain undergoing oxidative stress. *Ann Neurol* 32 Suppl:S22-7, 1992.

[23] Zaleska MM, Nagy K, Floyd RA. Iron-induced lipid peroxidation and inhibition of dopamine synthesis in striatum synaptosomes. *Neurochem Res* 14:597-605, 1989.

[24] Martin JB. Molecular basis of the neurodegenerative disorders. *N Engl J Med* 340:1970-80, 1999.

[25] Price DL, Tanzi RE, Borchelt DR, Sisodia SS. Alzheimer's disease: genetic studies and transgenic models. *Annu Rev Genet* 32:461-93, 1998.

[26] Farlow MR. Etiology and pathogenesis of Alzheimer's disease. *Am J Health Syst Pharm* 55 Suppl 2:S5-10, 1998.

[27] Cummings JL, Vinters HV, Cole GM, Khachaturian ZS. Alzheimer's disease: etiologies, pathophysiology, cognitive reserve, and treatment opportunities. *Neurology* 51:Suppl 1:S2-17, 1998.

[28] Carter J, Lippa CF. Beta-amyloid, neuronal death and Alzheimer's disease. *Curr Mol Med* 1:733-7, 2001.

[29] Hardy J, Gwinn-Hardy K. Genetic classification of primary neurodegenerative disease. *Science* 282:1075-9, 1998.

[30] Goedert M. Neurofibrillary pathology of Alzheimer's disease and other tauopathies. *Prog Brain Res* 117:287-306, 1998.

[31] Selkoe DJ. The genetics and molecular pathology of Alzheimer's disease: roles of amyloid and the presenilins. *Neurol Clin* 18:903-22, 2000.

[32] Farrer LA, Cupples LA, Haines JL, Hyman B, Kukull WA, Mayeux R, Myers RH, Pericak-Vance MA, Risch N, van Duijn CM. Effects of age, sex, and ethnicity on the association between apolipoprotein E genotype and Alzheimer disease. A meta-analysis. APOE and Alzheimer Disease Meta Analysis Consortium. *JAMA* 278:1349-56, 1997.

[33] Hensley K, Carney JM, Mattson MP, Aksenova M, Harris M, Wu JF, Floyd RA, Butterfield DA. A model for beta-amyloid aggregation and neurotoxicity based on free radical generation by the peptide: relevance to Alzheimer disease. *Proc Natl Acad Sci USA* 91:3270-4, 1994.

[34] Behl C, Davis JB, Lesley R, Schubert D. Hydrogen peroxide mediates amyloid beta protein toxicity. Cell 77:817-27, 1994.

[35] Kruman I, Bruce-Keller AJ, Bredesen D, Waeg G, Mattson MP. Evidence that 4-hydroxynonenal mediates oxidative stress-induced neuronal apoptosis. *J Neurosci* 17:5089-100, 1997.

[36] Mark RJ, Lovell MA, Markesbery WR, Uchida K, Mattson MP. A role for 4-hydroxynonenal, an aldehydic product of lipid peroxidation, in disruption of ion homeostasis and neuronal death induced by amyloid beta-peptide. *J Neurochem* 68:255-64, 1997.

[37] Springer JE, Azbill RD, Mark RJ, Begley JG, Waeg G, Mattson MP. 4-hydroxynonenal, a lipid peroxidation product, rapidly accumulates following traumatic spinal cord injury and inhibits glutamate uptake. *J Neurochem* 68:2469-76, 1997.

[38] Behl C, Davis J, Cole GM, Schubert D. Vitamin E protects nerve cells from amyloid beta protein toxicity. *Biochem Biophys Res Commun* 186:944-50, 1992.

[39] Lucca E, Angeretti N, Forloni G. Influence of cell culture conditions on the protective effect of antioxidants against beta-amyloid toxicity: studies with lazaroids. *Brain Res* 764:293-8, 1997.

[40] Shacter E. Protein oxidative damage. *Methods Enzymol* 319:428-36, 2000.

[41] Shacter E. Quantification and significance of protein oxidation in biological samples. *Drug Metab Rev* 32:307-26, 2000.

[42] Reznick AZ, Packer L. Oxidative damage to proteins: spectrophotometric method for carbonyl assay. *Methods Enzymol* 233:357-63, 1994.

[43] Stadtman ER, Berlett BS. Reactive oxygen-mediated protein oxidation in aging and disease. *Chem Res Toxicol* 10:485-94, 1997.

[44] Harris ME, Hensley K, Butterfield DA, Leedle RA, Carney JM. Direct evidence of oxidative injury produced by the Alzheimer's beta-amyloid peptide (1-40) in cultured hippocampal neurons. *Exp Neurol* 131:193-202, 1995.

[45] Harris ME, Wang Y, Pedigo NW Jr, Hensley K, Butterfield DA, Carney JM. Amyloid beta peptide (25-35) inhibits Na+-dependent glutamate uptake in rat hippocampal astrocyte cultures. *J Neurochem* 67:277-86, 1996.

[46] Hensley K, Carney J, Hall N, Shaw W, Butterfield DA. Electron paramagnetic resonance investigations of free radical-induced alterations in neocortical synaptosomal membrane protein infrastructure. *Free Radic Biol Med* 17:321-31, 1994.

[47] Butterfield DA, Howard B, Yatin S, Koppal T, Drake J, Hensley K, Aksenov M, Aksenova M, Subramaniam R, Varadarajan S, Harris-White ME, Pedigo NW Jr, Carney JM. Elevated oxidative stress in models of normal brain aging and Alzheimer's disease. *Life Sci* 65:1883-92, 1999.

[48] Hensley K, Hall N, Subramaniam R, Cole P, Harris M, Aksenov M, Aksenova M, Gabbita SP, Wu JF, Carney JM, Lovell M, Markesbery WR, Butterfield DA. Brain regional correspondence between Alzheimer's disease histopathology and biomarkers of protein oxidation. J Neurochem 65:2146-56, 1995.

[49] Pappolla MA, Chyan YJ, Omar RA, Hsiao K, Perry G, Smith MA, Bozner P. Evidence of oxidative stress and in vivo neurotoxicity of beta-amyloid in a transgenic mouse model of Alzheimer's disease: a chronic oxidative paradigm for testing antioxidant therapies in vivo. *Am J Pathol* 152:871-7, 1998.

[50] Smith MA, Hirai K, Hsiao K, Pappolla MA, Harris PL, Siedlak SL, Tabaton M, Perry G. Amyloid-beta deposition in Alzheimer transgenic mice is associated with oxidative stress. *J Neurochem* 70:2212-5, 1998.
[51] Good PF, Werner P, Hsu A, Olanow CW, Perl DP. Evidence of neuronal oxidative damage in Alzheimer's disease. *Am J Pathol* 149:21-8, 1996.
[52] Pappolla MA, Omar RA, Kim KS, Robakis NK. Immunohistochemical evidence of oxidative stress in Alzheimer's disease. *Am J Pathol* 140:621-8, 1992.
[53] Mecocci P, MacGarvey U, Beal MF. Oxidative damage to mitochondrial DNA is increased in Alzheimer's disease. *Ann Neurol* 36:747-51, 1994.
[54] Lovell MA, Ehmann WD, Butler SM, Markesbery WR. Elevated thiobarbituric acid-reactive substances and antioxidant enzyme activity in the brain in Alzheimer's disease. Neurology 45:1594-601, 1995.
[55] Subbarao KV, Richardson JS, Ang LC. Autopsy samples of Alzheimer's cortex show increased peroxidation in vitro. *J Neurochem* 55:342-5, 1990.
[56] Esposito E, Rotilio D, Di Matteo V, Di Giulio C, Cacchio M, Algeri S. A review of specific dietary antioxidants and the effects on biochemical mechanisms related to neurodegenerative processes. *Neurobiol Aging* 23:719-35, 2002.
[57] Rao G, Fisch L, Srinivasan S, D'Amico F, Okada T, Eaton C, Robbins C. Does this patient have Parkinson disease? *JAMA* 289:347-53, 2003.
[58] Lotharius J, Brundin P. Pathogenesis of Parkinson's disease: dopamine, vesicles and alpha-synuclein. *Nat Rev Neurosci* 3:932-42, 2002.
[59] Tanner CM. Is the cause of Parkinson's disease environmental or hereditary? Evidence from twin studies. *Adv Neurol* 91:133-42, 2003.
[60] Steece-Collier K, Maries E, Kordower JH. Etiology of Parkinson's disease: Genetics and environment revisited. *Proc Natl Acad Sci USA* 99:13972-4, 2002.
[61] Uversky VN, Fink AL. Amino acid determinants of alpha-synuclein aggregation: putting together pieces of the puzzle. *FEBS Lett* 522:9-13, 2002.
[62] Cole NB, Murphy DD. The cell biology of alpha-synuclein: a sticky problem? Neuromolecular Med 1:95-109, 2002.
[63] Chung KK, Dawson VL, Dawson TM. The role of the ubiquitin-proteasomal pathway in Parkinson's disease and other neurodegenerative disorders. *Trends Neurosci* 24(11 Suppl):S7-14, 2001.
[64] Koutsilieri E, Scheller C, Grunblatt E, Nara K, Li J, Riederer P. Free radicals in Parkinson's disease. *J Neurol* 249 Suppl 2:II1-5, 2002.
[65] Spina MB, Cohen G. Dopamine turnover and glutathione oxidation: implications for Parkinson disease. *Proc Natl Acad Sci USA* 86:1398-400, 1989.
[66] Oreland L, Gottfries CG. Brain and brain monoamine oxidase in aging and in dementia of Alzheimer's type. Prog Neuropsychopharmacol Biol Psychiatry 10:533-40, 1986.
[67] Olanow CW. Oxidation reactions in Parkinson's disease. *Neurology* 40(10 Suppl 3):suppl 32-7, 1990.
[68] Ito S, Fujita K. Conjugation of dopa and 5-S-cysteinyldopa with cysteine mediated by superoxide radical. Biochem. *Pharmacol* 31:2887–2889, 1982.
[69] LaVoie MJ, Hastings TG. Dopamine quinone formation and protein modification associated with the striatal neurotoxicity of methamphetamine: evidence against a role for extracellular dopamine. *J. Neurosci* 19:1484–1491, 1999.
[70] Xu J, Kao SY, Lee FJ, Song W, Jin LW, Yankner BA. Dopamine-dependent neurotoxicity of alpha-synuclein: a mechanism for selective neurodegeneration in Parkinson disease. *Nat Med* 8:600-6, 2002.
[71] Conway KA, Rochet JC, Bieganski RM, Lansbury PT Jr. Kinetic stabilization of the alpha-synuclein protofibril by a dopamine-alpha-synuclein adduct. *Science* 294:1346-9, 2001.
[72] Tabrizi SJ, Orth M, Wilkinson JM, Taanman JW, Warner TT, Cooper JM, Schapira AH. Expression of mutant alpha-synuclein causes increased susceptibility to dopamine toxicity. *Hum Mol Genet* 9:2683-9, 2000.
[73] Schapira AH, Cooper JM, Dexter D, Clark JB, Jenner P, Marsden CD. Mitochondrial complex I deficiency in Parkinson's disease. *J Neurochem* 54:823-7, 1990.
[74] Dexter DT, Carayon A, Javoy-Agid F, Agid Y, Wells FR, Daniel SE, Lees AJ, Jenner P, Marsden CD. Alterations in the levels of iron, ferritin and other trace metals in Parkinson's disease and other neurodegenerative diseases affecting the basal ganglia. *Brain* 114:1953-75, 1991.
[75] Dexter DT, Carter CJ, Wells FR, Javoy-Agid F, Agid Y, Lees A, Jenner P, Marsden CD. Basal lipid peroxidation in substantia nigra is increased in Parkinson's disease. *J Neurochem* 52:381-9, 1989.
[76] Ebadi M, Srinivasan SK, Baxi MD. Oxidative stress and antioxidant therapy in Parkinson's disease. *Prog Neurobiol* 48:1-19, 1996.

[77] Shoulson I. DATATOP: a decade of neuroprotective inquiry. Parkinson Study Group. Deprenyl And Tocopherol Antioxidative Therapy Of Parkinsonism. Ann Neurol 44:S160-6, 1998.
[78] Rowland LP. Amyotrophic lateral sclerosis. *Curr Opin Neurol* 7:310-5, 1994.
[79] Tandan R, Bradley WG. Amyotrophic lateral sclerosis: Part 1. Clinical features, pathology, and ethical issues in management. *Ann Neurol* 18:271-80, 1985.
[80] Leigh PN, Anderton BH, Dodson A, Gallo JM, Swash M, Power DM. Ubiquitin deposits in anterior horn cells in motor neurone disease. *Neurosci Lett* 93:197-203, 1988.
[81] Mezey E, Dehejia A, Harta G, Papp MI, Polymeropoulos MH, Brownstein MJ. Alpha synuclein in neurodegenerative disorders: murderer or accomplice? *Nat Med* 4:755-7, 1998.
[82] Cudkowicz ME, McKenna-Yasek D, Sapp PE, Chin W, Geller B, Hayden DL, Schoenfeld DA, Hosler BA, Horvitz HR, Brown RH. Epidemiology of mutations in superoxide dismutase in amyotrophic lateral sclerosis. *Ann Neurol* 41:210-21, 1997.
[83] Siddique T, Nijhawan D, Hentati A. Molecular genetic basis of familial ALS. Neurology 47(4 Suppl 2):S27-34, 1996.
[84] Gurney ME, Pu H, Chiu AY, Dal Canto MC, Polchow CY, Alexander DD, Caliendo J, Hentati A, Kwon YW, Deng HX. Motor neuron degeneration in mice that express a human Cu,Zn superoxide dismutase mutation. Science 264:1772-5, 1994.
[85] Beal MF, Ferrante RJ, Browne SE, Matthews RT, Kowall NW, Brown RH Jr. Increased 3-nitrotyrosine in both sporadic and familial amyotrophic lateral sclerosis. *Ann Neurol* 42:644-54, 1997.
[86] Crow JP, Sampson JB, Zhuang Y, Thompson JA, Beckman JS. Decreased zinc affinity of amyotrophic lateral sclerosis-associated superoxide dismutase mutants leads to enhanced catalysis of tyrosine nitration by peroxynitrite. *J Neurochem* 69:1936-44, 1997.
[87] Estevez AG, Crow JP, Sampson JB, Reiter C, Zhuang Y, Richardson GJ, Tarpey MM, Barbeito L, Beckman JS. Induction of nitric oxide-dependent apoptosis in motor neurons by zinc-deficient superoxide dismutase. *Science* 286:2498-500, 1999.
[88] Ischiropoulos H, Beckman JS. Oxidative stress and nitration in neurodegeneration: cause, effect, or association? *J Clin Invest* 111:163-9, 2003.
[89] Poduslo JF, Whelan SL, Curran GL, Wengenack TM. Therapeutic benefit of polyamine-modified catalase as a scavenger of hydrogen peroxide and nitric oxide in familial amyotrophic lateral sclerosis transgenics. *Ann Neurol* 48:943-7, 2000.
[90] Reinholz MM, Merkle CM, Poduslo JF. Therapeutic benefits of putrescine-modified catalase in a transgenic mouse model of familial amyotrophic lateral sclerosis. *Exp Neurol* 159:204-16, 1999.
[91] Vyth A, Timmer JG, Bossuyt PM, Louwerse ES, de Jong JM. Survival in patients with amyotrophic lateral sclerosis, treated with an array of antioxidants. *Neurol Sci* 139 Suppl:99-103, 1996.
[92] Davies S, Ramsden DB. Huntington's disease. *Mol Pathol* 54:409-13, 2001.
[93] Martin JB, Gusella JF. Huntington's disease. Pathogenesis and management. *N Engl J Med* 315:1267-76, 1986.
[94] Sharp AH, Ross CA. Neurobiology of Huntington's disease. Neurobiol Dis 3:3-15, 1996.
[95] Forno LS. Neuropathologic features of Parkinson's, Huntington's, and Alzheimer's diseases. *Ann N Y Acad Sci* 648:6-16, 1992.
[96] Bird ED. Chemical pathology of Huntington's disease. *Annu Rev Pharmacol Toxicol* 20:533-51, 1980.
[97] Martin JB, Beal MF. Huntington's disease and neurotoxins. *Ann N Y Acad Sci* 648:169-75, 1992.
[98] Gusella JF, Persichetti F, MacDonald ME. The genetic defect causing Huntington's disease: repeated in other contexts? *Mol Med* 3:238-46, 1997.
[99] Rosenblatt A, Margolis RL, Becher MW, Aylward E, Franz ML, Sherr M, Abbott MH, Lian KY, Ross CA. Does CAG repeat number predict the rate of pathological changes in Huntington's disease? *Ann Neurol* 44:708-9, 1998.
[100] Hackam AS, Singaraja R, Wellington CL, Metzler M, McCutcheon K, Zhang T, Kalchman M, Hayden MR. The influence of huntingtin protein size on nuclear localization and cellular toxicity. *J Cell Biol* 141:1097-105, 1998.
[101] Saudou F, Finkbeiner S, Devys D, Greenberg ME. Huntingtin acts in the nucleus to induce apoptosis but death does not correlate with the formation of intranuclear inclusions. *Cell* 95:55-66, 1998.
[102] Alam ZI, Halliwell B, Jenner P. No evidence for increased oxidative damage to lipids, proteins, or DNA in Huntington's disease. *J Neurochem* 75:840–6, 2000.
[103] Greco A, Minghetti L, Levi G. Isoprostanes, novel markers of oxidative injury, help understanding the pathogenesis of neurodegenerative diseases. *Neurochem Res* 25:1357–64, 2000.

Frontiers in Neurodegenerative Disorders and Aging: Fundamental Aspects, Clinical Perspectives and New Insights
T. Özben and M. Chevion (Eds.)
IOS Press, 2004

Fruit Polyphenolics and Signaling in the Aged Brain: Altering Motor and Cognitive Deficits

James A. Joseph, and Barbara Shukitt-Hale
USDA-HNRCA at Tufts University, 711 Washington Street, Boston, MA 02111 USA

Abstract: Although research involving the molecular biology of and the determination of the genetic mechanisms of aging involves elegant science associated with state-of-the-art techniques, it is evident that techniques useful in altering, reversing, or forestalling the deleterious effects of aging may be years away. Health care costs dictate that alternate approaches must be utilized to alter declines in aging, especially those involving neuronal function and behavior. Mechanistically, it appears that many of the changes with aging are the result of increased vulnerability to oxidative stress and inflammation, especially in the CNS. Research from our laboratory and others suggests that reducing this vulnerability may translate into improvements in cognitive and motor function, as well as in neuronal signaling. Numerous epidemiological studies have indicated that individuals who consume a diet containing high amounts of fruits and vegetables may prevent age-related disease such as Alzheimer Disease, and that this prevention may result from the potent antioxidant and anti-inflammatory properties of these fruits and vegetables. Research from our laboratory has suggested that dietary supplementation with fruit or vegetable extracts high in antioxidants (e.g., blueberry, spinach) can decrease the enhanced vulnerability to oxidative stress that occurs in aging and that these reductions are expressed as improvements in behavior. However, additional research has suggested multiple mechanisms in addition to those involving the antioxidant or anti-inflammatory properties of the polyphenolic compounds in these fruits and vegetables, the most important of which may be their ability to increase cellular signaling and neuronal communication. The present review discusses the beneficial properties of fruits such as berries with a view toward suggesting their useful application in reducing the deleterious effects of aging.

1. Introduction

There are very few of us who, as we were growing up, didn't hear Mom's familiar statement, "Eat your fruits and vegetables. They're good for you!" At the time we didn't realize how much Mom knew about what we should eat to stay healthy. Now it seems as though Mom's prophetic statement might not only be important for us, but may actually be important in reducing the tremendous health costs of aging populations, which are on the rise in many countries throughout the world, along with increases in all of the age-associated diseases (e.g., cancer, cardiovascular disease). Some of the most devastating of these diseases include those that involve the nervous system [e.g., Alzheimer's (AD) and Parkinson's (PD) diseases]. In the US, for example, by the year 2050, 30% of the total population will be over 65 years of age, and, given present trends, a large portion of this population will be exhibiting the common correlative motor and cognitive behavioral deficits that occur in aging. These deficits may occur even in the absence of specific age-related neurodegenerative diseases, but could act to exacerbate the symptoms. Thus, the aged brain may provide a sensitive environment for the development of neurodegenerative diseases such as AD and certain forms of PD. As an example, the interaction between the genetic changes in AD and this sensitive environment in aging may be perceived as a "soup," where the production of amyloid beta in association with apolipoprotein E gene polymorphisms 4/4 or 3/4 and mutations in presenilin-1 act upon an aging environment that shows increased vulnerability to oxidative stress and inflammation. While researchers throughout the world continue to explore methods to utilize genetic or molecular biological applications to alter the soup and prevent or reverse the changes in aging, it appears that any fruitful approaches are still years away. The question arises, then, as to whether nutritional methods might be employed today to accomplish this task and stem this inevitable decline into a health care nightmare.

In this brief review we will describe this aging "soup" by discussing motor, cognitive, and neuronal (e.g., signaling) deficits that occur in aging, showing how these deficits are related to increased vulnerability to oxidative stress (OS) and inflammation (INF) of the aged brain and determining the possible role of nutritional supplementation with fruits containing high amounts of polyphenols, such as anthocyanins, in reversing or forestalling these deficits.

2. Preparing the Soup: Vulnerability Increases to Oxidative Stress and Inflammation

It has been shown that not only is the CNS particularly vulnerable to OS, but this vulnerability increases during aging (see [1-2] for review). Cantuti-Castelvetri and colleagues [3] have shown that senescent rats exhibited significantly greater motor behavioral deficits and reduced tyrosine hydroxylase immunoreactivity (in pars compacta) than young rats following intra-nigral applications of dopamine (DA). Factors such as: increases in the ratio of oxidized to total glutathione [4], significant lipofuscin accumulation [5] with bcl-2 increases [6], increases in membrane lipid peroxidation [7], reduced glutamine synthetase [8], and reductions in redox active iron [5, 9] contribute to this vulnerability. Research has also shown that besides the factors discussed above, OS vulnerability in aging may be the result of three additional factors: a) alterations in the membrane microenvironment, b) differential vulnerability of neurotransmitter receptors, and c) alterations in calcium buffering ability. In the case of membranes and aging, indications are that age-related changes in the neuronal plasma membrane molecular structure and physical properties (e.g., increased rigidity) may increase vulnerability to oxidative stress and inflammation [1, 10]. Research also suggests that alterations in membrane lipids [11] and differential OS sensitivity among neurotransmitter receptor subtypes may increase vulnerability to OS and inflammation. Thus, modifications of membrane lipid composition with cholesterol (CHL) and sphingomyelin (SPH) to levels similar to those seen in neuronal membranes in aging dramatically increased the vulnerability of the cells to OS, as assessed by alterations in viability and impairments in calcium buffering [12].

It also appears that particular receptor subtypes may impart increases in vulnerability to oxidative stress and inflammation. We have found, for example, that muscarinic receptor subtypes (M1-M5), when transfected into COS-7 cells, determine the degree of sensitivity (decreases in calcium buffering or viability) of these cells to OS agents such as dopamine or amyloid beta [13-14]. Calcium buffering has been shown to be significantly reduced in senescence [15-17]. The consequences of such long-lasting increases in cytosolic calcium may involve cell death induced by several mechanisms (e.g., xanthine oxidase activation [18]) with subsequent pro-oxidant generation and loss of the functional capacity of the cell.

2.1 Inflammation

Recent evidence also suggests that, as we have discussed above with respect to OS, inflammatory events in the central nervous system play an important role in aging and AD [19-20]. For example, by middle age there is an increased glial fibrillary acid protein expression [21] that later, in the elderly, even occurs in the absence of an inflammatory stimulus [22]. It has also been reported that TNF-alpha (tumor necrosis factor) is produced in higher amounts during cytotoxic reactions in the elderly [23] and that neuronal inhibition of glial activities may be lost during aging [24]. Other studies have reported increases in TNF-alpha and IL-6 in the sera of aged mice and humans [25-26]. In fact, it has been suggested that the up-regulation of C-reactive protein may represent one factor in biologic aging [27].

2.2 Behavior

The alterations in memory deficits in aging are seen on cognitive tasks that require the use of spatial learning and memory [28], while alterations in motor function may include decreases in coordination, muscle strength and balance [29]. Indeed, these changes have been shown in many studies and appear to be expressed in both animals [28] and humans [30]. Alterations in memory appear to occur primarily in secondary memory systems and are reflected in the storage of newly acquired information [31]. Deficits in motor performance are thought to be the result of alterations in the striatal dopamine (DA) system. For example, the striatum shows marked neurodegenerative changes with age [31], and the cerebellum also shows age-related alterations [32]. Interestingly, there are changes in behavior with increases in oxidative stress and inflammation that parallel those seen in aging [33-34]. In this respect, we have shown that exposing young rats to particles of high energy and charge (HZE particles) disrupts the functioning of the dopaminergic system and dopamine-mediated behaviors, similar to the adverse behavioral and neuronal effects seen in aged animals [35-36]. In one set of these experiments, we have shown that whole-body exposure of rats to HZE particles, primarily 600 MeV or 1 GeV ^{56}Fe, impairs motor behavior [37], spatial learning and memory behavior [38], and amphetamine-induced conditioned taste aversion [39]. Associated with these findings were deficits in oxotremorine-enhancement of K^+-evoked DA release and carbachol stimulated GTPase activity that paralleled those seen in aging [36]. Therefore, the deficits induced by radiation are similar to those that occur during aging, are associated with free-radical damage, and support the hypothesis that these changes may share a common chemical/biological mechanism [37]. Another model used to produce oxidative stress involves exposing young rats to a normobaric hyperoxia environment of 100% oxygen (O_2) at 760 mm Hg (sea level pressure). We have shown that motor function, as measured by accelerating rotarod, wire suspension, small rod walk, and large rod walk, is impaired following 48 hours of 100% O_2 [33], as is cerebellar ß-adrenergic and striatal muscarinic receptor functioning [40]. Thus, it appears that insults such as OS may act to accelerate behavioral deficits similar to those seen in aging, and these findings, in conjunction with those discussed above, suggest that increased OS and possibly inflammatory sensitivity are ultimately expressed as behavioral decrements.

3. Stirring the Soup: Neuronal Signaling and Behavioral Deficits in Aging

In addition to the changes in calcium buffering discussed above, there are also changes in the sensitivity of several receptor systems, most notably: a) dopaminergic [41-42]; b) muscarinic [43-44]; c) opioid [45]; and d) adrenergic [46]. Additional research indicates that there are age-related alterations in calcium-sensitive signaling molecules associated with memory, especially the conversion of short- to long-term memory. These include:

a. Calcium-dependent PKCs (protein kinase C) PKAs, and Protein Tyrosine Kinases (PTKs) – There are several functions of calcium-dependent PKCs including the modulation of ion channels and receptor sensitivity and presynaptic neurotransmitter release [47]. However, two of the most important may be regulation of signaling and modulation of short- to long-term memory. Studies have shown that PKC activity is important in memory formation, particularly spatial memory [48-50], and that treatment with PKC inhibitors impairs memory formation [51]. It appears that training induces the calcium-induced translocation [52] of PKC from the soluble to the particulate subcellular fraction [53]. However, in aging, there appear to be alterations in this translocation [54], which are correlated with decrements in spatial memory [55]. Colombo and coauthors [52] showed that young rats with the best spatial memory performance also had the highest PKC in the particulate (i.e., membrane) fraction of the hippocampus and PKC-gamma in the soluble (i.e., cytosolic) fraction.

PKC may also: a) interact with several signaling molecules that are described below; b) alter the affinity of neuronal proteins [e.g., calmodulin (CaM)]; and c) be important for the subsequent stimulation of CaM-dependent enzymes, including CaM-dependent protein kinases (e.g., CaM II and IV) and CaM-dependent phosphatases (e.g., calcineurin). Thus, PKC does not operate in a vacuum and there is a great amount of cross-talk with other signaling molecules such as PKA and PTK in the initiation of memory formation and the conversion of short- to long-term memory. Evidence indicates that both PKA [56-58] and PTK (for review see [49]) may also be involved in this conversion. In the case of PTK this may be done through direct modulation of brain-derived nerve growth factor (BDNF) [59], where in aging, studies indicate that BDNF expression was reduced in several brain areas [59]. PKA appears to mediate long-term memory formation by participating in cAMP response element binding (CREB) activation through initiation of the mitogen activated protein kinase (MAPK) cascade. In addition, it also appears that cross-talk among these kinases may be important in modulating or regulating different signaling pathways at various stages of the network (for review see [49])

b. MAPK – A great deal of work has shown the importance of the MAPK cascade in proliferation and differentiation [60]. However, evidence is increasing that MAPK is critical in long-term memory formation through the activation of CREB. More specifically there is a great amount of data indicating that MAPKs are involved not only in hippocampal memory formation but also in memory modulation in other brain structures [61]. Moreover studies have indicated that the activation of these molecules is OS sensitive [62] and that they may serve as biochemical signal integrators and/or molecular coincidence detectors for modulating coordinated responses to extracellular signals in neurons [63]. Particularly important in this regard are the extracellular signal regulated kinases (ERK) 1/2, and the Jun kinases (JNKs). Studies have demonstrated the role of ERK signaling cascades in diverse types of learning and memory such as conditioned taste aversion [64], novel taste learning [65], spatial learning [66], and inhibitory avoidance [67]. Moreover, data also show that carbachol stimulation of M1-M4 MAChR-transfected COS-7 cells can activate ERK 1/2 using a signal transduction pathway similar to that operating in neurons, and that ERK-mediated responses can serve as a convergence site for MAChR activation and other neurotransmitter receptors [68].

In the case of aging, findings indicate that ERK activities were reduced in cortical brain slices of senescent rats (24 mo) without declines in the corresponding proteins [69]. In the hippocampus, a 20% decline in mRNA levels of ERK was observed in the CA3 region in the 12-month-old group as compared to the 3-month-old group [70]. An additional study showed that exposure of hippocampal slices from senescent mice expressing amyloid beta 1-42 produced a down-regulation of hippocampal ERK activity. Finally, preliminary findings from our laboratory indicate that these decrements in ERK activity in response to oxidative stress are area- and age-specific (see below).

c. CREB –There is a great deal of evidence to suggest that CREB is involved in the formation of memory and regulates the transcription of immediate early genes that, in turn, activate late response genes which ultimately subserve long-term memory (see [71-72] for reviews). Bourtchuladze and coauthors [73] have shown that CREB knockout mice were impaired in Morris water maze performance. CREB activity also has been shown to decline with age [74-75]. Conversely, Josselyn and coauthors [76] have shown that overexpression of CREB enhances the formation of long-term memory after massed training. Thus, it appears that losses in CREB activity may contribute to the declines in cognitive function that have been previously reported (see above).

4. Quenching the "Fire"

The findings discussed above suggest that increased vulnerability to OS and INF in the aged brain leads to reductions in neuronal signaling and behavior. Given these considerations it might be suggested that aging provides the fire for the "soup", and with the addition of genetic changes, such as those seen in AD, provides the fire that leads to toxicity and neuronal loss. If this is the case, then one approach to improving neuronal functioning might be to alter the neuronal environment and reduce the impact of the oxidative and inflammatory stressors. In recent years it is becoming increasingly apparent that one way to accomplish this is through diet. Numerous studies have suggested that diets in which there are high amounts of saturated fat and low quantities of fruits and vegetables may enhance the development of a host of what have become known as "life style" diseases (e.g., diabetes) that involve oxidative stress and inflammation (e.g., see [77] for review).

Therefore, in order to offset the deleterious effects of these insults, many people take antioxidant supplements that include Vitamins E and C, Ginkgo Biloba, and a host of others. However, recent work discussed below suggests that the combinations of antioxidants/anti-inflammatories found in fruits and vegetables may be very effective in quenching the fire of aging. Plants, including food plants (fruits and vegetables), synthesize a vast array of chemical compounds that are not involved in their primary metabolism. These 'secondary compounds' instead serve a variety of ecological functions directed, ultimately, toward enhancing the plant's survivability [78]. Interestingly, these compounds may be responsible for the multitude of beneficial effects that fruits and vegetables have on an array of health-related bioactivities, two of the most important of which may be their antioxidant and anti-inflammatory properties. Moreover, recent work discussed below also suggests that the polyphenolic compounds found in fruits and vegetables may actually directly influence neuronal communication. As pointed out above, this may be a critical factor in the positive benefits observed with respect to cognitive and motor behaviors. However, an important question becomes determining the choice of the fruit or vegetable to test in an aging model, since there are over 4000 polyphenolic compounds that are widespread in fruits, vegetables, nuts, seeds, and grains. To make these determinations we utilized fruits and vegetables identified as being high in antioxidant activity via the Oxygen Radical Absorbance Capacity Assay (ORAC) [79-81] and showed that long-term feeding (from 6 to 15 months of age; F344 rats) with a supplemented AIN-93 diet [strawberry extract or spinach extract (1-2% of the diet) or vitamin E (500 IU)] retarded age-related decrements in cognitive or neuronal function [82]. Results indicated that the supplemented diets could prevent the onset of age-related deficits in several indices (e.g., cognitive behavior, Morris water maze performance) [82].

In a subsequent experiment [15], we found that dietary supplementation (for 8 weeks, supplemented at 2% of the diet) with spinach, strawberry or blueberry (BB) extracts in an AIN-93 defined diet was effective in reversing age-related deficits in neuronal and behavioral (cognitive) function in aged (19 mo) F344 rats. However, only the BB-supplemented group exhibited improved performance on tests of motor function. Specifically, the BB-supplemented group displayed improved performance in rod walking and accelerating rotarod tasks, while none of the other supplemented groups differed from control on these tasks. Several other experiments conducted since then (in preparation) have indicated that primarily only the animals supplemented with blueberries, cranberries or purple grape juice (10-50% as a liquid) have consistently shown improvements in motor behavior.

Rodents in all diet groups, but not the control group in this study [15], showed improved working memory (short-term memory) performance in the Morris water maze, demonstrated as one-trial learning following a 10 min retention interval. We also observed significant increases in several indices of neuronal signaling (e.g., muscarinic receptor sensitivity), and found that BB diet reversed age-related losses in Ca^{45} buffering capacity. These findings were replicated in a subsequent study that employed a more natural based diet (NIH 31) [83]. However, it was clear from these supplementation studies [15, 83] that the significant effects of BB supplementation on both motor and cognitive behavior were due to a multiplicity of actions, in addition to those involving antioxidant and anti-inflammatory activity.

Interestingly, an examination of reactive oxygen species (ROS) production in the brain tissue obtained from animals in the various diet groups indicated that the striata obtained from all of the supplemented groups exhibited significantly lower ROS levels (by assaying DCF; 2',7'-dichlorofluorescein diacetate) than the controls [15]. However, on further examination it did not appear to be of sufficient magnitude to account for the host of beneficial effects exhibited by the BB-supplemented animals. We have since found that brain tissue taken from BB-supplemented animals shows greater protection against both oxidative and inflammatory stressors that are applied in vitro than tissue taken from control animals.

Nevertheless, from these findings, it was becoming increasingly clear that although the fruit and vegetable extracts offered some antioxidant/anti-inflammatory protection, those properties were only the tip of the proverbial iceberg, especially in light of the myriad of interactions possible among the polyphenolics present in the blueberries. The literature suggests, for example, that flavonoids can have potent effects on cell signaling. As examples, delphinidin inhibits endothelial cell proliferation and cell cycle progression by ERK 1/2 activation [84], while grape seed proanthocyanidin can reduce ischemia reperfusion-induced activation of JNK-1 and C-Jun and reduce cardiomyocyte apoptosis [85]. Additional research indicates that phytochemicals can regulate multiple signaling pathways in a selective manner at the level of transcription, especially those concerned with MAP kinase [86].

With respect to aging, in a recent study [87] APP/PS1 transgenic mice, which express amyloid beta plaques in regions such as the hippocampus, were given BB supplementations beginning at four months of age (2% of the diet as in [15]) and continuing to 12 months of age. The mice were then tested for their performance in a Y-maze. The results revealed an interesting dichotomy in the BB-supplemented animals between Y maze performance and indices of brain pathology. It appeared that although BB supplementation did not affect amyloid beta production or deposition, the supplementation seemed to have prevented the deficits in Y-maze performance seen in the transgenic animals fed the control diets. However, it appeared that instead of altering plaque formation or deposition, the BB supplementation enhanced several important signaling parameters including striatal carbachol-stimulated GTPase, hippocampal ERK and hippocampal PKC. Interestingly, except for the findings with respect to GTPase, there were no reductions in these parameters (ERK, PKC) in the non-supplemented APP/PS1 mice. The changes in striatal carbachol-stimulated GTPase activity were significantly correlated with Y-maze performance, while there was a trend toward a significant correlation with PKC. It is possible that the correlation between Y-maze performance and ERK would have been significant with a larger N ($r = 0.34$). Thus, since some of these indices were also correlated with Y-maze performance, it is clear that BB supplementation may facilitate behavioral performance by enhancing neuronal communication.

While it could be construed that the signaling increases were the indirect result of increases in antioxidant/anti-inflammatory activities, an additional study [88] with BB-supplemented young rats showed that performance on several behavioral parameters was significantly correlated with ERK or PKC activity. Moreover, Andres-Lacueva and colleagues [89] have shown that the brain is permeable to dietary polyphenols (e.g, anthocyanins) from the blueberries. The number of anthocyanins were positively correlated with behavioral performance on a water maze [89]. Therefore, these findings suggest that some of these anthocyanins are able to enter the brain and can influence behavior. It may be that the beneficial behavioral effects observed with the blueberries may directly affect neuronal communication.

5. Neurogenesis

One other component that may be affected by blueberry supplementation is neuronal plasticity. While neurons and glia of the mature central nervous system are believed to be generated primarily during early postnatal life, it is now known that the brain exhibits much more plasticity than was once thought. Formation of new neurons has been shown in different areas of the brain such as the hippocampus [90] throughout the life span. However, despite this continuous proliferation, neurogenesis decreases with age [91].

Importantly, it appears that this proliferation can be altered. During the past several years, studies have identified various factors that can up-regulate [92-99] or down-regulate [91, 100-101] the production and survival of hippocampal neurons developed during adulthood. For example, it has been shown that rearing animals in an enriched environment [93, 97, 102] can alter the rate of neurogenesis decline seen during aging, possibly by enhancing the survival rate of these cells [99, 103-104]. Since it appears that the rate of neurogenesis is plastic, it might be possible that one other aspect of neuronal communication modified by blueberry supplementation is the rate of growth and proliferation of new neurons. To this end it has been shown that newly generated neurons in the hippocampus modulate some types of hippocampal-dependent memory [105]. Additionally, in preliminary experiments in our laboratory [106], we have shown that the rate of neurogenesis increases in the dentate gyrus (hippocampal associated memory control area) of blueberry-supplemented old animals. Moreover, these increases were negatively correlated with the number of errors that these rats made on a radial arm water maze task (e.g., working memory errors, $r = -0.65$, $p < 0.05$). Additional data indicate that the putative increases in neurogenesis of these animals were associated with ERK enhancement.

Taken together these findings, which suggest that blueberries, and possibly other fruits and vegetables, may directly affect signaling and neuronal communication, are extremely important, since they indicate for the first time that nutrition may be utilized not only as an adjunct to traditional medical treatment to prevent nervous system disorders, but rather also to increase neuronal function so that more conventional treatments (for AD or PD) may be more effective. More work is needed, of course, but we are approaching the time when medicine and nutrition may become important partners for quenching the fires of brain aging. Perhaps we have even been here before, but it has been lost in antiquity.

2000 BC – Here, eat this berry.
1000 BC – That berry is heathen. Here, say this prayer.
AD 1850 – That prayer is superstition. Here, drink this potion.
AD 1940 – That potion is snake oil. Here, swallow this pill.
AD 1985 – That pill is ineffective. Here take this vaccine.
The "New" millennium – That vaccine doesn't work anymore. Here, eat this berry.

References

[1] Joseph JA, Denisova N, Fisher D, Bickford P, Prior R, Cao G. Age-related neuro-degeneration and oxidative stress: putative nutritional intervention. *Neurol Clin* (1998) 16:747-755.

[2] Joseph JA, Denisova NA, Fisher D, Shukitt-Hale B, Bickford P, Prior R, Cao G. Membrane and receptor modifications of oxidative stress vulnerability in aging: Nutritional considerations. *Ann NY Acad Sci* (1998) 854:268-276.

[3] Cantuti-Castelvetri I, Shukitt-Hale B, Joseph JA. Dopamine neurotoxicity: age-dependent behavioral and histological effects. *Neurobiol Aging* (2003) 24(5):697-706.

[4] Olanow CW. An introduction to the free radical hypothesis in Parkinson's disease. *Ann Neurol* (1992) 32:S2-S9.

[5] Gilissen EP, Jacobs RE, Allman, JM. Magnetic resonance microscopy of iron in the basal forebrain cholinergic structures of the aged mouse lemur. *J Neurol Sci* (1999) 168:21-27.

[6] Sadoul R. Bcl-2 family members in the development and degenerative pathologies of the nervous system. *Cell Death Differ* (1998) 5:805-815.

[7] Yu BP. Cellular defenses against damage from reactive oxygen species. *Physiol Rev* (1994) 76:139-162.

[8] Carney JM, Smith CD, Carney AM, Butterfield DA. Aging- and oxygen-induced modifications in brain biochemistry and behavior. *Ann NY Acad Sci* (1994) 738:44-53.

[9] Savory J, Rao, JK, Huang Y, Letada PR, Herman MM. Age-related hippocampal changes in Bcl-2:Bax ratio, oxidative stress, redox-active iron and apoptosis associated with aluminum-induced neurodegeneration: increased susceptibility with aging. *Neurotox* (1999) 20:805-817.

[10] Joseph JA, Shukitt-Hale B, Denisova NA, Martin A, Perry G, Smith MA. Copernicus revisited: Amyloid beta in Alzheimer's disease. *Neurobiol Aging* (2001) 22:131-146.

[11] Denisova NA, Erat SA, Kelly JF, Roth GS. Differential effect of aging on cholesterol modulation of carbachol stimulated Low-Km GTPase in striatal synaptosomes. *Exp Gerontol* (1998) 33:249-265.

[12] Denisova NA, Fisher D, Provost M, Joseph JA. The role of glutathione, membrane sphingomyelin, and its metabolites in oxidative stress-induced calcium "dysregulation" in PC12 cells. *Free Radic Biol Med* (1999) 27(11-12):1292-1301.

[13] Joseph JA, Fisher DR, Strain J. Muscarinic receptor subtype determines vulnerability to oxidative stress in COS-7 cells. *Free Radic Biol Med* (2002) 32:153-161.

[14] Joseph JA, Fisher DR Muscarinic receptor subtype determines vulnerability to amyloid beta toxicity in transfected cos-7 cells. *J Alz Dis* (2003) 5(3):197-208.

[15] Joseph JA, Shukitt-Hale B, Denisova NA, Bielinski D, Martin A, McEwen, JJ, Bickford, PC. Reversals of age-related declines in neuronal signal transduction, cognitive and motor behavioral deficits with blueberry, spinach or strawberry dietary supplementation. *J Neurosci* (1999) 19:8114-8121.

[16] Landfield PW, Eldridge JC. The glucocorticoid hypothesis of age-related hippocampal neurodegeneration: role of dysregulated intraneuronal Ca^{2+}. *Ann NY Acad Sci* (1994) 746:308-321.

[17] Pottorf WJ, Duckles SP, Buchholz JN. Aging and calcium buffering in adrenergic neurons. *Auton Neurosci* (2002) 96(1):2-7.

[18] Cheng Y, Wixom P, James-Kracke MR, Sun AY. Effects of extracellular ATP on Fe^{2+}-induced cytotoxicity in PC-12 cells. *J Neurochem* (1994) 66:895-902.
[19] Wilson CJ, Finch CE, Cohen HJ. Cytokines and cognition--the case for a head-to-toe inflammatory paradigm. *J Am Geriatr Soc* (2002) 50(12):2041-2056.
[20] Prolla TA, Mattson MP. Molecular mechanisms of brain aging and neurodegenerative disorders: lessons from dietary restriction. *Trends Neurosci* (2001) 24(11 Suppl):S21-31.
[21] Rozovsky I, Finch CE, Morgan TE. Age-related activation of microglia and astrocytes: in vitro studies show. *Neurobiol Aging* (1998) 19:97-103.
[22] McGeer PL, McGeer EG. The inflammatory response system of the brain: implications for therapy of Alzheimer and other neurodegenerative diseases. *Brain Res Rev* (1995) 21:195-218.
[23] Chang HN, Wang SR, Chiang SC, Teng WJ, Chen ML, Tsai JJ, Huang DF, Lin HY, Tsai YY. The relationship of aging to endotoxin shock and to production of TNFa. *J Gerontol* (1996) 51:M220-M222.
[24] Chang RC, Chen W, Hudson P, Wilson B, Han DS Hong JS. Neurons reduce glial responses to lipopolysaccharide (LPS) and prevent injury of microglial cells from over-activation by LPS. *J Neurochem* (2001) 76:1042-1049.
[25] Spaulding CC, Walford RL, Effros RB. Calorie restriction inhibits the age-related dysregulation of the cytokines TNF-alpha and IL-6 in C3B10RF1 mice. *Mech Ageing Dev* (1997) 93:87-94.
[26] Volpato S, Guralnik JM, Ferrucci L, Balfour J, Chaves P, Fried LP, Harris TB. Cardiovascular disease, interleukin-6, and risk of mortality in older women: the women's health and aging study. *Circulation* (2001) 103:947-953.
[27] Kushner I. C-reactive protein elevation can be caused by conditions other than inflammation and may reflect biologic aging. *Cleve Clin J Med* (2001) 68:535-537.
[28] Shukitt-Hale B, Mouzakis G, Joseph JA. Psychomotor and spatial memory performance in aging male Fischer 344 rats. *Exp Gerontol* (1998) 33:615-624.
[29] Joseph JA, Bartus RT, Clody DE, Morgan D, Finch C, Beer B, Sesack S. Psychomotor performance in the senescent rodent: Reduction of deficits via striatal dopamine receptor up-regulation. *Neurobiol Aging* (1983) 4:313-319.
[30] West RL. An application of pre-frontal cortex function theory to cognitive aging. *Psych Bull* (1996) 120:272-292.
[31] Joseph JA. The putative role of free radicals in the loss of neuronal functioning in senescence. *Integ Physiol Behav Sci* (1992) 27:216-227.
[32] Bickford P. Motor learning deficits in aged rats are correlated with loss of cerebellar noradrenergic function. *Brain Res (1993)* 620:133-138.
[33] Shukitt-Hale B. The effects of aging and oxidative stress on psychomotor and cognitive behavior. *Age* (1999) 22:9-17.
[34] Hauss-Wegrzyniak B, Vraniak P, Wenk GL. The effects of a novel NSAID on chronic neuroinflammation are age dependent. *Neurobiol Aging* (1999) 20:305-313.
[35] Joseph JA, Erat S, Rabin BM. CNS effects of heavy particle irradiation in space: Behavioral implications. *Adv Space Res* (1998) 22:209-216.
[36] Joseph JA, Shukitt-Hale B, McEwen JJ, Rabin BM. CNS-induced deficits of heavy particle irradiation in space: the aging connection. *Adv Space Res* (2000) 25:2057-2064.
[37] Joseph JA, Hunt WA, Rabin BM, Dalton TK. Possible "accelerated striatal aging" induced by ^{56}Fe heavy-particle irradiation: Implications for manned space flights. *Radiat Res* (1992) 130:88-93.
[38] Shukitt-Hale B, Casadesus G, McEwen JJ, Rabin BM, Joseph, JA. Spatial learning and memory deficits induced by exposure to iron-56-particle radiation. *Radiat Res* (2000) 154:28-33.
[39] Rabin BM, Joseph JA, Erat S. Effects of exposure to different types of radiation on behaviors mediated by peripheral or central systems. *Adv Space Res* (1998) 22:217-225.
[40] Bickford PC, Chadman K, Williams B, Shukitt-Hale B, Holmes D, Taglialatela G, Joseph J. Effect of normobaric hyperoxia on two indexes of synaptic function in Fischer 344 rats. *Free Radic Bio Med* (1999) 26:817-824.
[41] Joseph JA, Berger RE, Engel BT, Roth G S. Age-related changes in the nigrostriatum: A behavioral and biochemical analysis. *J Gerontol* (1978) 33:643-649.
[42] Levine MS, Cepeda C. Dopamine modulation of responses mediated by excitatory amino acids in the neostriatum. *Adv Pharmacol* (1998) 42:724-729.
[43] Egashira T, Takayama F, Yamanaka Y. Effects of bifemelane on muscarinic receptors and choline acetyltransferase in the brains of aged rats following chronic cerebral hypoperfusion induced by permanent occlusion of bilateral carotid arteries. *Jap J Pharmacol* (1996) 72:57-65.
[44] Joseph JA, Kowatch MA, Maki T, Roth GS. Selective cross activation /inhibition of second messenger systems and the reduction of age-related deficits in the muscarinic control of dopamine release from perfused rat striata. *Brain Res* (1990) 537:40-48.

[45] Kornhuber J, Schoppmeyer K, Bendig C, Riederer P. Characterization of [3H] pentazocine binding sites in post-mortem human frontal cortex. *J Neural Trans* (1996) 3:45-53.
[46] Gould TJ, Bickford P. Age-related deficits in the cerebellar beta-adrenergic signal transduction cascade in Fischer 344 rats. *J Pharmacol Exp Therapeu* (1997) 281:965-971.
[47] Haydon PG, Man-Son-Hing H, Doyle RT, Zoran M. FMRFamide modulation of secretory machinery underlying presynaptic inhibition of synaptic transmission requires a pertussis toxin-sensitive G-protein. *J Neurosci* (1991) 11(12):3851-3860.
[48] Leahy JC, Luo Y, Kent CS, Meiri KF, Vallano ML. Demonstration of presynaptic protein kinase C activation following long-term potentiation in rat hippocampal slices. *Neurosci* (1993) 52:563-574.
[49] Micheau J, Riedel G. Protein kinases: which one is the memory molecule? *Cell Molec Life Sci* (1999) 55:534-548.
[50] Colombo PJ, Gallagher M. Individual differences in spatial memory among aged rats are related to hippocampal PKCgamma immunoreactivity. *Hippocampus* (2002) 12(2):285-289.
[51] Serrano PA, Beniston DS, Oxonian MG, Rodriguez WA, Rosenzweig MR, Bennett EL. Differential effects of protein kinase inhibitors and activators on memory formation in the 2-day-old chick. *Behav Neural Biol* (1994) 61:60-72.
[52] Colombo PJ, Wetsel W, Gallagher MG. Spatial memory is related to hippocampal subcellular concentrations of calcium-dependent protein kinase C isoforms in young and aged rats. *Proc Nat Acad Sci USA* (1997) 94:1495-1499.
[53] Van der Zee EA, Compaan JC, Bohus B, Luiten PG. Alterations in the immunoreactivity for muscarinic acetylcholine receptors and colocalized PKC gamma in mouse hippocampus induced by spatial discrimination learning. *Hippocampus* (1995) 5:349-362.
[54] Battaini F, Elkabes S, Bergamaschi S, Ladisa V, Lucchi L, De Graan PN, Schuurman T, Wetsel WC, Trabucchi M, Govoni S. Protein kinase C activity, translocation, and conventional isoforms in aging rat brain. *Neurobiol Aging* (1995) 16:37-148.
[55] Fordyce DE, Wehner JM. Effects of aging on spatial learning and hippocampal protein kinase C in mice. *Neurobiol Aging* (1993) 14:309-317.
[56] Nguyen PV, Kandel ER. A macromolecular synthesis-dependent late phase of long-term potentiation requiring cAMP in the medial perforant pathway of rat hippocampal slices. *J Neurosci* (1996) 16:3189-3198.
[57] Nguyen PV, Kandel ER. Brief theta-burst stimulation induces a transcription-dependent late phase of LTP requiring cAMP in area CA1 of the mouse hippocampus. *Learn Mem* (1997) 4:230-243.
[58] Rosenzweig MR, Bennett EL, Colombo PJ, Lee DW, Serrano PA. Short-term, intermediate-term, and long-term memories. *Behav Brain Res* (1993) 57:193-198.
[59] Boxall AR, Lancaster B. Tyrosine kinases and synaptic transmission. *Eur J Neurosci* (1998) 10:2-7.
[60] Graves JD, Campbell JS, Krebs EG. Protein serine/threonine kinases of the MAPK cascade. *Ann N Y Acad Sci* (1995) 766:320-343.
[61] Sgambato V, Pages C, Rogard M, Besson MJ, Caboche J. Extracellular signal-regulated kinase (ERK) controls immediate early gene induction on corticostriatal stimulation. *J Neurosci* (1998) 18:8814-8825.
[62] Zhang L, Jope RS. Oxidative stress differentially modulates phosphorylation of ERK, p38 and CREB induced by NGF or EGF in PC12 cells. *Neurobiol Aging* (1999) 20:271-278.
[63] Sweatt JD. Memory mechanisms: the yin and yang of protein phosphorylation. *Curr Biol* (2001) 11:R391-394.
[64] Berman DE, Hazvi S, Rosenblum K, Seger R, Dudai Y. Specific and differential activation of mitogen-activated protein kinase cascades by unfamiliar taste in the insular cortex of the behaving rat. *J Neurosci* (1998) 18:10037-10044.
[65] Swank MW, Sweatt JD. Increased histone acetyltransferase and lysine acetyltransferase activity and biphasic activation of the ERK/RSK cascade in insular cortex during novel taste learning. *J Neurosci* (2001) 21:3383-3391.
[66] Selcher JC, Atkins CM, Trzaskos JM, Paylor R, Sweatt JD. A necessity for MAP kinase activation in mammalian spatial learning. *Learn Mem* (1999) 6:478-490.
[67] Schafe GE, Nadel NV, Sullivan GM, Harris A, LeDoux JE. Memory consolidation for contextual and auditory fear conditioning is dependent on protein synthesis, PKA, and MAP kinase. *Learn Mem* (1999) 6:97-110.
[68] Rosenblum K, Futter M, Jones M, Hulme EC, Bliss TV. ERKI/II regulation by the muscarinic acetylcholine receptors in neurons. *J Neurosci* (2000) 20:977-985.
[69] Zhen X, Uryu K, Cai G, Johnson GP, Friedman E. Age-associated impairment in brain MAPK signal pathways and the effect of restriction in Fischer 344 rats. *J Gerontol A Biol Sci Med Sci* (1999) 54:B539-548.

[70] Simonyi A, Murch K, Sun GY. Extracellular signal-regulated kinase 2 mRNA expression in the rat brain during aging. *Neurochem Res* (2003) 28(9):1375-1378.
[71] Lamprecht R. CREB message to remember. *Cell Mol Life Sci* (1999) 55:554-563.
[72] Mazzucchelli C, Brambilla R. Ras-related and MAPK signaling in neuronal plasticity and memory formation. *Cell Mol Life Sci* (2000) 57:604-611.
[73] Bourtchuladze R, Frenguelli B, Blendy J, Cioffi D, Schutz G, Silva AJ. Deficient long-term memory in mice with a targeted mutation of the cAMP-responsive element-binding protein. *Cell* (1994) 79(1):59-68.
[74] Matsumoto A. Age-dependent changes in phosphorylated cAMP response element-binding protein immunoreactivity in motoneurons of the spinal nucleus of the bulbocavernosus of male rats. *Neurosci Lett* (2000) 279(2):117-120.
[75] Gozal D, Row BW, Kheirandish L, Liu R, Guo SZ, Qiang F, Brittian KR. Increased susceptibility to intermittent hypoxia in aging rats: changes in proteasomal activity, neuronal apoptosis and spatial function. *J Neurochem* (2003) 86(6):1545-1552.
[76] Josselyn SA, Shi C, Carlezon WA Jr, Neve RL, Nestler EJ, Davis M. Long-term memory is facilitated by cAMP response element-binding protein overexpression in the amygdala. *J Neurosci* (2001) 21:2404-2412.
[77] Weisburger JH. Lifestyle, health and disease prevention: the underlying mechanisms. *Eur J Cancer Prev* (2002 Aug) 11 Suppl 2:S1-7.
[78] Parr AJ, Bolwell GP. Phenols in the plant and in man. The potential for possible nutritional enhancement of the diet by modifying the phenols content or profile. *J Sci Food Agric* (2000) 80:985–1012.
[79] Cao G, Sofic E, Prior RL. Antioxidant capacity of tea and common vegetables. *J Agric Food Chem* (1996) 44:3426-3431.
[80] Prior RL, Cao G, Martin A, Sofic E, McEwen J, O'Brien C, Lischner N, Ehlenfeldt M, Kalt W, Krewer G, Mainland M. Antioxidant capacity as influenced by total phenolic and anthocyanin content, maturity and variety of Vaccinium species. *J Agric Food Chem* (1998) 46:2586-2593.
[81] Wang H, Cao G, Prior R. Total antioxidant capacity of fruits. *J Agric Food Chem* (1996) 44:701-705.
[82] Joseph JA, Shukitt-Hale B, Denisova NA, Prior RL, Cao G, Martin A, Taglialatela G, Bickford PC. Long-term dietary strawberry, spinach or vitamin E supplementation retards the onset of age-related neuronal signal-transduction and cognitive behavioral deficits. *J Neurosci* (1998) 18:8047-8055.
[83] Youdim KA, Shukitt-Hale B, Martin A, Wang H, Denisova N, Joseph, JA. Short-term dietary supplementation of blueberry polyphenolics: Beneficial effects on aging brain performance and peripheral tissue function. *Nutr Neurosci* (2000) 3:383-397.
[84] Martin S, Favot L, Matz R, Lugnier C, Andriantsitohaina R. Delphinidin inhibits endothelial cell proliferation and cell cycle progression through a transient activation of ERK-1/-2. *Biochem Pharmacol* (2003) 65:669-675.
[85] Sato M, Bagchi D, Tosaki A, Das DK. Grape seed proanthocyanidin reduces cardiomyocyte apoptosis by inhibiting ischemia/reperfusion-induced activation of JNK-1 and C-JUN. *Free Radic Biol Med* (2001) 31:729-737.
[86] Frigo DE, Duong BN, Melnik LI, Schief LS, Collins-Burow BM, Pace DK, McLachlan JA, Burow ME. Flavonoid phytochemicals regulate activator protein-1 signal transduction pathways in endometrial and kidney stable cell lines. *J Nutr* (2002) 132:1848-1853.
[87] Joseph JA, Arendash G, Gordon M, Diamond D, Shukitt-Hale B, Morgan D. Blueberry supplementation enhances signaling and prevents behavioral deficits in an Alzheimer disease model. *Nutr Neurosci* (2003) 6:153-163.
[88] Shukitt-Hale B, McEwen JJ, Szprengiel A, Joseph JA. Effect of age on the radial arm water maze - a test of spatial learning and memory. *Neurobiol Aging* (2004) 25:223-229.
[89] Andres-Lacueva C, et al. (in preparation)
[90] Gage FH, Kempermann G, Palmer TD, Peterson DA, Ray J. Multipotent progenitor cells in the adult dentate gyrus. *J Neurobiol* (1998) 36:249-266.
[91] Kuhn HG, Dickinson-Anson H, Gage FH. Neurogenesis in the dentate gyrus of the adult rat: age-related decrease of neuronal progenitor proliferation. *J Neurosci* (1996) 16:2027-2033.
[92] Kee NJ, Preston E, Wojtowicz JM. Enhanced neurogenesis after transient global ischemia in the dentate gyrus of the rat. *Exp Brain Res* (2001) 136:313-320.
[93] Kempermann G, Brandon EP, Gage FH. Environmental stimulation of 129/SvJ mice causes increased cell proliferation and neurogenesis in the adult dentate gyrus. *Curr Biol* (1998) 8:939-942.
[94] Kempermann G, Kuhn HG, Gage FH. Experience-induced neurogenesis in the senescent dentate gyrus. *J Neurosci* (1998) 18:3206-3212.

[95] Lee J, Duan W, Long JM, Ingram DK, Mattson MP. Dietary restriction increases the number of newly generated neural cells, and induces BDNF expression, in the dentate gyrus of rats. *J Mol Neurosci* (2000) 15:99-108.

[96] Nacher J, Rosell DR, Alonso-Llosa G, McEwen BS. NMDA receptor antagonist treatment induces a long-lasting increase in the number of proliferating cells, PSA-NCAM-immunoreactive granule neurons and radial glia in the adult rat dentate gyrus. *Eur J Neurosci* (2001) 13:512-520.

[97] Nilsson M, Perfilieva E, Johansson U, Orwar O, Eriksson PS. Enriched environment increases neurogenesis in the adult rat dentate gyrus and improves spatial memory. *J Neurobiol* (1999) 39:569-578.

[98] Tanapat P, Hastings NB, Reeves AJ, Gould E. Estrogen stimulates a transient increase in the number of new neurons in the dentate gyrus of the adult female rat. *J Neurosci* (1999) 19:5792-5801.

[99] Van Praag H, Christie BR, Sejnowski TJ, Gage FH. Running enhances neurogenesis, learning, and long-term potentiation in mice. *Proc Natl Acad Sci USA* (1999) 96:13427-13431.

[100] Cameron HA, Gould E. Adult neurogenesis is regulated by adrenal steroids in the dentate gyrus. *Neurosci* (1994) 61:203-209.

[101] Cameron HA, McEwen BS, Gould E. Regulation of adult neurogenesis by excitatory input and NMDA receptor activation in the dentate gyrus. *J Neurosci* (1995) 15:4687-4692.

[102] Kempermann G, Gage FH. Experience-dependent regulation of adult hippocampal neurogenesis: effects of long-term stimulation and stimulus withdrawal. *Hippocampus* (1999) 9:321-332.

[103] Ambrogini P, Cuppini R, Cuppini C, Ciaroni S, Cecchini T, Ferri P, Sartini S, Del Grande P. Spatial learning affects immature granule cell survival in adult rat dentate gyrus. *Neurosci Lett* (2000) 286:21-24.

[104] Gould E, Reeves AJ, Fallah M, Tanapat P, Gross CG, Fuchs E. Hippocampal neurogenesis in adult Old World primates. *Proc Natl Acad Sci USA* (1999) 96:5263-5267.

[105] Shors TJ, Miesegaes G, Beylin A, Zhao M, Rydel T, Gould E. Neurogenesis in the adult is involved in the formation of trace memories. *Nature* 410, (2001) 410:372-376.

[106] Casadesus G, in preparation.

Frontiers in Neurodegenerative Disorders and Aging: Fundamental Aspects, Clinical Perspectives and New Insights
T. Özben and M. Chevion (Eds.)
IOS Press, 2004

Oxidative stress in Alzheimer's Disease. Effectiveness of Treatment with Antioxidants.

José Viña, Ana Lloret, Rafael Ortí, Dolores Alonso
Departments of Physiology, Preventive Medicine, and Neurology. Faculty of Medicine. Valencia.

Abstract: The free radical theory of aging postulates that free radicals are critical in causing damage associated with aging and age associated diseases. Mitochondria are important as causative agents and as targets of free radicals. Azheimers´s disease is associated with oxidative stress which can be followed in vivo by determining biomarkers such as plasma lipoperoxide formation or the oxidation of blood glutathione. We have found that Alzheimer´s patients show an increased lipoperoxide formation and an oxidation of blood glutathione. Moreover, the oxidation of glutathione is related to the cognitive status of the patients. Treatment with vitamin E resulted in an improved cognitive performance only of those patients in which if acted as an antioxidant. Thus the effect of vitamin E on Alzheimer's disease patients shows considerable variations both in its antioxidant function and in its capacity to improve cognitive functions. Epidemiological studies that aim to test the effect of antioxidants on given functions should be accompanied by determination of the patient´s antioxidant status

1. The mitochondrial theory of ageing

Ageing is characterised by a progressive accumulation of changes with time, which are responsible for an increased probability of disease and death. Many theories have been put forward to explain ageing. In fact, more than a hundred have been published (for a review, see 1). One of the most prominent of such theories is the free radical theory of ageing which was postulated by Harman in 1956 (2). This theory postulates that oxygen free radicals are involved in damage associated with ageing. The theory was further refined by Miquel and co-workers in the 80's (3). These authors postulated that mitochondria were key organelles to generate reactive oxygen species in ageing. They were also essential targets of the damage caused by these oxygen species (3). A critical feature of this theory is that it suggests the possibility of intervention either by preventing formation of free radicals or minimising damage by administration of antioxidants. Many of these antioxidants have shown beneficial effects to prevent age-associated damage to cells and, more important, to lower the incidence of age-associated diseases. Of the various antioxidants available, great attention has been paid to antioxidant vitamins, particularly vitamin E, and to natural extracts rich in flavonoids such as *ginkgo biloba*. Quite recently the role of oestrogens, and phytoestrogens has been underlined.

Address for correspondence: Prof José Viña. Dpt° de Fisiología Facultad de Medicina
Av. Blasco Ibáñez, 17 E46011 – Valencia, Spain.

2. Neuronal damage is increased in cells from central nervous system when compared with cells from other tissues

A key feature of any theory of ageing is that it might explain the fact that post-mitotic cells, i.e. cells that do not divide any more, suffer more damage than mitotic ones. In fact, mitosis appears to have a regenerating role in preventing age-associated accumulation of damage. Figure 1 shows that DNA from brain mitochondria exhibits a much higher level of the oxidised base 8-hydroxy-deoxyguanine than hepatic mitochondrial DNA. Moreover, it also shows that oxidative damage to mitochondrial DNA is very significantly increased in ageing. Oxidative damage to brain mitochondrial DNA is more than twofold higher than that of hepatic mitochondrial DNA (4). This may have clinical importance. Indeed, age-associated diseases occur primarily in organs which contain mainly post-mitotic cells. The central nervous system is a paradigmatic example. Many age-associated diseases are related to it. For instance, evidence of oxidative stress has been documented in Parkinson's (5) and in Alzheimer's disease (6).

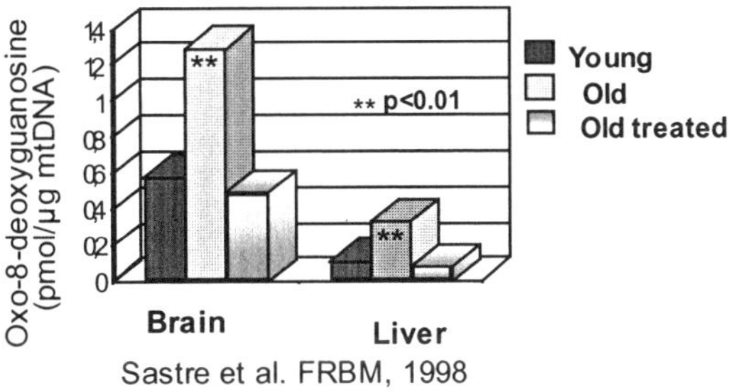

Figure 1. Effect of age and treatment with EGb 761 on oxidative damage to mitochondrial DNA

3. Role of mitochondrial oxidative stress in disease

Free radicals are involved in the pathophysiology of many diseases. (For a review see 7) Cardiovascular disease is a clear example of this. We have recently shown that oxidative stress occurs in diabetes due to the activation of xanthine oxidase (8). In some diseases, both mitochondrial and extra mitochondrial oxidative stress are important to explain pathophysiology. For instance, we have found that in AIDS, there is an absence of cystathionase, an critical enzyme for the maintenance for normal glutathione levels (9) but also that treatment with antiretroviral agents causes mitochondrial oxidative stress (10). Thus, preventing or at least minimising oxidative stress is an important strategy in the treatment of several diseases. In this chapter we shall deal with the importance of antioxidant treatment in neurological diseases and in particular in Alzheimer's disease.

4. Oxidative stress, antioxidants and Alzheimer's disease: Background

The fact that there is oxidative stress in Alzheimer's disease has been recognised for a few years. In 1991, Stadtman and co-workers (11) reported that there is excess brain protein oxidation in Alzheimer's disease (11). Moreover, Floyd and co-workers reported that beta-amyloid aggregation might cause free radical generation which is relevant to Alzheimer's disease. The group of George Perry and Mark Smith have reported on several occasions that oxidative stress is indeed involved in the pathogenesis of this disease. In fact, they suggested that all factors involved in Alzheimer's disease are related to oxidative stress (12). In this context it is critical that there is an iron accumulation in Alzheimer's disease. This in turn is the source of redox generated free radicals (13). However, St George-Hyslop reviewed evidence showing that damage caused by beta amyloid peptide might be caused not only from the extracellular space but also from inside cells (14). Moreover, and it will be relevant in the context of the present chapter, Cecchi and co-workers (15) showed that oxidative stress in Alzheimer's disease can be detected in peripheral cells and not only in neuronal cells. Therefore, evidence has largely accumulated showing that oxidative stress is a key event in the onset and development of Alzheimer's disease.

Three key studies have been published showing that treatment with vitamin E is effective in Alzheimer's disease. In fact, Sano *et al.* (16) reported results of a controlled trial showing that vitamin E is an effective treatment of Alzheimer's disease. This is a critical paper. It showed for the first time that vitamin E could be a treatment and not just a mechanism for prevention of Alzheimer's disease See Figure 2). Moreover, in 2002, two major papers appeared published in JAMA in which the role of dietary intake of antioxidants and the risk of Alzheimer's disease was investigated. Both studies concluded that an increased intake of vitamin E lowers the risk of Alzheimer's disease (17, 18).

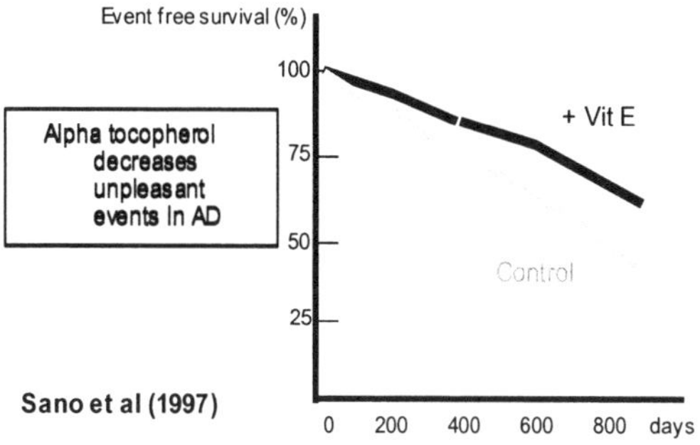

Figure 2. Vitamin E as treatment of Alzheimer's Disease

5. Aim of the study

The aim of the present study was to test whether systemic oxidative stress occurs in Alzheimer's disease patients. We also checked if decreasing oxidative stress by oral administration of antioxidants improved cognitive function in these patients. A critical aim of this study was to determine if improvement in antioxidant redox status in Alzheimer's disease patients correlated with improvement in cognitive function in the patients. Work by the group of Azzi (19) showed that vitamin E has several functions apart from its antioxidant function. Therefore, the observed beneficial effects of vitamin E on Alzheimer's disease patients could be due not to its antioxidant properties, but rather to other functions related to cell signalling. We thus examined the possible relationship between the antioxidant effect of administration of vitamin E to Alzheimer's disease patients and its beneficial effects in improving cognitive function in these patients.

6. Glutathione redox status and Alzheimer's disease

Glutathione redox status (mainly represented by the GSSG/GSH ratio) is an index of oxidative stress (20). We have tested this in several pathophysiological situations in which blood glutathione is affected. For instance, we found that oxidation of blood glutathione correlates with the increased lactate levels observed in exercise (21). In a similar fashion, we found that oxidation of mitochondrial glutathione in ageing (22) or in apoptosis (23) correlates with oxidative damage to mitochondrial DNA (see Figure 3). We thus measured the GSSG/GSH ratio in Alzheimer's disease patients at the onset of the study and found that Alzheimers´s patients had a higher level of blood glutathione oxidation than the age-matched controls (see Figure 4). Moreover, when cognitive function of these patients was assessed, using several methods but we will only report here results using the minimental state examination test, we found that blood glutathione oxidation correlates with cognitive function in these patients. Thus, it appears that systemic oxidative stress correlates well with cognitive function in Alzheimer's disease patients.

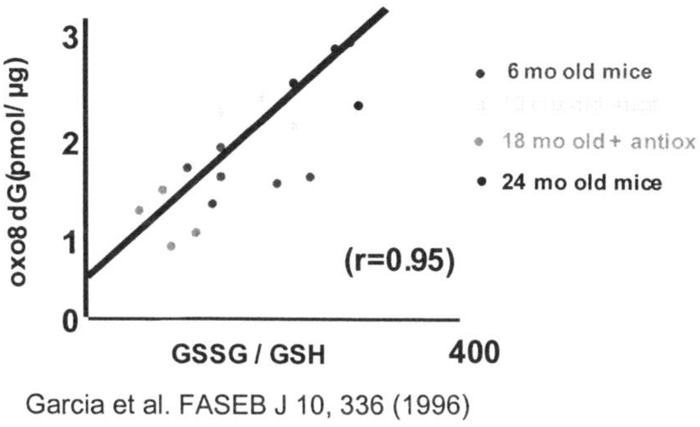

Figure 3. Relationship between DNA and glutathione oxidation

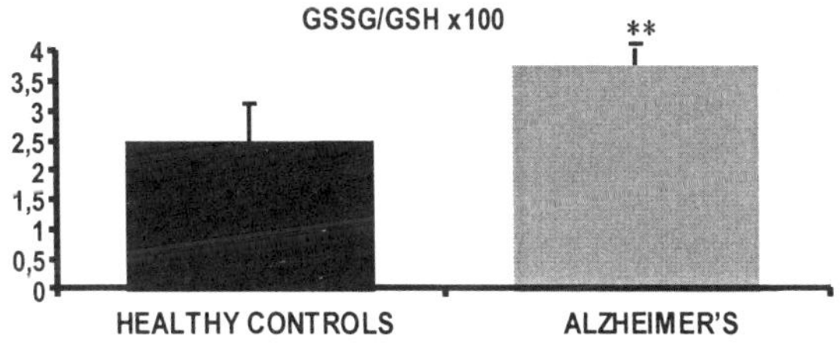

Figure 4. Glutathione redox status in controls and in Alzheimer's patients

Vitamin E is a useful treatment for Alzheimer's disease, but its effects show interindividual variations. Figure 5 shows that vitamin E is useful to improve cognitive performance in Alzheimer's disease patients. This confirms the results previously published by Sano and co-workers (16). We also determined the effect of vitamin E on blood lipid peroxidation in these patients. The latter was determined as malondialdehyde formed from plasma lipid peroxides. The malondialdehyde-thiobarbiturate adduct was separated and determined by high performance liquid chromatography. **Figure 5** shows that Alzheimer's disease patients had a higher level of plasma malondialdehyde and an increased oxidation of blood glutathione when compared with controls.

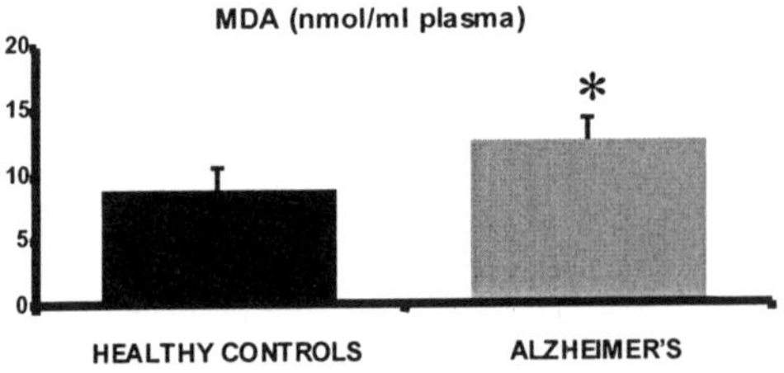

Figure 5. Lipid hydroperoxides (as MDA) in controls and in Alzheimer's

Treatment with vitamin E significantly improved cognitive performance of Alzheimer's disease patients after six months of treatment. It also ameliorated systemic oxidative stress as determined by blood glutathione redox ratio. However, the response to vitamin E showed significant interindividual variations. Not all patients responded equally to vitamin E. Some patients did not show a significant reduction of the glutathione redox ratio upon treatment with vitamin E. In these same patients vitamin E did not significantly increase cognitive performance. Figure 6 shows that changes in glutathione redox ratio and in cognitive performance were directly related. A decrease in the oxidation state of the patient correlated with an increase in cognitive performance as determined by the minimental state examination score. A possible explanation for this is that the rate of absorption of vitamin E also shows great interindividual variations (24). Thus, the same dose of vitamin E will not result in a similar antioxidant effect *in vivo*. These results strongly suggest the idea that the beneficial effect of vitamin E in cognition in Alzheimer's disease patients is related to its antioxidant properties and not to other roles of this vitamin in cell signalling.

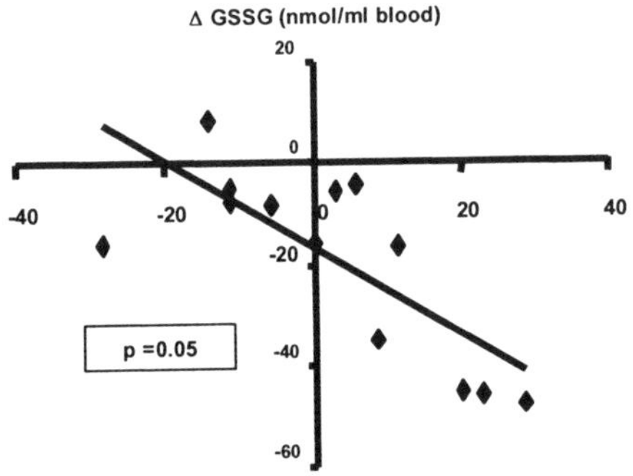

Figure 6. Relationship between Δ GSSG and Δ MMSE in AD patients treated with vitamin E

7. Concluding remarks

The results reported here show that Alzheimer's disease causes a systemic oxidative stress which is more pronounced when cognitive functions of the patient are more severely impaired. They also confirm that vitamin E can be considered as a treatment of Alzheimer's disease.

In our view, the most important conclusion of these studies is, however, that the effect of vitamin E on Alzheimer's disease patients shows considerable variations both in its antioxidant function and in its capacity to improve cognitive functions. These results go along the line of the thoughts of Halliwell (25) who suggested that, in epidemiological studies that aim to test the effect of antioxidants on given functions (i.e. the incidence of cardiovascular diseases, giving antioxidants such as vitamin E should be accompanied by determination of the antioxidant status. Abundant evidence is mounting showing the fact that there is great interindividual variation between the systemic antioxidant effect of oral antioxidants. The results reported here are an example of such variation.

References

[1] Medvedev ZA (1990). "An attempt at a rational classification of theories of ageing." Biol Rev Camb Philos Soc. **65**(3):375-98

[2] Harman, D. (1956). "Aging: a theory based on free radical and ratiation chemistry." J. Gerontol **11**: 298-300.

[3] Miquel, J., A. C. Economos, et al. (1980). "Mitochondrial role in cell aging." Exp Gerontol **15**(6): 575-91.

[4] Sastre, J., A. Millan, et al. (1998). "A Ginkgo biloba extract (EGb 761) prevents mitochondrial aging by protecting against oxidative stress." Free Radic Biol Med **24**(2): 298-304.

[5] Gotz, M. E., A. Freyberger, et al. (1990). "Oxidative stress: a role in the pathogenesis of Parkinson's disease." Journal of Neural Transmission. Supplementum **29**: 241-249.

[6] Cross CE, Halliwell B, Borish ET et al. (1987). "Oxygen radicals and human disease." Ann Intern Med. **107**:526-545.

[7] Free radicals, oxidative stress and antioxidants. Pathological and physiological significance. Ozben, T. editor. Plenum Press. New York and London. 1998.

[8] Desco MC, Asensi M, Marquez R et al. (2002) "Xanthine oxidase is involved in free radical production in type 1 diabetes: protection by allopurinol." Diabetes **51**:1118-1124

[9] Martin JA, Sastre J, De la Asuncion JG et al. (2001) "Hepatic gamma-cystathionase deficiency in patients with AIDS." JAMA **285**:1444-1445

[10] De la Asuncion JG, del Olmo ML, Sastre J et al. (1998) "AZT treatment induces molecular and ultrastructural oxidative damage to muscle mitochondria. Prevention by antioxidant vitamins." J Clin Invest. **102**:4-9.

[11] Stadman, E. R. (1992). "Protein oxidation and aging." Science **257**: 1220-1224.

[12] Smith MA, Perry G, Richey PL et al. (1996) "Oxidative damage in Alzheimer's." Nature. **382**:120-121.

[13] Smith MA, Harris PL, Sayre LM, Perry G. (1997) "Iron accumulation in Alzheimer disease is a source of redox-generated free radicals." Proc Natl Acad Sci U S A. 94:9866-9868

[14] St. George-Hyslop PH. (2000) "Piecing together Alzheimer's " Sci. Am. **283**: 52-59.

[15] Cecchi C, Latorraca S, Sorbi S et al. (1999) "Gluthatione level is altered in lymphoblasts from patients with familial Alzheimer's disease." Neurosci Lett. **275**:152-154

[16] Sano M, Ernesto C, Thomas RG et al. (1997) "A controlled trial of selegiline, alpha-tocopherol, or both as treatment for Alzheimer's disease. The Alzheimer's Disease Cooperative Study." N Engl J Med. **336**:1216-1222

[17] Morris MC, Evans DA, Bienias JL et al. (2002) "Dietary intake of antioxidant nutrients and the risk of incident Alzheimer disease in a biracial community study." JAMA. **287**:3230-3237

[18] Engelhart MJ, Geerlings MI, Ruitenberg A et al. (2002) "Dietary intake of antioxidants and risk of Alzheimer disease." JAMA. **287**:3223-3229

[19] Azzi A, Ricciarelli R, Zingg JM. (2002) "Non-antioxidant molecular functions of alpha-tocopherol (vitamin E)." FEBS Lett. **519**:8-10

[20] Asensi M, Sastre J, Pallardo FV, et al. (1999) "Ratio of reduced to oxidized glutathione as indicator of oxidative stress status and DNA damage." Methods Enzymol. **299**:267-76.

[21] Sastre, J., M. Asensi, et al. (1992). "Exhaustive physical exercise causes oxidation of glutathione status in blood: prevention by antioxidant administration." The American Journal of Physiology **263**(2): R992-R995

[22] García de la Asunción, J., A. Millán, et al. (1996). "Mitochondrial glutathione oxidation correlates with age-associated oxidative damage to mitochondrial DNA." FASEB J **10**(2): 333-8.

[23] Esteve JM, Mompo J, Garcia de la Asunción J et al. (1999) "Oxidative damage to mitochondrial DNA and glutathione oxidation in apoptosis: studies in vivo and in vitro." FASEB J **13**(9):1055-64.

[24] Roxborough HE, Burton GW, Kelly FJ. (2000) "Inter- and intra-individual variation in plasma and red blood cell vitamin E after supplementation." Free Radic Res. **33**:437-445

[25] Halliwell B. The antioxidant paradox. (2000) Lancet. **355**: 1179-1180.

Mitogen-Activated Protein Kinase Pathways in Nervous System and Alzheimer Disease

Xiongwei Zhu, Gemma Casadesus, Hyoung-gon Lee, George Perry, Mark A. Smith
Institute of Pathology, Case Western Reserve University, Cleveland, Ohio, USA;

Abstract: Given the fact that mitogen-activated protein kinase (MAPK) pathways play critical roles in regulating almost all cellular processes from gene expression to cell death, and that all three major MAPK pathways, i.e., extracellular signal-regulated kinase (ERK) pathway, c-Jun N-terminal kinase/stress-activated protein kinase (JNK/SAPK) pathway, and p38 pathway, are activated in susceptible neurons in Alzheimer disease, the importance of these pathways in the disease pathogenesis ahs become increasingly recognized. In this review we discuss some salient progress of the role of MAPK in Alzheimer disease after reviewing the general organization and biological function of MAPK pathways.

1. Introduction

Alterations in gene expression and enzyme activity, induced by extracellular stimuli/stress, are mediated through the interplay of multiple signaling pathways. Among these are the highly conserved mitogen-activated protein kinase (MAPK) pathways, which are the central mediators that propagate signals from the membrane to the nucleus. All eukaryotic cells posses multiple MAPK pathways, each of which is preferentially activated by distinct sets of stimuli, to allow cells to respond coordinately/synergistically to multiple divergent inputs. Given that MAPK pathways play important roles in almost all cellular processes in response to a variety of stimuli in both physiological and pathophysiological conditions, specifically in neuronal cells and the nervous system, and that most aspects of cellular function and process are altered in chronic disease conditions of the nervous system such as AD, it is of particular interest and importance to explore what roles MAPKs play in the pathophysiology of AD [1].

2. Components and Organization of MAPK Pathways

MAPKs comprise a group of serine/threonine kinases, which are activated through multiple protein kinases in response to extracellular stimuli by dual phosphorylation at conserved threonine and tyrosine residues [2]. The MAPK module is composed of at least three kinases that establish a sequential activation pathway. The top kinase of the three-kinase module is a MAPK kinase kinase (MKKK). The MKKK are serine/threonine kinases that, when activated, phosphorylate the next kinase in the module, a MAPK kinase (MKK). The MKKs are kinases that recognize and phosphorylate a Thr-X-Tyr motif in the activation loop of MAPK, which define MKK as dual-specificity kinases. MAPKs are the final kinases in the three-kinase module and phosphorylate substrates on serine and threonine residues. The vast majority of defined substrates of MAPKs are transcription factors. However, MAPK can also phosphorylate many other substrates including protein kinases, phospholipases, and cytoskeleton-associated proteins such as τ protein [3].

Based on the sequence similarity, mechanisms of upstream regulation, and to a lesser extent, substrate specificity, MAPK pathways can be divided into several subgroups amongst which extracellular signal regulated kinases (ERK) 1 and 2, c-Jun N-terminal kinase (JNK)/stress-activated protein kinase (SAPK), and p38 are the three best characterized [4].

3. Biological Function of MAPK Pathways

3.1 Gene Expression

One of the most explored functions of the MAPK signaling module is the regulation of gene expression in response to extracellular stimuli [5]. As a matter of fact, the vast majority of MAPK substrates are transcription factors [3]. However, MAPKs not only serve as information highways between the plasma membrane and the nuclear proteins that control gene expression but also amplify and integrate various cell-surface-generated signals to exert a more complex control of gene expression. For example, JNK/SAPK phosphorylates c-Jun and thereby enhances its ability to activate transcription without affecting DNA binding [6]. ERKs 1 and 2 phosphorylate Ets transcription factors such as TCF/Elk1 and CREB that are involved in the induction of *fos* genes, whose products form heterodimers with Jun proteins to form activation protein 1 (AP-1) complexes [5]. Also, ERKs 1 and 2 can phosphorylate cytoplasmic kinase RSK90, which in turn enters the nucleus and phosphorylates c-Fos [7]. The p38 proteins phosphorylate and enhance the activity of MEF2C and related family members, and the MEF2 family of transcription factors have an important role in mediating c-Jun induction by serum [8].

3.2 Proliferation Regulation and Cell Cycle Control

ERKs 1 and 2 are activated by mitogens in all cells and a common view is that they are essential shared elements of mitogenic signaling [2]. For example, expression of constitutively active components of the ERK pathway causes cell transformation [9] and prolonged activation and nuclear retention of ERKs is required for transcription of cyclin D1 [10], suggesting a mechanism for ERK-mediated enhancement of cell cycle entry. JNK/SAPK may also have a role in mitogenic signaling and in T cells, the JNK/SAPK pathway stimulates proliferation by inducing IL-2 expression [11]. Also, several lines of evidence suggest that JNK/SAPK plays an important role in tumor cells [12]. The involvement of p38 in cell growth became apparent when a slower proliferation of cultured mammalian cells was observed after the cells were treated with the p38 inhibitor, SB203580 [13]. Also, p38 activation induced by bFGF is specifically required for the proliferative response to bFGF and p38 can reverse the Rb-mediated repression of E2F1, which is necessary for the expression of many genes that are required for cell cycle progression. Further, p38 is the first kinase outside of the CDK family that is shown to regulate the function of Rb protein *in vivo* [14]. There is also evidence indicating a negative role for p38 in cell proliferation such as inhibition of cyclin D1 [10], which would therefore, inhibit cell cycle progression. Thus, p38 activity likely exerts a positive effect at certain stages of cell cycle and an inhibitory one at others.

3.3 Differentiation

All three MAPK pathways have also been implicated in cell differentiation. For example, sustained ERK activation leads to differentiation of PC12 cells [15] and the p38 pathway is both sufficient and necessary for SKT6 differentiation into haemoglobinised cells [16]. GTPase-deficient Gα16 and Gαq induce persistent JNK/SAPK activation and cause PC12 cell differentiation [17].

3.4 Inflammation

p38 plays an important role in inflammation [18] since the activation of the p38 pathway is essential for the production of pro-inflammatory cytokines such as IL-1β, TNF-α and IL-6, as well as the induction of COX-2, iNOS and adherent proteins such as VCAM-1 and many other inflammatory related molecules. In addition to these, the p38 pathway plays a regulatory role in the proliferation and differentiation of cells of the immune system. In fact, in addition to p38, lipopolysaccharide (LPS) also activates ERK1/2 and JNK/SAPK and all of these components are required for the biosynthesis of TNF-α [19], which suggests that other MAPK pathways may also have a role in the inflammatory response.

3.5 Cell Survival and Cell Death

By and large, activation of ERKs has been linked to cell survival while JNK/SAPK and p38 activation are linked to induction of apoptosis [20]. However, this is an oversimplification and the actual roles of each MAPK pathway are highly cell-type and context dependent.

Activation of the ERK pathway may provide protection against apoptosis in some cell types. In PC-12 cells, withdrawal of NGF led to the inhibition of ERK1/2 and cell death [20], while constitutive activation of ERK1/2 in these cells inhibits apoptosis. Additionally, blockage of ERK1/2 activation prevents protection against TNF-α-induced apoptosis that is mediated by FGF-2 in L929 cells [21]. However, the ERK pathway may be positively involved in cell death as indicated by the observation that ERK activation facilitates apoptosis in activation-induced T cell death [22] and the inhibition of MEK1 activity inhibits Fas-induced apoptosis [23].

A pro-apoptotic function has been established for JNK activation in many cases. Inhibition of JNK/SAPK by introduction of dominant negative mutants of JNK1, its downstream target c-Jun, or its upstream activator MKK4, shows that JNK/SAPK is necessary for apoptosis in the response to growth factor withdrawal, stress, DNA damage, and ligation of Fas on the cell surface [24]. It seems that JNK-induced apoptosis partially depends on the induction of death cytokines, such as the Fas ligand [25], whose promoter contains an AP-1 site, explaining the dependence on c-Jun phosphorylation. However, in some cases, the activation of JNK/SAPK may act to promote survival or growth. The strongest evidence for this is derived from the analysis of compound mutant $jnk1^{-/-}jnk2^{-/-}$ embryos that exhibit increased apoptosis within the developing forebrain [26].

Ample evidence suggests a correlation between the activation of the p38 pathway and apoptosis. Such a correlation is based on the concomitant activation of p38 and apoptosis induced by a variety of factors including NGF withdrawal and Fas ligation [18]. However, additional evidence suggests an opposite role likely also exists since inhibition of p38 activity also inhibits sodium salicylate-induced FS-4 fibroblast apoptosis [27] and TL1-induced bovine pulmonary artery endothelial cell apoptosis [28].

4. ERK Pathway in Nervous System

In brain, strong evidence suggests that ERKs are important components of activity-dependent signaling cascades within neurons and that modulation of their activity may be required for both synaptic plasticity and learning and memory [29]. Activity-dependent changes in neuronal function are predominantly mediated by elevation in intracellular calcium levels, a process in which the Ras-ERK cascade has been widely implicated as a major target for calcium signaling, particularly through stimulation of a specific GEF, RasGRF [30], or via tyrosine kinases such as Src or Pyk2 [31]. *In vivo* studies have demonstrated that multiple diverse stimuli, such as electroconvulsive seizure [32], corticostriatal stimulation [33], circadian rhythmicity [34] and opioid withdrawal [35], can induce selective ERK activation within discrete brain regions, which underscores the importance of ERK signaling in the regulation of neuronal function. Accumulating data have identified a prominent role for ERKs in long-term potentiation (LTP), the molecular mechanism that underlies learning and memory. LTP-inducing stimuli could specifically increase expression of ERK2 and B-Raf in the hippocampus, and ERKs are essential for hippocampal LTP induction [36]. Additional roles for ERKs in dentate gyrus LTP [37] and long-term depression (LTD) [38] in cerebellar purkinje neurons have also been described, which may reflect a requirement of ERK-dependent, CREB-mediated, gene expression [39]. Behavioral studies in rodents provide more compelling and direct evidence for an ERK-dependent role in learning and memory [40, 41], in which behavioral performance was associated with increased ERK activity, and inhibition of ERK signaling specifically impaired learning.

5. ERK Pathway and AD

ERK is activated in a number of pathophysiologically relevant conditions. For example, ERK activation specifically occurs in the rat hippocampus after bicucullin-induced seizures and ischemia [42, 43]. This activation of ERK is NMDA receptor- and calcium influx-dependent. Also, ERK activation plays a direct mechanistic role in 6-OHDA toxicity which may contribute to the dopaminergic neuronal cell death that occurrs in Parkinson disease (PD) [44].

Given that ERKs play a significant role in hippocampus-related learning and memory, it is conceivable that disease conditions, such as AD, which involve the hippocampus and affect learning and memory, involves the ERK pathway. In fact, relevant to AD, strong evidence demonstrated that ERK is activated in AD and activated ERK is found specifically in intracytoplasmic punctuate structures and intracellular NFTs, mainly in a subpopulation of neurons exhibiting early tau deposition [45-47]. The abnormal activation of upstream activators in the ERK pathways, including active Ras, SOS/Grb2, and MEK1/2 [45, 48-50], and downstream effector, S6K [51], are also reported in AD compared to control cases which lends further credence to the notion that the entire pathway is altered in AD. Given that ERK can phosphorylate the τ protein *in vitro* and *in vivo* in a PHF-τ manner [52-55], the colocalization of ERK with phospho-tau demonstrated by immunocytochemical studies and fluorescence resonance energy transfer studies suggest that ERK may play important roles in the phosphorylation of tau in AD [45-47, 56].

It is clearly demonstrated that Aβ is toxic to cultured neurons. Whether Aβ leads to ERK activation and whether ERK activation contributes to Aβ cytotoxicity are not clear. There are some contradictory results concerning the effects of Aβ on the ERK pathway in cultured cells [54, 57-60] which may be due to the relatively high basal level activity of ERK in neuronal cultures and relatively small effect that Aβ may have on the ERK pathway. However, it is reported that increased Aβ levels can lead to ERK activation in a brain slice model and a transgenic mouse model [61, 62]. Therefore, the aberrant activation of the ERK pathway in neurons by physiological levels of Aβ may serve as a molecular basis for the disruption in memory accompanying AD.

Numerous studies showed that the ERK pathway plays an important role in AβPP processing and secretion. The activation of ERK leads to an increased secreted form of AβPP [63, 64] which in turn further activates ERK, forming a positive feed-forward loop [65]. Additional evidence also showed that ApoE and presenilins interact with the ERK pathway [66, 67]. Given the requirement of ERK activation for multiple functions of AD-related proteins and its critical role in learning and memory, the precise control of the ERK pathway is critical. The decline of the regulation on the ERK pathway during aging, as evidenced by the declined responsiveness of ERK to extracellular stimuli, may account for the development of cognitive impairment in AD.

6. JNK/SAPK Pathway in Neuronal Death and Neurodegeneration

Although the expression and activity of JNK/SAPK and JKK proteins under basal conditions [68], and the activation of JNK/SAPKs by non-noxious environmental stimuli [69] strongly argues for a physiological role of JNK/SAPKs in the nervous system, not much is known about the function and activation of JNK/SAPKs under physiological conditions. However, JNK/SAPK may be involved in neuronal regeneration and neuroplasticity [70], since JNK/SAPKs are activated under regenerative conditions in the peripheral nervous system and activated by electroconvulsive seizures, an animal model for neuroplasticity and treatment of depression [71].

There is a great deal of evidence in support of a role for the JNK/SAPK pathway in regulating cell death in neurons. For example, JNK/SAPK is activated in PC12 cells upon NGF withdrawal [20] and, in a dopaminergic cell line, NM9D, 6-hydroxydopamine induces activation of JNK/SAPK and apoptosis [72].

The apoptotic actions of JNK/SAPKs in the adult brain were first demonstrated in JNK3 knockout mice whose hippocampal neurons were protected against excitotoxic death. JNK/SAPK activation is implicated in the processes leading to neuronal death following nerve fiber lesions, ischemia and seizure [73]. Damage of dopaminergic neurons of substantia nigra compacta (SNC) by axon transection in the adult rat brain results in strong activation of JNK/SAPKs and c-Jun phosphorylation that precede and parallel the nigral cell death [74]. JNK1 is activated in cortex and hippocampus of rats that have been treated with kanic acid to induce seizures [75]. Further, CEP-1347, a specific inhibitor of JNK /SAPKpathway, is neuroprotective in a number of *in vivo* models [76]. Therefore, taken together, these studies show that JNK/SAPK is a potent effector of apoptosis and degeneration of neurons *in vitro* and in brain [77].

7. JNK Pathway and AD

In relation to AD, several lines of evidence demonstrated the direct involvement of the JNK/SAPK pathway: JNK/SAPK is activated in degenerating neurons in AD [47, 78-81] and is redistributed, from nuclei to the cytoplasm, in a manner that correlates with the progression of the disease such that phospho-JNK/SAPK is exclusively associated with neurofibrillary alterations in severe AD cases [78]; additionally, c-Jun, downstream of JNK/SAPK is induced and co-localizes with TUNEL labeling [82] and we recently demonstrated that c-Jun is also activated in AD [83]; moreover, Cdc/42/Rac and JKK1, the upstream activators of JNK/SAPK, are also activated in AD [84, 85]. Further, JNK/SAPK can phosphorylate tau protein in a manner similar to that found for tau in AD (PHF-τ) [86-89].

The effect of Aβ on the JNK/SAPK pathway is well explored. Neurons treated with Aβ show increased c-Jun expression [90]; More importantly, JNK/SAPK is activated by Aβ by two-three folds in different neuronal cultures and Aβ-induced JNK/SAPK activation mediates Aβ toxicity [57, 91-93]. These *in vitro* findings are further supported by *in vivo* studies that neurons from c-Jun null mice are resistant to Aβ toxicity [94], that JNK/SAPK activation is localized to amyloid deposits within neurites containing phospho-tau in mice double transgenic for AβPP (K670N/M671L) and PS1 (P264L) [95] and that activation of the JNK/SAPK pathway mediates the effects of Aβ on LTP and cell death in hippocampus *in vivo* [96]. However, the mechanism by which Aβ induces JNK/SAPK activation is largely unanswered but it seems that some oxidative event is involved. JNK/SAPK is also implicated in the modulation of AβPP metabolism since JNK3 induces robust phosphorylation of Thr668 within the carboxy-terminus of AβPP [97], which regulates the function and metabolism of AβPP; Furthermore, JIP1b, the JNK/SAPK scaffolding protein, strongly binds to the cytoplasmic domain of AβPP [98-100]. Although by and large, JNK/SAPK activation is associated with subsequent apoptosis and its activation by Aβ *in vitro* leads to cell death, it may not necessarily lead to cell death *in vivo*. Therefore, its *in vivo* role still needs to be established.

8. p38 in Nervous System and AD

The p38 pathway can be activated by a variety of extracellular stimuli including growth factors such as GM-CSF, FGF, NGF, IGF, VEGF and PDGF, heat shock, cell stretching, pro-inflammatory cytokines and oxidative stress, which can lead to a variety of cellular responses including cell growth, cell cycle, cell death, cell differentiation and inflammation [73]. The role of p38 seems highly cell type and stimuli dependent.

p38 also plays an important role in neurodegeneration in some animal models [73]. For example, the role of the p38 pathway in CNS have beeen explored in studies of ischemia and the mechanisms by which p38 modulates outcome may be attributed to their temporal/spatial and cellular distribution following ischemia [101]. Following bilateral common carotid occlusion with reperfusion in gerbils, p38 is increased as is mitogen-activated protein kinase-activated protein kinase 2 (MAPKAPK-2) activity over 4 days [102]. p38 has also been evaluated over several time points following permanent middle cerebral arteral occlusion and robust expression at 24 hours in the peri-infarct region [103]. The timing of MAPK expression in this study suggests that p38 may be involved in the subsequent cell death that follows ischemia. Inhibition of p38 MAPK has been shown to be neuroprotective following permanent focal stroke in the rat [104].

The role of p38 in AD is not well explored although an increase in the p38 level and activity in AD brain tissue had been described [105, 106]. Both p38 and active p38 are increased and localized to neurofibrillary tangles and senile plaques neurites in AD [105, 106]. Moreover, the immediate upstream activator, MKK6, is also activated and similarly localized in AD [107]. The p38 pathway is primarily activated by cellular stress including oxidative stress [3] which is a prominent feature in AD. The activation of p38 pathway can transducer the oxidative stress signaling leading to the induction of iNOS and HO-1 [108, 109], which are also induced in AD. Therefore we suspect that p38 is likely activated by oxidative stress in AD. Similar to ERK and JNK, p38 is also able to phopshorylate tau protein *in vitro* [110, 111], but whether it is the case *in vivo* is not clear [1]. The effect of Aβ on p38 is controversial in cultured cells with conflicting observation being reported [57, 91, 112] and no conclusive *in vivo* observation is available [1].

Acknowledgement

Work in author's laboratory is supported by NIH (NS38648), Alzheimer's Association (NIRG-02-3923)

References

[1] Zhu, X., et al., The MAPK Pathways in Alzheimer's Disease. NeuroSignals, 2002. 11: p. 270-281.
[2] Robinson, M.J. and M.H. Cobb, Mitogen-activated protein kinase pathways. Curr Opin Cell Biol, 1997. 9(2): p. 180-6.
[3] Kyriakis, J.M. and J. Avruch, Mammalian mitogen-activated protein kinase signal transduction pathways activated by stress and inflammation. Physiol Rev, 2001. 81(2): p. 807-69.
[4] Chang, L. and M. Karin, Mammalian MAP kinase signalling cascades. Nature, 2001. 410(6824): p. 37-40.
[5] Treisman, R., Regulation of transcription by MAP kinase cascades. Curr Opin Cell Biol, 1996. 8(2): p. 205-15.
[6] Kallunki, T., et al., c-Jun can recruit JNK to phosphorylate dimerization partners via specific docking interactions. Cell, 1996. 87(5): p. 929-39.
[7] Frodin, M. and S. Gammeltoft, Role and regulation of 90 kDa ribosomal S6 kinase (RSK) in signal transduction. Mol Cell Endocrinol, 1999. 151(1-2): p. 65-77.
[8] Han, J., et al., Activation of the transcription factor MEF2C by the MAP kinase p38 in inflammation. Nature, 1997. 386(6622): p. 296-9.
[9] Oka, H., et al., Constitutive activation of mitogen-activated protein (MAP) kinases in human renal cell carcinoma. Cancer Res, 1995. 55(18): p. 4182-7.
[10] Lavoie, J.N., et al., Cyclin D1 expression is regulated positively by the p42/p44MAPK and negatively by the p38/HOGMAPK pathway. J Biol Chem, 1996. 271(34): p. 20608-16.
[11] Hsueh, Y.P. and M.Z. Lai, c-Jun N-terminal kinase but not mitogen-activated protein kinase is sensitive to cAMP inhibition in T lymphocytes. J Biol Chem, 1995. 270(30): p. 18094-8.
[12] Xu, X., et al., Constitutively activated JNK is associated with HTLV-1 mediated tumorigenesis. Oncogene, 1996. 13(1): p. 135-42.
[13] Ziegler-Heitbrock, H.W., et al., In vitro desensitization to lipopolysaccharide suppresses tumour necrosis factor, interleukin-1 and interleukin-6 gene expression in a similar fashion. Immunology, 1992. 75(2): p. 264-8.

growth factor (bFGF) [27, 28]. Most of these factors mediate their cellular effects through the activation of the Ras-dependent mitogen-activated protein kinase pathway (MAPK) (Zhu et al., 2002). The small G-protein Ras is a proto-oncogene that is involved in the regulation of the G0/G1 transition of the cell cycle through co-operation with cyclin D1. Not surprisingly, given the early appearance of cell cycle changes, Ras is elevated in very early stage of the disease, preceding both neurofibrillary pathology and the formation of amyloid plaques [29, 30] and co-localizes with cell cycle markers such as $p16^{INK4a}$ suggesting that Ras mediates downstream ectopic mitotic signalling [31]. The findings that Grb2 and SOS-1, upstream activators of Ras-MAPK pathway, are also altered in cases of AD in comparison to age-matched controls not only confirms the involvement of Ras but also further suggests that a signal derived from the cell surface contributes to a stimulus for neurons in AD to re-enter the cell cycle [32]. Importantly, members of MAPK pathway downstream to Ras such as Raf, MEK1/2 and ERK1/2 are all activated in AD compared to control cases [33-36] and like Ras, ERK activation is a very early event [37]. Further, the activation of ERK pathway is linked to alterations that affect cell cycle control such as phosphorylation of c-Myc in AD [38].

4. Genetic Factors and Mitotic Regulation

Genetic-linkage studies have established that mutations in at least three genes, the amyloid-beta precursor protein (AβPP) and the two homologous genes, presenilin 1 and presenilin 2 (PS1 and PS2) are associated with early-onset AD [39]. Although all these mutations inevitably lead to increased Aβ production, the exact mechanism(s) by which mutations in these genes are involved in AD pathogenesis remains elusive. Interestingly, although the precise function of each of these proteins is still unknown; one common feature is that these proteins seem to play a role in cell cycle control.

AβPP is a single-pass membrane protein expressed at the cell surface with a short C-terminal region located in the cytoplasm [40]. The proteolytic processing of this protein gives rise to the Aβ peptide and the soluble N-teminal ectodomain (sAPP). It is notable that in *in vitro* studies, the mitogenic activity of AβPP and its proteolytic fragments (i.e., Aβ peptide and sAβPP) has been demonstrated [10, 41-45]. For example, Aβ promotes the activation of a mitotic cycle in cultured differentiated neurons which even enter the S phase and start the replication of DNA [43], consistent with the *in vivo* finding that DNA is successfully replicated in some of the susceptible neurons in AD [10]. sAPP function as an epithelial growth factor and induces a two- to three-fold increases in the rate of cell proliferation and cell migration [44, 45]. Further, cell surface AβPP possess a neurite-promoting activity, co-localizes with adhesion plaque components and participates in synaptic recycling, suggesting that it can function as a receptor to transduce signals from the extracellular matrix to the interior of the cell [46]. Most interestingly, Fe65 and AβPP-BP1, the presumative adaptor proteins that interact with the C-terminus of AβPP and may transduce the downstream signal, are involved in cell cycle regulation [46-48]: AβPP-BP1 is a cell cycle protein that normally regulates negatively the progression of cells into the S phase and regulates positively into mitosis [46, 47]. Therefore, an overexpression of AβPP-BP1 may push neurons into S phase [46, 47], causing DNA sythesis and aberrant expression of cdc2/cyclin B1, as is observed in susceptible neurons in AD [5]. Strikingly, the other adaptor, Fe65, a nuclear protein, regulates negatively G1 to S phase cell cycle progression by inhibiting the key S phase enzymes, thymidylate synthase (TS) [48]. Therefore, it is conceivable that AβPP may act as a cell surface receptor to

relay cell cycle-related signals. The overexpression or mutation of AβPP may therefore push neurons into an aberrant cell cycle and, in support of this hypotheses, FAD mutants of AβPP have a greater capacity to drive DNA synthesis than expression of wild AβPP [46, 47].

Human presenilin (PS) protein 1 and 2 are approximately 67% homologous. PS1 is required for the proteolytic processing of Notch and AβPP, molecules that play pivotal roles in cell-fate determination during development and AD pathogenesis, respectively. Interestingly, the majority of reports indicate that presenilins are localized to the endoplasmic reticulum (ER) and Golgi, consistent with secondary structure predictions of a multiple trans-membrane protein [49]. However, some reports have indicated that presenilins are localized to the cell surface and also to the centromere and centrosome of dividing cells [50]. The binding of presenilins of centromeres and centrosomes have led to speculations that presenilins are involved in chromosome segregation and cell division. Notably, by BrdU labelling studies of transfected HeLa cells, it has been shown that the overexpression of both PS1 and PS2 proteins resulted in G1 phase arrest of the cell cycle [51, 52] which may be due to the decrease in Cdk4 activity and retinoblastoma tumor suppressor protein phosphorylation that correlated with decreased levels of β-catenin and cyclin D1 [53]. Overexpression of FAD PS1/2 mutants further increase cell cycle arrest compared to wild-type PS1/2 and the degree to which the different FAD PS1 mutants inhibited cell cycle progression correlates somewhat with the age of AD onset induced by the mutations in carrier [52]. Conversely, PS1 deficiency results in accumulation of cytosolic β-catenin, leading to a β-catenin/lymphoid enhancer factor-1 (LEF)-dependent increase in cyclin D1 transcription and accelerated entry into the S phase of the cell cycle in keratinocytes [54]. Consistent with a key role in cell cycle control, PS1 knockout mice that are rescued through neuronal expression of human PS1 transgene develop spontaneous cancers [55]. Furthermore, impaired cell cycle control of neuronal precursor cells in the neocortical primordium with significantly prolonged length of S-phase is demonstrated in PS1-deficient mice [56]. These compelling evidence suggest that PS1/2 play an important role in cell cycle control.

5. Conclusion

While it is clear that mitotic apparatus are altered in degenerating neurons in AD, whether these cells trigger cell death by re-entering cell cycle or whether these are simply epiphenomena when cells die is still under debate. However, given that alterations in mitotic apparatus and signalling are very early event in the disease process, and that both AβPP and PS1/2 are cell cycle regulators, the former may be the case. The next important question is why neurons die if they attempt to re-enter cell cycle. One possibility is that they may lack the ability to complete a full and successful cell cycle due to their unique features such as lifetime accumulation of unrepaired lesions in the silent genes [57]. An alternative explanation is that the re-sensitization of the cell cycle apparatus in these permanently differentiated cells may require so much adaptation potential which renders these cells extremely vulnerable to other insults such as oxidative damage [37]. For example, overexpression or mutation of AβPP or PS 1/2 that may push neurons into an aberrant cell cycle [46, 47, 52] also significantly enhanced neuronal vulnerability to hydrogen peroxide [58-61], reduction of trophic factors [62, 63], UV irradiation, and staurosporine [60, 64]. Whatever the mechanism, targeting aberrant mitotic control offers a novel therapeutic avenue for this disease.

Acknowledgement

Work in author's laboratory is supported by NIH (NS38648), Alzheimer's Association (NIRG-02-3923)

References

[1] Grana, X. and E.P. Reddy, Cell cycle control in mammalian cells: role of cyclins, cyclin dependent kinases (CDKs), growth suppressor genes and cyclin-dependent kinase inhibitors (CKIs). Oncogene, 1995. 11: p. 211-219.
[2] Sherr, C.J., G1 phase progression: cycling on cue. Cell, 1994. 79(4): p. 551-5.
[3] Meikrantz, W. and R. Schlegel, Apoptosis and the cell cycle. J Cell Biochem, 1995. 58(2): p. 160-74.
[4] Raina, A.K., et al., Cyclin' toward dementia: cell cycle abnormalities and abortive oncogenesis in Alzheimer disease. J Neurosci Res, 2000. 61(2): p. 128-33.
[5] Zhu, X., A.K. Raina, and M.A. Smith, Cell cycle events in neurons. Proliferation or death? Am J Pathol, 1999. 155(2): p. 327-9.
[6] McShea, A., et al., Abnormal expression of the cell cycle regulators P16 and CDK4 in Alzheimer's disease. Am J Pathol, 1997. 150(6): p. 1933-9.
[7] Nagy, Z., M.M. Esiri, and A.D. Smith, Expression of cell division markers in the hippocampus in Alzheimer's disease and other neurodegenerative conditions. Acta Neuropathol (Berl), 1997. 93(3): p. 294-300.
[8] Nagy, Z., et al., Cell cycle markers in the hippocampus in Alzheimer's disease. Acta Neuropathol (Berl), 1997. 94(1): p. 6-15.
[9] Smith, T.W. and C.F. Lippa, Ki-67 immunoreactivity in Alzheimer's disease and other neurodegenerative disorders. J Neuropathol Exp Neurol, 1995. 54(3): p. 297-303.
[10] Yang, Y., D.S. Geldmacher, and K. Herrup, DNA replication precedes neuronal cell death in Alzheimer's disease. J Neurosci, 2001. 21(8): p. 2661-8.
[11] Vincent, I., et al., Aberrant expression of mitotic cdc2/cyclin B1 kinase in degenerating neurons of Alzheimer's disease brain. J Neurosci, 1997. 17(10): p. 3588-98.
[12] Ogawa, O., et al., Ectopic localization of phosphorylated histone H3 in Alzheimer's disease: a mitotic catastrophe? Acta Neuropathol (Berl), 2003. 105(5): p. 524-8.
[13] Busser, J., D.S. Geldmacher, and K. Herrup, Ectopic cell cycle proteins predict the sites of neuronal cell death in Alzheimer's disease brain. J Neurosci, 1998. 18(8): p. 2801-7.
[14] McShea, A., et al., Abnormal expression of the cell cycle regulators P16 and CDK4 in Alzheimer's disease. Am J Pathol, 1997. 150(6): p. 1933-9.
[15] Zhu, X., et al., Neuronal CDK7 in hippocampus is related to aging and Alzheimer disease. Neurobiol Aging, 2000. 21(6): p. 807-13.
[16] Vincent, I., et al., Mitotic phosphoepitopes precede paired helical filaments in Alzheimer's disease. Neurobiol Aging, 1998. 19(4): p. 287-96.
[17] Connor, B., et al., Trk receptor alterations in Alzheimer's disease. Brain Res Mol Brain Res, 1996. 42(1): p. 1-17.
[18] Crutcher, K.A., et al., Detection of NGF-like activity in human brain tissue: increased levels in Alzheimer's disease. J Neurosci, 1993. 13(6): p. 2540-50.
[19] Allen, S.J., et al., Normal beta-NGF content in Alzheimer's disease cerebral cortex and hippocampus. Neurosci Lett, 1991. 131(1): p. 135-9.
[20] Bowen, R.L., et al., Elevated luteinizing hormone expression colocalizes with neurons vulnerable to Alzheimer's disease pathology. J Neurosci Res, 2002. 70(3): p. 514-8.
[21] Birecree, E., et al., Immunoreactive epidermal growth factor receptors in neuritic plaques from patients with Alzheimer's disease. J Neuropathol Exp Neurol, 1988. 47(5): p. 549-60.
[22] Styren, S.D., et al., Epidermal growth factor receptor expression in demented and aged human brain. Brain Res, 1990. 512(2): p. 347-52.
[23] Masliah, E., et al., PDGF is associated with neuronal and glial alterations of Alzheimer's disease. Neurobiol Aging, 1995. 16(4): p. 549-56.
[24] Fenton, H., et al., Hepatocyte growth factor (HGF/SF) in Alzheimer's disease. Brain Res, 1998. 779(1-2): p. 262-70.

[25] Connor, B., et al., Insulin-like growth factor-I (IGF-I) immunoreactivity in the Alzheimer's disease temporal cortex and hippocampus. Brain Res Mol Brain Res, 1997. 49(1-2): p. 283-90.

[26] Tham, A., et al., Insulin-like growth factors and insulin-like growth factor binding proteins in cerebrospinal fluid and serum of patients with dementia of the Alzheimer type. J Neural Transm Park Dis Dement Sect, 1993. 5(3): p. 165-76.

[27] Stopa, E.G., et al., Basic fibroblast growth factor in Alzheimer's disease. Biochem Biophys Res Commun, 1990. 171(2): p. 690-6.

[28] Gomez-Pinilla, F., B.J. Cummings, and C.W. Cotman, Induction of basic fibroblast growth factor in Alzheimer's disease pathology. Neuroreport, 1990. 1(3-4): p. 211-4.

[29] Gartner, U., et al., Induction of p21ras in Alzheimer pathology. Neuroreport, 1995. 6(10): p. 1441-4.

[30] Gartner, U., M. Holzer, and T. Arendt, Elevated expression of p21ras is an early event in Alzheimer's disease and precedes neurofibrillary degeneration. Neuroscience, 1999. 91(1): p. 1-5.

[31] Luth, H.J., et al., Aberrant expression of nNOS in pyramidal neurons in Alzheimer's disease is highly co-localized with p21ras and p16INK4a. Brain Res, 2000. 852(1): p. 45-55.

[32] McShea, A., et al., Signal transduction abnormalities in Alzheimer's disease: evidence of a pathogenic stimuli. Brain Res, 1999. 815(2): p. 237-42.

[33] Zhu, X., et al., Distribution, levels, and activation of MEK1 in Alzheimer's disease. J Neurochem, 2003. 86(1): p. 136-42.

[34] Ferrer, I., et al., Phosphorylated map kinase (ERK1, ERK2) expression is associated with early tau deposition in neurones and glial cells, but not with increased nuclear DNA vulnerability and cell death, in Alzheimer disease, Pick's disease, progressive supranuclear palsy and corticobasal degeneration. Brain Pathol, 2001. 11(2): p. 144-58.

[35] Pei, J.J., et al., Up-regulation of mitogen-activated protein kinases ERK1/2 and MEK1/2 is associated with the progression of neurofibrillary degeneration in Alzheimer's disease. Brain Res Mol Brain Res, 2002. 109(1-2): p. 45-55.

[36] Perry, G., et al., Amyloid precursor protein in senile plaques of Alzheimer disease. Lancet, 1988. 2(8613): p. 746.

[37] Zhu, X., et al., Differential activation of neuronal ERK, JNK/SAPK and p38 in Alzheimer disease: the 'two hit' hypothesis. Mech Ageing Dev, 2001. 123(1): p. 39-46.

[38] Ferrer, I., et al., Phosphorylated c-MYC expression in Alzheimer disease, Pick's disease, progressive supranuclear palsy and corticobasal degeneration. Neuropathol Appl Neurobiol, 2001. 27(5): p. 343-51.

[39] Hardy, J., Amyloid, the presenilins and Alzheimer's disease. Trends Neurosci, 1997. 20(4): p. 154-9.

[40] Selkoe, D.J., Amyloid beta-protein and the genetics of Alzheimer's disease. J Biol Chem, 1996. 271(31): p. 18295-8.

[41] Schubert, D., et al., Amyloid beta protein precursor is a mitogen. Biochem Biophys Res Commun, 1989. 162(1): p. 83-8.

[42] Milward, E.A., et al., The amyloid protein precursor of Alzheimer's disease is a mediator of the effects of nerve growth factor on neurite outgrowth. Neuron, 1992. 9(1): p. 129-37.

[43] Copani, A., et al., Mitotic signaling by beta-amyloid causes neuronal death. Faseb J, 1999. 13(15): p. 2225-34.

[44] Hoffmann, J., et al., A possible role for the Alzheimer amyloid precursor protein in the regulation of epidermal basal cell proliferation. Eur J Cell Biol, 2000. 79(12): p. 905-14.

[45] Schmitz, A., et al., The biological role of the Alzheimer amyloid precursor protein in epithelial cells. Histochem Cell Biol, 2002. 117(2): p. 171-80.

[46] Neve, R.L., D.L. McPhie, and Y. Chen, Alzheimer's disease: a dysfunction of the amyloid precursor protein(1). Brain Res, 2000. 886(1-2): p. 54-66.

[47] Chen, Y., et al., The amyloid precursor protein-binding protein APP-BP1 drives the cell cycle through the S-M checkpoint and causes apoptosis in neurons. J Biol Chem, 2000. 275(12): p. 8929-35.

[48] Bruni, P., et al., Fe65, a ligand of the Alzheimer's beta-amyloid precursor protein, blocks cell cycle progression by down-regulating thymidylate synthase expression. J Biol Chem, 2002. 277(38): p. 35481-8.

[49] Kovacs, D.M., et al., Alzheimer-associated presenilins 1 and 2: neuronal expression in brain and localization to intracellular membranes in mammalian cells. Nat Med, 1996. 2(2): p. 224-9.

[50] Dewji, N.N. and S.J. Singer, Cell surface expression of the Alzheimer disease-related presenilin proteins. Proc Natl Acad Sci U S A, 1997. 94(18): p. 9926-31.

[51] Janicki, S.M. and M.J. Monteiro, Presenilin overexpression arrests cells in the G1 phase of the cell cycle. Arrest potentiated by the Alzheimer's disease PS2(N141I)mutant. Am J Pathol, 1999. 155(1): p. 135-44.

[52] Janicki, S.M., S.M. Stabler, and M.J. Monteiro, Familial Alzheimer's disease presenilin-1 mutants potentiate cell cycle arrest. Neurobiol Aging, 2000. 21(6): p. 829-36.
[53] Prat, M.I., et al., Presenilin 1 overexpressions in Chinese hamster ovary (CHO) cells decreases the phosphorylation of retinoblastoma protein: relevance for neurodegeneration. Neurosci Lett, 2002. 326(1): p. 9-12.
[54] Soriano, S., et al., Presenilin 1 negatively regulates beta-catenin/T cell factor/lymphoid enhancer factor-1 signaling independently of beta-amyloid precursor protein and notch processing. J Cell Biol, 2001. 152(4): p. 785-94.
[55] Xia, X., et al., Loss of presenilin 1 is associated with enhanced beta-catenin signaling and skin tumorigenesis. Proc Natl Acad Sci U S A, 2001. 98(19): p. 10863-8.
[56] Yuasa, S., et al., Impaired cell cycle control of neuronal precursor cells in the neocortical primordium of presenilin-1-deficient mice. J Neurosci Res, 2002. 70(3): p. 501-13.
[57] Nouspikel, T. and P.C. Hanawalt, When parsimony backfires: neglecting DNA repair may doom neurons in Alzheimer's disease. Bioessays, 2003. 25(2): p. 168-73.
[58] Marques, C.A., et al., Neurotoxic mechanisms caused by the alzheimer's disease-linked swedish APP mutation: Oxidative stress, caspases and JNK pathway. J Biol Chem, 2003.
[59] Eckert, A., et al., Elevated vulnerability to oxidative stress-induced cell death and activation of caspase-3 by the Swedish amyloid precursor protein mutation. J Neurosci Res, 2001. 64(2): p. 183-92.
[60] Deng, G., C.J. Pike, and C.W. Cotman, Alzheimer-associated presenilin-2 confers increased sensitivity to apoptosis in PC12 cells. FEBS Lett, 1996. 397(1): p. 50-4.
[61] Nakajima, M., et al., Deficiency of presenilin-1 increases calcium-dependent vulnerability of neurons to oxidative stress in vitro. J Neurochem, 2001. 78(4): p. 807-14.
[62] Leutz, S., et al., Reduction of trophic support enhances apoptosis in PC12 cells expressing Alzheimer's APP mutation and sensitizes cells to staurosporine-induced cell death. J Mol Neurosci, 2002. 18(3): p. 189-201.
[63] Guo, Q., et al., Alzheimer's PS-1 mutation perturbs calcium homeostasis and sensitizes PC12 cells to death induced by amyloid beta-peptide. Neuroreport, 1996. 8(1): p. 379-83.
[64] Xu, X., et al., Wild-type but not Alzheimer-mutant amyloid precursor protein confers resistance against p53-mediated apoptosis. Proc Natl Acad Sci U S A, 1999. 96(13): p. 7547-52.

Frontiers in Neurodegenerative Disorders and Aging:
Fundamental Aspects, Clinical Perspectives and New Insights
T. Özben and M. Chevion (Eds.)
IOS Press, 2004

Putative Mechanisms of Apoptosis Related to Redox Unbalance

Luisa Rossi, Katia Aquilano, Giuseppe Filomeni, Marco F. Lombardol, Giuseppe Rotilio and Maria R. Ciriolo
Department of Biology, University of Rome "Tor Vergata"
Via della Ricerca Scientifica 1, 00133, Rome, Italy. rotilio@bio.uniroma2.it

Abstract: Intracellular redox state unbalance is responsible for induction of apoptosis triggered by several stimuli. In fact, many signal transducers and executors of apoptosis are redox-sensitive. In this chapter the mechanisms by which oxidants such as ROS, RNS, sulfhydryl-reactive compounds and redox metals induce apoptosis through activation of redox-signalling pathways are outlined. Moreover, the involvement of these processes in some pathological conditions is also pointed out.

1. Apoptosis: An active mode of programmed death

Rotilio, G.

Apoptosis is a morphologically distinct form of cell death that is designed to rapidly remove unwanted and potentially dangerous cells. During development, apoptosis plays a key role in removing surplus cells of the developing embryo. In addition, the inappropriate regulation of apoptosis is associated with a variety of diseases including cancer, AIDS, neurodegenerative diseases and ischemic stroke [1].

Apoptosis is characterized by an ordered sequence of events that can be roughly summarized in:

1. Induction by a chemical or physical stimulus.
2. Activation of the cell-suicide program through induction of gene transcription and death-related protein activities.
3. Removal of apoptotic cell through macrophages or neighbouring cell phagocytic-activity without inflammation.

These events comprise many other biochemical processes including changes in calcium and pH homeostasis, translocation and activation of several proteins, induction of phosphorylative process and alteration of cellular structures. Moreover, various and several are the effectors of these events, which represent the molecular basis of apoptosis, while specific pathways of induction are dependent on cell type, nature of stimulus and availability of peculiar molecular factors.

During the past decade, rapid progress has been made in identifying some of the molecules that are responsible for the regulation and execution of apoptosis. The existence of a cell-suicide program was originally proposed on the basis of the typical and common morphological changes characterizing apoptotic cell (plasma membrane blebs, cell shrinkage, chromatin condensation, protein aggregates and apoptotic bodies formation). From these studies emerged the importance of an unusual class of proteases, termed caspases (cysteine proteases that specifically cleave at an aspartate residue) [2]. Caspases function in apoptosis and/or cytokine processing. Among the 14 different classes that have been discovered so far, caspase-3, -6, and -7 (*executers*) are directly involved in proteolysis of cellular macromolecules leading to cell death, whereas caspase-2, -8, -9, and -10 (*initiators*) are fundamental in the commitment of apoptosis, as they activate executer caspases. The remaining classes are involved in inflammatory response.

To date, at least three distinct pathways of induction of apoptosis have been characterized (Figure 1).

The first is that induced by T killer lymphocytes on tumoral or viral-infected cells. In this case, the apoptotic process is associated with perforin-mediated membrane alteration and granzyme B activation, which leads to direct activation of caspases [1].

The second apoptotic pathway is triggered by chemical and physical stresses including UV and γ radiations, growth factors withdrawal, hypoxic conditions and pro-oxidant agents. In this case p53, the "guardian of genome", is the most important protein in cell response. p53 regulates the activation of gene transcription following DNA damage [3]. It induces protein repair by increasing heat shock proteins (Hsps), modulates cell cycle progression by p21, the inhibitor of cyclin-dependent kinases. This factor is able to induce cell cycle arrest, which can be followed either by the recovery of cell division – when DNA damaged is repaired – or by the induction of caspase-dependent apoptosis – when damage becomes irreversible. p53-dependent apoptotic pathway leads to a characteristic cascade of events with the involvement of mitochondria-sited proteins.

The last apoptotic pathway is that mediated by the so-called "death receptors" including tumour necrosis factor (TNF), Fas (APO1/CD95) and TNF-related apoptosis inducing ligand (TRAIL) [4]. These receptors are transmembrane proteins that, upon extracellular ligand binding, are able to trimerize and to recruit adaptor proteins and caspases-8 in the intracellular domain. Pro-caspases-8 and the death effector domain of intermediate adaptor proteins form a complex at the receptor site called the death inducing signal complex (DISC), which finally leads to caspases-8 auto-cleavage and activation.

1.1 The intrinsic death signal: the "mitochondrial pathway"

Recently, our understanding of how mammals regulate caspases activation has improved by the evidence of an alternative route involving mitochondria (Figure 1). In this pathway, cellular stresses including DNA damage, heat shock and oxidative stress result in caspases activation through the release of caspases-activating factors from the mitochondrial intermembrane space. Several evidences have suggested that cytochrome *c* can be released from the intermembrane space into the cytosol where it drives the assembly of a high-molecular weight caspases-activating complex termed *apoptosome* [5]. For the complete formation of the apoptosome, ATP (or dATP), cytochrome *c*, pro-caspase-9, and Apaf-1 (Apoptotic Protease Activating Factor 1) are needed. Binding of cytochrome *c* to Apaf-1 promotes oligomeritation of the latter and recruitment of pro-caspases-9 into a multimeric Apaf-1/pro-caspase-9 complex that results in caspases-9 activation.

To activate Apaf-1 and realize its death-promoting activity cytochrome *c* must leave mitochondria and enter the cytosol. The most important event associated with apoptosis is uncoupling of the mitochondrial oxidative phosphorylation that gives rise to the loss of transmembrane mitochondrial potential ($\Delta\Psi_m$), a decrease in ATP formation, and an increase in ROS production [6]. This has been often associated with the opening of mitochondrial permeability transition (PT) pore or megachannel, thus suggesting that during apoptosis, the release of cytochrome *c* might occur via this route. Recent studies showed that PT depends on the opening of a multimolecular pore named Mithocondrial permeability transition pore (MPTP) [7]. MPTP is localized as a join multi-protein complex between the two mitochondrial membranes. The voltage-dependent anion channel (VDAC) and the adenine nucleotide translocator (ANT) represent the nucleus of the pore structure and are sited at the external and internal mitochondrial membranes respectively. Both proteins possess a vital role for the cell: VDAC guarantees a free passage of low molecular weight compounds to the cytoplasm, whereas ANT transports ATP outside of the matrix exchanging it with cytosolic-produced ADP. However, the ability of mitochondria to maintain transmembrane potential during the initial stages of cytochrome *c* release argues that this phenomenon does not require PT opening. Instead, it suggests a specific permeabilization of the outer mitochondrial membrane. In this regard, a growing body of evidence now suggests that members of the Bcl-X_L family play a key role in promoting cytochrome *c* release upon different apoptotic stimuli [8].

Bcl-2 represents the most studied negative regulator of apoptosis of the Bcl-X_L superfamily; it is a 26-kDa protein firstly characterized in transformed B lymphocytes, where its overexpression was associated with protection against cell death mediated by different stimuli. However, Bcl-2 is only one of the numerous members of related proteins, some of which prevent apoptosis (such as BclX_L and Bcl-2 itself), whereas others induce cell death (such as Bax and Bid). Owing to their high homology, these proteins can form homo- or hetero-dimers; thus, the final decision between death and survival depends on the relative concentration of the two classes of proteins within the cell. Particularly in vertebrates, the pro-apoptotic member Bax freely inserts into the mitochondrial outer membrane and, by conformational rearrangement, forms homopolymers that have the capacity to generate pores in mitochondrial membranes [9]. However, it remains to be demonstrated whether apoptosis-associated cytochrome *c* release occurs via Bax-associated pores.

Once the apoptosome is assembled, cell is not yet committed to death, in fact, bacterial proteins, IAPs (inhibitor of apoptosis proteins), have been found to inhibit programmed cell death downstream apoptosome assembly, and recently a mammalian cytosolic isoform has also been characterized [10]. IAPs seem to directly inhibit initiator and executor caspases, not allowing apoptosis to proceed. In addition, heat shock proteins (Hsps) have recently been found to negatively interact within the apoptotic machinery. The capability of Hsp70 to interact and recruit Apafl, and of Hsp27 to bind cytochrome *c*, in order to prevent apoptosome oligomerization, have been demonstrated [11, 12]; furthermore, it has been suggested that also Hsp90 can inhibit apoptosome formation even if mechanisms through which it could act remain still unclear. Although the cell is equipped with a variety of molecular factors that counteract the apoptotic program, this process still occurs. Several hypotheses are suggested in order to explain this phenomenon, among which the best understood refocuses attention on mitochondria. A novel pro-apoptotic mitochondrial protein, Smac (the second mitochondria-derived activator of caspases), or its murine homologue DIABLO (direct IAP-binding protein with low pI), has been described to be released from mitochondria during apoptosis and appears to act by neutralizing IAPs function [9]. This leads to a multistep process in which the result of the interaction between cytosolic (IAPs) and mitochondrial (Smac/DIABLO and cytochrome *c*) proteins on caspases activation can induce or inhibit apoptosis.

A novel molecular process, which might connect the receptor- and the mitochondrial-mediated pathways, has been discovered [13]. Bid, a pro-apoptotic member of the Bcl-X_L superfamily, is a small protein that functions downstream of activation of death receptors upon its proteolytic cleavage mediated by caspase-8. The active truncated form of Bid (t-Bid) translocates to the mitochondrial membrane where it can induce the oligomerization of Bax. The latter event might promote the release of cytochrome *c* into the cytosol and the activation of caspase-9.

Besides the caspase-dependent apoptosis, mitochondria seem to play a central role also in the caspase-independent process [14]. AIF (apoptosis inducing factor) and endonuclease G are proteins that are released into the cytosol upon apoptogenic stimuli, but in contrast to cytochrome *c* and Smac/DIABLO, they do not trigger activation of caspases. The flavoprotein AIF shows the capability to induce DNA condensation by translocating into the nucleus; however, its action seems to involve also a mitochondria-dependent response by the induction of cytochrome c release. On the other hand, endonuclease G is a protein physiologically involved in the replication of mitochondrial DNA, which, upon apoptogenic stimulus, is translocated into the nucleus and activates DNA fragmentation.

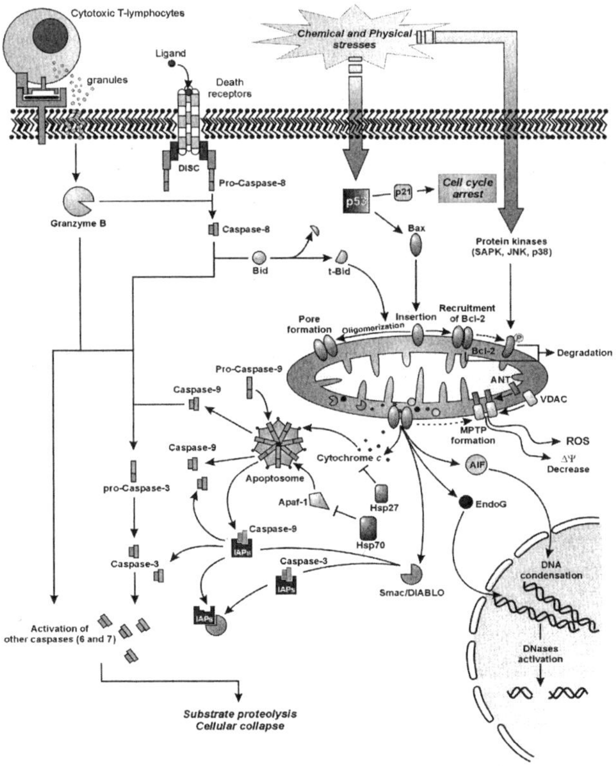

Figure1. Extrinsic and intrinsic pathways characterizing apoptosis

2. Reactive oxygen and nitrogen species in pathophysiological events

Aquilano, K. and Ciriolo, M.R.

In the past two decades, research in the field of free radicals and oxidative stress has exponentially raised. The intensity of research in this area is documented by a large amount of publications and by the evidence that researchers are continuously approaching this study. This phenomenon may be the result of the recent widely accepted knowledge that free radicals are not only dangerous species but, at low concentration, have been designed by evolution to participate in the maintenance of cellular homeostasis. This notion derives from the evidence that cells constantly generate free radicals both as waste products of aerobic metabolism and in response to a large variety of stimuli. Once produced free radicals could lead to activation/inhibition of redox-regulated transcription factors that in turn stimulate/abrogate the expression of genes involved in several cell functions. Nevertheless, free radicals and other reactive species have been traditionally considered as toxic molecules able to induce a random oxidative damage. Growing evidence suggests that in many instances the production of radical species is tightly regulated and their downstream targets very specific. This concept was finely demonstrated with the discovery of Moncada and co-workers that the free radical nitric oxide (NO) was the "endothelium derived relaxing factor" [15]. NO was found to be synthesized in a very controlled fashion and it was even found to bind haemoglobin and soluble guanylate cyclase as part of a previously unknown vasoregulatory mechanism [16]. Moreover, being NO a gaseous molecule, the mechanism through which it exerts its physiological action is peculiar and is quite different from that of other messengers. Due to the high diffusibility and permeability, NO is not transported through membrane carriers or pores and, on the basis of its chemistry, it can exert its function without interacting with intra- or extra-cellular receptors. At physiological concentrations, NO is actually implicated in several processes including fecundation [17], embriogenesis [18], modulation of neurotrasmission [19], vasodilatation [20], inflammatory response [21]. Moreover, it is considered a molecule that can protect some cells from apoptosis induced by many different types of stimuli [22]. These findings were greatly surprising and largely gave new emphasis on the studies of possible physiological roles of other reactive molecules in cellular signal transduction. Actually, studies of the past few years have demonstrated that reactive oxygen and nitrogen species (ROS and RNS) actively participate in several cell-signalling pathways as physiological "second messengers" in cell growth and differentiation.

2.1 Sources of reactive oxygen and nitrogen species

Among radicals, those derived from O_2 are the most frequent reactive species to be physiologically produced. Due to the triplet ground state, O_2 is preferentially reduced by subsequent monoelectronic addition resulting in intermediate reactive oxygen species (ROS) such as superoxide radical ($O_2^{\cdot-}$), hydrogen peroxide (H_2O_2) and hydroxyl radical ($OH^{\cdot}$). The major physiological sources of ROS, is represented by mitochondria during the phosphorylative process, where O_2 is reduced to H_2O by cytochrome *c* oxidase. This enzyme retains all partially reduced intermediates until full reduction is achieved; thus, production of ROS through reduction of O_2 at the level of cytochrome *c* oxidase is practically absent. Nevertheless, about 2% of electrons carried by the mitochondrial electron transport chain can escape from this pathway and pass directly to O_2, generating $O_2^{\cdot-}$. Oxidative phosphorylation in mitochondria depends on four electron transporting complexes (I-IV) and one H^+-translocating ATP synthase complex. Two of these complexes were shown to be responsible for the majority of the $O_2^{\cdot -}$ generated by mitochondria probably by a non enzymatic mechanism: complex I, the NADH-ubiquinone oxidoreductase, and complex III, the ubiquinol-cytochrome c oxidoreductase [23]. Ubisemiquinone species (UQ_{10}) generated in the course of electron transport reactions donate electrons to O_2 and provide a constant source of $O_2^{\cdot -}$:

$$UQ_{10}^{\cdot -} + O_2 \rightarrow O_2^{\cdot -} + UQ_{10}$$

Other minor but not less important sources of ROS exist intracellularly that include a variety of cellular enzymes. Among these, NADPH oxidase is a multicomponent enzyme, which represents one of the most abundant sources of ROS in phagocytes [24]. In non-stimulated cells, its components are in different subcellular compartments with the flavocytochrome subunits, $gp91^{phox}$ and $gp22^{phox}$ in the plasma membrane and the $p47^{phox}$/ $p67^{phox}$ /$p40^{phox}$ subunits in the cytosol as a complex. Upon phagocytosis or stimulation with soluble agents, the cytosolic components and the small GTPase Rac1/Rac2 translocate to the plasma membrane to bind the flavocytochrome, which is the final oxidase, transferring one electron from NADPH to oxygen to form $O_2^{\cdot -}$. The formation of ROS by non-phagocytic cells also involves membrane-localized NADPH oxidases. In fact, *phox* components have been identified in several cell types such as smooth muscle cells, fibroblasts, and endothelial cells [25]. Sources of ROS are also several flavin- and metal-containing enzymes that use O_2 as a substrate including xantine oxidase, monoamino- and amino-acid oxidases and cycloxygenase [26].

NO is formed endogenously by a family of NADPH-dependent enzymes, the nitric oxide synthases (NOSs). Three quite distinct isoforms of NOS have been identified: nNOS (also known as Type I, NOS-I or NOS-1) being the isoform first found (and predominating) in neuronal tissue; iNOS (also known as Type II, NOS-II or NOS-2) being the isoform which is inducible in a wide range of cells and tissues; eNOS (also known as Type III, NOS-III or NOS-3) being the isoform first found in vascular endothelial cells. They are products of different genes, with different localization, regulation, catalytic properties and inhibitor sensitivity. These isoforms have also been differentiated because of their constitutive (eNOS and nNOS) in opposition to inducible (iNOS) expression. All NOS isoforms function as homodimers and catalyze a two-step oxidation of the amino acid L-arginine to citrulline and NO *via* the intermediate compound N-hydroxy-L-arginine (Figure 2).

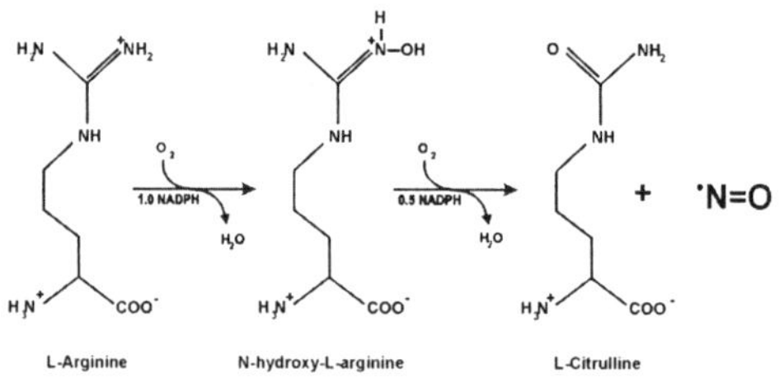

Figure 2. Synthesis of NO by nitric oxide synthases

NOSs monomers exhibit a bidomain structure in which an N-terminal oxygenase domain containing binding sites for haem, tetrahydrobiopterin and L-arginine is linked by a calmodulin-recognition site to a C-terminal reductase domain that contains binding sites for FAD, FMN and NADPH. Activation of NOSs may occur upon different stimuli and requires the binding of BH_4, FAD, FMN and haem [27]. Once produced, NO can exist in different chemical forms ($NO^{\cdot}$, NO^- and NO^+) and thus has a wide-ranging degree of chemical reactivity and functions in a variety of different biological roles [28].

2.2 ROS- and RNS-mediated cell damage

Being highly reactive ROS and RNS can interact in a non-specific way with a wide range of macromolecules including proteins, carbohydrates, lipids and DNA thus leading to the alteration and impairment of function of all cellular components (Figure 3).

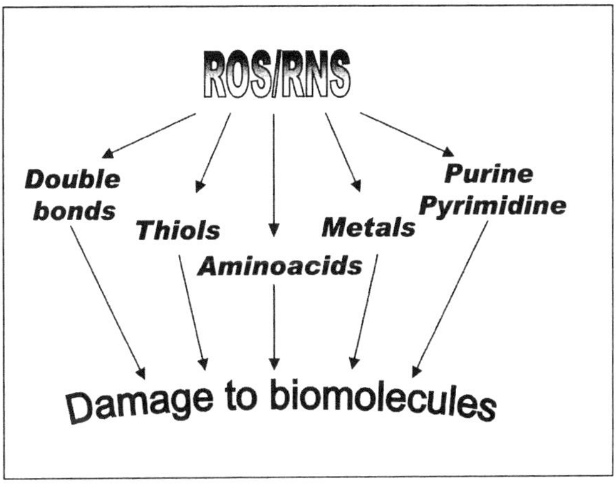

Figure 3. Biochemical targets of ROS and RNS

Free radicals cause DNA lesions, which have been shown to be both cytotoxic and mutagenic and appear to be responsible for substantial mutational load inside the cell. In fact, it has been estimated that 10,000 oxidative DNA lesions are produced per human genome per cell per day [29]. In particular, ROS can alter the purine and pyrimidine bases and the deoxyribose sugar, and cleave the phosphodiester DNA backbone. A number of stable products derive from DNA lesions including stable oxidized bases such as 8-oxoguanine, 8-oxoadenine, cytosine glycole and thymine glycole which are the most important because they can lead to biological consequences. DNA damages produced by free radical attack are repaired by the ubiquitous DNA repair process called base excision repair that include: i) DNA N-glycosylases that recognize damaged purines and pyrimidines; ii) 5' apurinic endonucleases that process strand breaks and sites of base loss; iii) DNA polimerases and iv) DNA ligases [30]. If the lesion is readily repaired, but an incorrect or non-cognate base is inserted, the lesion is potentially mutagenic. On the other hand, if the lesion blocks DNA polymerase, owing to failure in hydrogen bond or to the induced distortion of DNA helix, it is potentially lethal. In fact, when lesions persist in DNA, they can cause a multitude of cellular problems including arrest or induction of transcription, activation of specific signal transduction pathways, replication errors, and genomic instability. These molecular changes are observed in both cancer and aging supporting the notion that persistent DNA damage in the genome might be causative of these conditions.

Reactions of free radicals with proteins result in the oxidation of various amino acid side chains, often leading to a loss of protein function. The sulfur-containing amino acids cysteine and methionine are highly susceptible to oxidative damage. Methionine is easily oxidized to methionine sulfoxide [31], while oxidation of sulfhydryl groups of cysteine residues often results in the formation of intra- or intermolecular disulfide bridges [32]. Both these modifications can be reversed by the enzymes methionine sulfoxide reductase and protein disulfide isomerases, which reverse the formation of non-native disulfide bridges. Oxidation of aromatic amino acids can give rise to various hydroxyl derivatives, while that of some other amino acids such as lysine, arginine, proline, or threonine residues may yield carbonyl derivatives. In addition to modification of amino acid side chains, oxidation reactions can also mediate fragmentation of polypeptide chains [33, 34]. Another major consequence of protein oxidation is the formation of protein aggregates, which are often toxic to cells if allowed to accumulate [35]. Oxidative modifications of proteins may occur also under nitrosative stress. In this context, NO-derived reactive species are responsible of nitration and nitrosylation [36, 37]. The former refers to the binding of an NO_2 group to a tyrosine or tryptophan residue, whereas the latter refers to the binding of a NO group to a transition metal or cysteine residue. Among all known amino acid modifications, only nitrosylation, formation of disulfide bridges and methionine sulfoxide can be enzymatically reverted. Further products of methionine oxidation as well as nitration of tyrosine and tryptophan cannot be directly repaired and must be selectively removed by proteolytic systems in order to prevent the accumulation of non-functional damaged proteins [38].

ROS insult most commonly results in lipid peroxidation and consequently in a number of breakdown products that display a large variety of damaging actions. A primary effect of lipid peroxidation is the decrease of membrane fluidity, which alters membrane properties and can significantly disrupt membrane-bound proteins. Among the breakdown products of lipid peroxides, aldehydic molecules have been implicated as causative agents of cytotoxic processes [39]. As well as ROS, aldehydes by-products are relatively stable and can diffuse within the cytosol or even escape from the cell and attack targets far from the site of the original event. In fact, conserving high reactivity, aldheydes may act as mutagens, inactivate enzymes, or operate as endogenous fixative, reacting with proteins and nucleic acids to form heterogeneous cross-links. For this reason, they are considered as ultimate mediators of toxic effects elicited by oxidative stress.

2.3 Antioxidant defence

As consequence of physiological reactive species generation, each cell is equipped with an extensive antioxidant system to counteract their harmful properties either directly by interception or indirectly through reversal of oxidative damage. The antioxidant defence system of the cell is very intricate as it is present in each cell compartment and is disposed to scavenge all reactive species. Essentially, the antioxidant defence can be divided into enzymatic and non-enzymatic.

The latter group is characterized by a large set of molecules that can attenuate or completely block oxidative insults induced by ROS. These antioxidant species can be divided into two different classes: i) non thiolic compounds, such as vitamin C, or diene-containing molecules (vitamin E, β-carotene, polyphenols), which are able to delocalise the positive charge formed by the reaction with radicals; ii) sulfur-containing compounds, such as glutathione and thioredoxin, which can act as donors of reducing equivalents either directly or by the catalysis of specific enzymes.

The enzymatic antioxidant defence system is composed by a variety of proteins among which catalase, glutathione peroxidase and superoxide dismutase (SOD) are the most representative [40]. Catalase is a haem-containing enzyme, which is primarily localized in peroxisomes and is highly efficient in catalyzing the dismutation of H_2O_2 in O_2 and H_2O. Glutathione peroxidase is a selenium-containing enzyme and is localized in cytosol and mitochondria. This enzyme, using the redox cycle of glutathione, catalyzes the reduction of H_2O_2 and of organic hydroperoxides.

SOD represents the most important member of the enzymatic defence system against ROS in particular against $O_2^{\cdot-}$ which is efficiently disproportionated to H_2O_2 and H_2O. The evidence that SOD is fundamental for life derives from the observations that it is an ubiquitary enzyme which, in mammals, exists in three distinct isoforms: copper,zinc SOD (SOD1), extracellular SOD (ECSOD), manganese SOD (SOD2). In addition, another form, which contains iron (FeSOD), has been found only in bacteria and plants. Similarly to SOD1 also ECSOD contains Zn and has Cu in its catalytic centre. ECSOD is the most recently discovered and exists as a homotetramer of 135 KDa molecular weight with high affinity for heparin. ECSOD was first detected in human plasma, lymph, ascites, and cerebrospinal fluids [41]. The SOD2 has manganese as a cofactor and exists as a homotetramer with the individual subunit of about 23 KDa [42]. In aerobic cells, it is considered the first line of defence against mitochondria-derived oxyradicals as it is exclusively localized in this compartment [43]. Moreover, it has been shown that SOD2 plays a major role in promoting cellular differentiation and carcinogenesis [44] and in protecting against hyperoxia-induced pulmonary toxicity [45].

SOD1 is a homodimeric enzyme with a molecular mass of about 32 KDa, which is responsible for about 90% of the total SOD activity as it is present at a surprisingly high concentration (1 μM). Hence, in addition to the high catalytic efficiency, removal of $O_2^{\cdot-}$ occurs promptly even at very low concentrations of the radical, under any physiological conditions of pH and simultaneous presence of competing molecules [46]. Although, considered primarily a "cytosolic" enzyme, SOD1 has also been identified in mitochondria, peroxisomes, lysosomes and nucleus. For this reason it can be considered the most important member of the defence system against $O_2^{\cdot-}$. SOD1 is extensively distributed in a variety of cells and its expression, at least in cytosol, is quite stable so that its activity is often considered as an internal control of SOD1 gene expression. Even though SOD1 is considered to be constitutively expressed, its mRNA levels can be dramatically regulated in response to a wide array of mechanical, chemical, and biological stimuli (such as heat shock, UV and X-irradiation, heavy metals, hydrogen peroxide, nitric oxide) [47]. Synthesis of SOD1 mRNA can be also stimulated by the presence of metal ions, considered potent source for ROS, through the metal responsive element in SOD1 gene [48]. However, regulation of SOD1 gene transcription, in response to several stimuli, can be cell type-dependent. For instance, it has been found that in keratinocytes mRNA levels of SOD1 are up-regulated after exposure to NO flux [49]. Conversely, in neuroblastoma cells, NO insult does not induce increase in SOD1 expression [50]. In these context, it is worth to mention that SOD1 may represent also a protective factor against NO toxicity since this enzyme, by scavenging $O_2^{\cdot-}$, simultaneously prevent the formation of an higher reactive species, peroxynitrite ($ONOO^-$), which derives from the encounter of $O_2^{\cdot-}$ with NO. As matter of fact, macrophages are highly resistant, whereas, neuroblastoma cells are greatly sensitive to NO and are committed to apoptotic cell death failing in preventing $ONOO^-$ formation. When in neuroblastoma cells SOD1 is overexpressed, a significant protection against NO toxicity, confirming the assumption that SOD1 plays a pivotal role in counteracting NO harmful effects [50].

Among cellular compartments, mitochondria are the most equipped with antioxidants because, as previously reported, $O_2^{\cdot-}$ generation during electrons transport is an incessant physiological event. Mitochondria actually possess an efficient and extensive defence system composed of both enzymatic and nonenzymatic antioxidants: SOD, glutathione peroxidase, glutathione reductase, glutathione, vitamins E and C, thiol peroxidases. As previously mentioned, $O_2^{\cdot-}$ produced by the respiratory chain is readily dismutated by the SOD2 and SOD1 in the matrix and in the intermembrane space respectively [51]. As result of the dismutase activity, production of H_2O_2 is significantly high in this compartment but it is efficiently detoxified by glutathione peroxidase and catalase. It is not surprising that phenomena related to ROS production such as apoptosis, degenerative processes, or aging derive from impairment and/or loss of mitochondrial antioxidants or from the mitochondria damage alone.

2.4 ROS and RNS as redox regulators of apoptosis

The importance of ROS in taking part to the activation of the cell death program of apoptosis was understood from the discovery that they were highly produced after TNF-α-induced cell killing [52]. During this process, ROS accumulation was found to precede all the morphological and biochemical alterations typical of apoptosis. However, in other cases, ROS increase may be a side effect rather than a causal effect of the phenomena accompanying the apoptotic process. For example, release of cytochrome *c* in cytosol causes the impairment of the mitochondrial respiratory chain thus leading to the accumulation of ROS and the increase of the oxidation state of the apoptotic cells. In most cases, ROS trigger the apoptotic program oxidatively altering cellular components and/or activating the mitochondrial pathway. Alternatively, the increase of ROS produces unbalance of the redox state and the consequent activation of redox-sensitive factors (Fas, p53, HSF-1, NFκB) which can orchestrate, in addition to apoptosis, a number of processes such as inflammatory reactions, growth and differentiation pathways. In this section, the role of NO in the regulation of the apoptotic program will be discussed, while the aspects regarding the involvement of ROS and redox state will be described in section 4.

Differently from ROS, that are primarily considered pro-apoptotic molecules, NO has a dual role in the apoptotic process that strongly depends on its concentration [53]. Although firstly recognized as a physiological molecule with beneficial functions, NO was principally studied because of its cytotoxic properties. When produced at non-physiological concentrations, NO may induce cell death by apoptosis as well as driving an apoptotic response into a necrotic one. The cytotoxicity of NO mostly derives from its encounter with $O_2^{\cdot-}$ to form $ONOO^-$ [54]. This specie is far more reactive and damaging of its precursors and can diffuse freely intra- and inter-cellularly thus acting as a powerful oxidant. In fact, $ONOO^-$ rapidly reacts with DNA, lipids of cell membranes and proteins at the level of tyrosine or thiol groups.

However, NO may be responsible of cell damage by other pathways. In fact, it reacts with O_2 to produce reactive oxides of nitrogen, which may be formed preferentially within lipid membranes. Moreover, NO enhances the toxic effects caused by H_2O_2 or reacts rapidly with other radicals formed during oxidative stress, such as lipid peroxides.

To study the toxic properties of NO, several NO donors have been now synthesized. Among these, the most used is *S*-nitosoglutathione (GSNO), as it has been proposed to be present inside the cell as physiological and rapidly available store of NO. The reaction between glutathione and NO has been suggested to be catalysed by ceruloplasmin, a multicopper oxidase, involved in iron metabolism [55]. Upon NO insult with GSNO or with others NO donors, cells undergo cell cycle arrest and, consequently, apoptosis [50, 56]. These phenomena are characterised by an early induction of p53 protein, which is a sensor of DNA damage. Induction of cell cycle arrest in G1 phase is dependent on the transcriptional activation of p53 target genes such as p21 that is an inhibitor of cyclin-dependent kinases and thereby blocks cell cycle progression. NO-mediated apoptosis is characterized by the activation of the mitochondrial pathway. It involves the degradation of Bcl-2 and translocation of Bid or Bax from cytosol to mitochondria, where they may possibly form a pore through which cytochrome *c* may be exported to the cytosol. Indeed, in neuroblastoma cells, apoptosis elicited by NO treatment is executed by cytochorome *c*-mediated activation of downstream caspase-3. Activation of caspase-3 is also responsible for cleavage of p21 that is a critical point in order to make irreversible the apoptotic process elicited by the p53-mediated response to DNA damage [50, 56]. In addition, NO may exert its cytotoxic effects through the binding to cytochrome *c* oxidase and inhibition of its activity. This condition may lead to the disruption of the mitochondrial transmembrane potential, which in turn opens the permeability transition pore and permit the release of small pro-apoptotic molecules [57]. Overall, these factors may function as signals of mitochondrial impairment and strengthen the NO apoptotic response.

One of the well-known properties of NO is to bind to the haem group of target proteins especially of haemoglobin, soluble guanylate cyclase and cytochrome *c* oxidase whose functions clearly have been demonstrated to be regulated by endogenous haem nitrosylation. Recently, the possibility of haem nitrosylation of cytochrome *c* has been dissected, since cytochrome *c* has no free cysteines, and therefore, its haem iron is the most probable nitrosylation target [58]. Haem of guanylate cyclase and cytochrome *c* oxidase is 5-coordinated and this greatly accelerates NO binding. Haem of cytochrome *c* is instead 6-coordinated. However, cytochrome *c* undergoes a conformational change during apoptosis that may result in a 5-coordinated haem [59] favouring the increase of the reactivity of cytochrome *c* with NO. Because the haem edge of cytochrome *c* is involved in its association with Apaf-1 [60], it is possible that haem nitrosylation of cytochrome *c* facilitates apoptosome formation and thereby stimulates caspase-3 activation and consequently execution of the apoptotic process.

It is now widely demonstrated that NO, when produced at low concentration, may exert an inhibitory action at different levels of the apoptotic machinery. Owing to its capacity to react with thiol groups, it can block catalytically active cysteine residue of caspases. The thiol of cysteine at the catalytic site of these proteases is susceptible to redox modification and can be effectively modified by *S*-nitrosylation in the presence of NO. Among the 14 isoforms of caspases, only caspase-3, -8 and -9 have been found to be *S*-nitrosylated and this process occurs with a stoichiometry of 1:1 [61-63]. NO, *in vivo*, readily reacts with molecular oxygen and transition metal ions such as Fe and Cu. Therefore, the capacity of NO to *S*-nitrosylate caspases will depend on the abundance of those molecules and the availability of other thiol targets such as glutathione and free cysteines. *S*-nitrosylating species can be generated by the interaction of NO with Fe-sulfur complex. The reaction product of NO and iron-sulfur complexes, dinitrosyl-iron complexes, has been shown to carry out *S*-nitrosylation. It has been also demonstrated that NO may act as an anti-apoptotic factor through an indirect action, being potentially able to interact with transcription factors and favor the expression of several cytoprotective genes including HSP70 and HSP32. NO can also regulate the protein levels of Bcl-2 family proteins. In fact, NO donor elevates Bcl-2 expression both at the mRNA and protein levels and prevents apoptotic cell death through the inhibition of cytochrome *c* release from the intermembrane space into cytosol. Moreover, recent findings support the idea that NO inhibits apoptosis downstream of cytochrome *c* release by directly blocking caspase-9 activation. As well as for caspase-3, NO appears to inhibit caspase-9 directly, likely by nitrosylating its inactive procaspase form.

2.5 ROS and RNS in neurodegeneration

Oxidative and nitrosative stress occur when massive production of ROS and RNS overwhelms the antioxidant capacity of the cell and redox homeostasis is altered. Both oxidative and nitrosative stress are implicated in the pathogenesis of several diseases including AIDS, Huntington's, Parkinson's, Alzheimer's disease, amyotrophic lateral sclerosis (ALS) and retinal degenerative disorders (for details on some of this disease see section 3). Evidently, the brain is particularly vulnerable and this is not surprising as the central nervous system is highly aerobic, contains a high level of substrates easily oxidizable (e.g. membrane polyunsatured lipids), an inherently augmented flux of RNS and ROS generated during neurochemichal reactions (e.g. dopamine oxidation and NOS activity). Moreover, it possesses low levels of antioxidant defences (e.g. SOD, catalase, glutathione and peroxidases) and, for this reason the alteration of the function of antioxidant enzymes is often associated with the occurrence of neurodegenerative processes. Here is described the role of SOD1 in neurodegeneration with particular attention to amyotrophic lateral sclerosis (ALS).

The past decade has brought us new evidence of involvement of SOD1 in a number of diseases and pathologies: ALS, Down's syndrome, and premature aging are probably just some of the pathological conditions that develop as consequence of an altered SOD1 activity and ROS concentration. The SOD1 gene encoding for SOD1 has been localized to chromosome 21 (region 21q22) in humans [64]. Human chromosome 21 has been studied intensely because of the association between Down's syndrome and trisomy 21. Although patients with Down's syndrome show a 50% increase in SOD activity due to higher levels of SOD1 protein, the role of this enzyme in this pathology remains uncertain. The increased dosage of SOD1 gene associates with some symptoms of Down's syndrome, such as the pathological abnormalities of tongue neuromuscular junctions [65].

On the other hand, SOD1 has been involved in ALS, also known as Lou Gehrig's disease. This lethal disease is characterized by the persistent degeneration of both upper and lower motor neurons. Most cases (90-95%) of ALS are sporadic, whereas remaining cases are familial (FALS) and the best documented of these are due to inherited mutations in SOD1 gene. Up to date over 100 distinct mutations of SOD1 have been found in FALS patients and they consist mostly in a single amino acid substitution. A smaller group of mutations is characterized by the deletions and truncations of the full-length wild type protein. Although only 2% of patients with ALS and 10-15% with FALS have mutations in the SOD1 gene, the discovery of these mutations by Rosen et al. in 1993 provided the first molecular insight into the pathogenesis of this disease [66].

From this discovery, several theories have been proposed to explain the mechanism of motor neurons death caused by mutations in SOD1 enzyme. One hypothesis is that mutations in the SOD1 gene may impair enzyme activity that in turn could lead to the impairment of defence against $O_2^{\cdot -}$ and consequently to its accumulation. This theory was dismissed when SOD1 bearing the mutations were overexpressed in mice, resulting in motor neuron disease despite the elevated SOD1 activity [67]. Moreover, complete inactivation of SOD1 in "knock-out" mice did not cause any motor neuron abnormalities, although they exhibited increasing embryonic lethality and reduced fertility in females [68]. For this reasons, an opposite theory was proposed where a gain-of-function rather than loss of activity may be involved in the pathogenesis of ALS. On the basis of these hypotheses, SOD1 may acquire new properties in addition to catalytic removal of $O_2^{\cdot -}$ in dependence on the type of mutation. Up to date the causes of motor neurons death are not clear and some studies point to the hypothesis of oligomerization in which mutant SOD1 proteins are or become misfolded and consequently aggregate into increasingly high-molecular-weight species leading to toxic proteinaceous inclusions. On the other hand, the occurrence of oxidative stress may be caused by loss of dismutase or enhanced peroxidase activity or exposure of copper at the active site of mutant SOD1 [69]. Either way, the dominant mutations in SOD1 most likely play a key role in the pathogenesis of ALS in which the neurodegenerative process is most probably due to the commitment of apoptotic cell death. In fact, neurodegeneration in ALS is associated with glutamate-mediated excitotoxicity and abnormal regulation of calcium [70], DNA fragmentation, caspase activation, and altered expression of Bcl-2 family members [71] that are hallmarks of apoptosis.

The emerging theory to explain the commitment to apoptosis in motor neurons of ALS patients is the occurrence of oxidative and/or nitrosative stress. In fact, in both *in vivo* and *in vitro* models of ALS as well as in patients oxidative damage to proteins, lipids and DNA has been detected [72-74]. Moreover, also the activation of microglia was found, which produces large amounts of O_2^{-}, NO and $ONOO^{-}$ thus leading to the formation of nitrosative-damaged molecules such as nitrosylated proteins. Accumulation of nitrosylated proteins was also found as a consequence of enhanced nitrosylation by the catalysis of mutant SOD1 or increased NO production mostly due to up-regulation of the Ca^{2+}-dependent enzymes, iNOS and nNOS [73].

Although the theory of occurrence of oxidative stress has been widely accepted at least for some mutants, the involvement of NO is still controversial. Cellular models of FALS are now widely used in order to understand the molecular pathways underlying the involvement of ROS and RNS in mutant SOD1-linked neurodegeneration [50, 74, 75]. In particular, neuroblastoma cells transfected with G93A SOD1 mutant, which is associated with the most severe form of FALS, are used. In this experimental model, production of ROS is significantly increased, in spite of the high efficiency of the mutant in removing $O_2^{\cdot -}$, as consequence of gain of peroxidase activity by the mutated enzyme [50, 74]. A concurrent accumulation of oxidatively damaged molecules, as protein carbonyls and lipid peroxides, are observed. In this model, NO production does not increase but rather an augmented turnover of nNOS protein has been found [76]. These data are in contrast with the results obtained in other models, where instead an increase in nitrosylated proteins is found [73]. Oxidatively damaged proteins are cleared by proteolytic systems among which proteasome is the most specific one. It can be activated or inhibited by ROS in dependence on their concentration. Moreover, when activated, proteasome also regulates nNOS turnover, thus reducing the risk of nitrosative stress. It has been demonstrated that proteasome plays a fundamental role in cell survival of neuroblastoma cells carrying pro-oxidant G93A SOD1 mutant owing to its action on oxidized proteins accumulation as chemical inhibition of proteasome leads to RNS- and ROS-mediated neuronal death (Figure 4). Similarly, treatment with a high NO flux induces apoptosis in neuroblastoma cells carrying the G93A SOD1 mutant [50].

Paradoxically, SOD1 mutants associated with less severe form of FALS are defective in dismutase activity. Among these, the H46R SOD1 mutant consists in the substitution of histidine 46 of the active site with an arginine residue. It has been demonstrated that neuroblastoma cells expressing this mutant, unexpectedly, are protected from NO-mediated toxicity in spite of the impairment of SOD1 activity and the raise of ROS concentration [56]. These cells possess a higher content of glutathione, as protective factor, which counteracts NO toxicity by forming *S*-nitrosoglutathione, a far less reactive compound with respect to NO-derived radicals. As matter of fact, only chemical depletion of glutathione increases susceptibility to NO challenge. On the contrary, when exposed to oxyradical-generating species, such as *t*-butylhydroperoxide or paraquat, neuroblastoma cells carrying the H46R SOD1 mutant, are committed to apoptotic or necrotic cell death. These results confirm the role played by SOD1 as the major intracellular radical scavenger, as far as oxygen radicals are concerned, because, even though H46R SOD1 expressing cells have higher GSH content, this is not sufficient to counteract ROS toxicity.

Taken together these findings suggest that the mechanisms underlying ALS occurrence are far to be elucidated and are further complicated by the fact that the life expectancy after the onset of symptoms shows a remarkable degree of variations with respect to the mutations. In fact, on the basis of the type of mutation, SOD-linked FALS may acquire an as yet unidentified property more or less harmful [70].

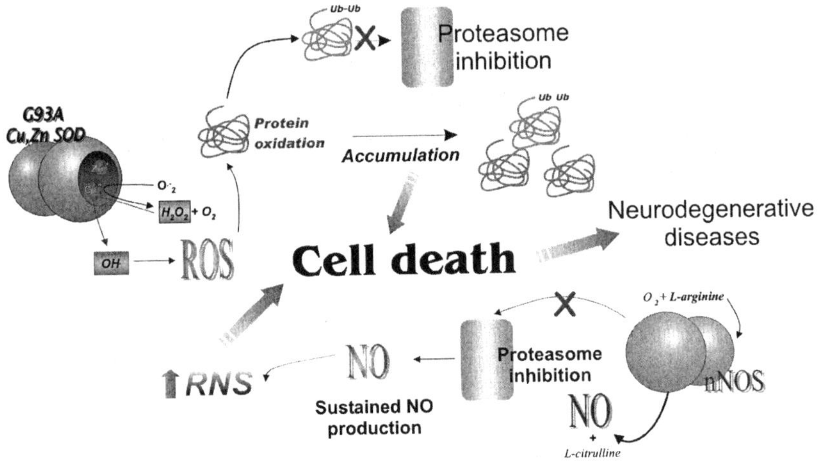

Figure 4. Schematic model of neuronal death in a cellular model of FALS

3. Copper-related neurodegeneration

Lombardo, M.F. and Rossi, L.

3.1 Copper metabolism and distribution

Copper is a transition metal and it has been established since 1928 as an essential nutrient for animals. Despite its low concentration, this metal plays a very important role: it can donate and accept electrons at physiological concentration and, thus, it is present in the active site of several enzymes in different metabolic pathways. All organisms require copper as a catalytic cofactor for biological processes such as iron transport, peptide hormone production, pigmentation, blood clotting and normal cell growth and development [77]. In particular, copper is a component of Cytochrome *c* Oxidase (Cytox), which catalyses the reduction of oxygen to water, an essential step in cellular respiration and of the SOD1 that plays a key role in the cellular response to oxidative stress catalyzing the dismutation of superoxide to hydrogen peroxide. The decreased activity of these two enzymes can lead to a pro-oxidant status, particularly in the mitochondria.

However, copper redox properties, so important for life, can also be dangerous when this metal escapes cellular homeostatic control: copper free ions are able to enhance ROS production. In particular, free reduced copper can be produced in the reaction between oxidized copper and $O_2^{\cdot -}$:

$$\mathbf{O_2^{\cdot -} + Cu^{+2} \rightarrow O_2 + Cu^{+1}}$$

Then, reduced copper can react with H_2O_2 to form $OH^{\cdot}$ in the so called "Fenton reaction":

$$\mathbf{H_2O_2 + Cu^{+1} \rightarrow OH^- + OH^{\cdot} + Cu^{+2}}$$

The sum of these two reactions is the metal catalysed reaction between H_2O_2 and $O_2^{\cdot -}$ (Haber-Weiss reaction):

$$\begin{array}{l}\mathbf{O_2^{\cdot -} + Cu^{+2} \rightarrow O_2 + Cu^{+1}}\\ \mathbf{H_2O_2 + Cu^{+1} \rightarrow OH^- + OH^{\cdot} + Cu^{+2}}\\ \hline \mathbf{O_2^{\cdot -} + H_2O_2 \rightarrow OH^- + OH^{\cdot} + O_2}\end{array}$$

It gives rise to the powerful oxidant $OH^{\cdot}$, which induces dramatic oxidative changes to proteins, lipids and nucleic acids, seriously impairing their biological function.

While the intracellular copper total concentration is between 0.01 and 0.1mM, the intracellular free copper ions concentration is very low (about 10^{-18} M) [78]. It is evident that intracellular copper is bound to several proteins (chaperons, carriers and enzymes) and that the cells have developed dedicated components and sophisticated mechanisms to acquire and maintain adequate copper concentration [78, 79]. Those proteins have been found in yeasts at the beginning, but later their homologues have been found in humans too.

Copper passively enters into the cell by a high affinity membrane carrier: the protein Ctr1 (Km ≈1-5 μM) [80]. Ctr 1 is expressed at low levels in brain and perturbations of its expression particularly affects brain copper level and copper enzyme activities, indicating that this protein plays a crucial role for copper acquisition and development of central nervous system CNS [81].

Copper is present in all subcellular compartments: nucleus, mitochondria, lysosomes, endoplasmic reticulum and cytosol. It has been demonstrated by studies on yeast that there are at least three independent copper-delivery pathways: delivery to mitochondria for Cytox activity, to the cytosolic milieu for SOD1, and to the secretory pathway [78, 79]. Copper transporters, the so-called "copper chaperones", share the same motif of copper binding (MXCXXC); they may be low-molecular weight soluble proteins, but also membrane proteins, showing ATP-binding sites and multiple copper binding domains.

Deliver of copper to mitochondria is particularly important for Cytox activity and respiration. Cytox subunit I and II are mitochondrially encoded and require a total of three copper ions as co-factors (Cu_A and Cu_B sites): therefore they must be metallated within the mitochondria. Copper delivery to Cytox seems to be a very complex process mediated by several copper-binding proteins (Cox 17, the integral proteins of the mitochondrial inner membrane Sco1, Sco2 and Cox 11); new ones are under continuous discovery. They all appear to be essential for Cytox assembly and function. Cox 17 is a putative shuttle that binds and carries copper from cytosol, fundamental for copper delivery to the Cu_A site of Cytox [82]; Cox 11, is an essential protein for the formation of Cu_B site of Cytox [83]; Sco2 mutations are associated with Cytox deficiency and cardioencephalomyopathy in humans [84].

Copper delivery to SOD1 is mediated by a specific protein: CCS (Copper Chaperone for Superoxide dismutase) [85]. One of domains of CCS is similar to one found in SOD1 and this makes possible the physical interaction between the two proteins which are supposed to form an eterodimer during the exchange of the copper ion [79]. Copper deficiency causes an overexpression of CCS, probably due to a slower protein turnover [86], maybe in order to optimise the transfer of the residual copper within the cytosolic milieu. Furthermore, CCS has also a role in the intracellular localization of SOD1: in fact, a small fraction of this enzyme is located in the intermembrane space of mitochondria (IMS) [51, 87]. It has been suggested that the apo-SOD1 would be able to cross the mitochondrial outer membrane but, after CCS-mediated copper transfer, it would stabilize in the IMS.

Copper-carrier proteins have been identified in the secretory pathway too: the Atox1 soluble chaperone donates copper to the highly homologous copper-transporting ATPases, ATP7 A and B, which are located at the membrane of the trans-Golgi network [88]. Atox1-deficient cells accumulate high levels of intracellular copper: metabolic studies indicated that this defect was caused because of impaired cellular copper efflux. This copper chaperone plays a critical role in perinatal copper homeostasis: Atox1-deficient mice show developmental abnormalities [89].

ATP7A presents eight transmembrane alpha-helix domains, an ATP-binding domain at the C-terminus, a phosphatase domain, six copper-binding motifs at the N-terminus. Both C- and N-terminus are cytosolic. One of the eight transmembrane alpha-helixes presents a motif CPC that is probably involved in copper transport across the membrane [79, 90].

ATP7B shares 55% of homology with ATP7A. Both of them can actively pump copper into the lumen of Golgi where this metal is loaded onto nascent secretory copper-proteins; they are also important for intracellular copper concentration control: under high copper concentration these proteins leave the *trans*-Golgi network to re-distribute to the plasma membrane where they pump copper out of the cell [91]. The importance of ATP7A/B in the control of intracellular copper concentration is evidenced by two inherited pathologies: the X-linked Menkes' disease (MD), due to mutations to the *ATP7A* gene or *MNK* [92], and the autosomic recessive Wilson's disease (WD), due to mutations to the *ATP7B* gene or *WND* [93]. The phenotypes of these two pathologies are justified by the different patterns of expression of ATP7A and ATP7B. The former is expressed predominantly in intestine, placenta, brain and kidney; the latter in liver and hardly in brain. Therefore, at the physiological level we can see that ATP7A is important for copper transfer from intestinal cells to the blood and the whole organisms, while ATP7B is important for biliary copper excretion. Thus, mutations of MNK result in systemic copper deficiency, while mutations of WND result in systemic copper overload. Indeed, MD and WD represent the effect of two opposite situations in copper imbalance: copper deficiency and copper excess, respectively. Interestingly, both these diseases are characterized by oxidative damage and neurodegeneration.

3.2 Altered copper homeostasis and/or copper handling are linked to neurodegeneration

In the latest years there has been a growing interest in studying neurodegenerative diseases associated with altered copper homeostasis or with its aberrant chemistry. Copper can directly induce oxidative stress when it is in excess or improperly bound, causing protein fragmentation and/or aggregation, in those that are defined as "conformational neurodegenerative diseases" [77].

As mentioned above (section 2), CNS is particularly sensitive to damage induced by ROS. Oxidative stress may represent the trigger of programmed cell death, which has been suggested as the mechanism underlying the slow elimination of neural cells in many *in vivo* and *in vitro* models, during development of the CNS as well as in human neurodegenerative diseases [94]. Interestingly, the mitochondrion seems to be the subcellular compartment mostly affected in this kind of pathologies: it can be the mediator of apoptotsis and its progressive impairment could explain their slow progression [95].

Neurodegeneration associated with excess copper is best represented by WD. This disease is biochemically characterized by accumulation of copper in the liver and brain of affected patients, due to impaired biliary excretion of this metal [96]. The age of onset of WD ranges from the age of 9 years up to 50. Diagnosis mainly relies on hepatic dysfunction; indeed, at the earliest stage of the disease, copper accumulates in the cytosol of hepatocytes inducing hepatocytes necrosis, followed by increased copper release into the bloodstream leading to hemolysis. Eventually, copper levels increase in other organs such as kidney, brain and cornea. In the latter, copper accumulation produces pigmented rings (Kayser-Fleisher rings), which represent the hallmark of the latest stage of the disease. WD patients may display neurological symptoms that arise only when copper concentration becomes elevated in the cerebrospinal fluid [97]. Moreover, upon D-penicillamine (a copper chelator) therapy, the neurological signs diminish together with copper concentration in the cerebrospinal fluid, underlining the correlation of neurological signs and increased brain copper concentrations [98]. In brain, deposition of copper occurs in the basal ganglia resulting in gliosis and neuronal loss. Progressive neurodegeneration leads to neurological symptoms including tremors, dystonia, slurring of speech, rigidity. Behavioural disturbances are also present with changes of personality, depression and schizophrenia [96].

Other neurodegenerative diseases, such as ALS, Alzheimer's disease (AD), Parkinson's disease (PD) and prion diseases, are associated with copper aberrant chemistry and/or handling, and are indicated as "conformational" diseases because they are characterized by protein misfolding and/or aggregation. However, the relationship between protein oxidation/aggregation and neurodegeneration remains unclear. Redox metals, such as copper, iron, as well as redox-inactive zinc, could drive the generation of strong oxidants and nitrating agents, and/or could be directly involved in the aggregation process of proteins. Furthermore, the translocation of aggregated peptides to the mitochondrial membrane has been suggested to cause mitochondrial damage, thus playing an important role in triggering or perpetuating neurodegeneration [99].

ALS is a neurodegenerative disease, characterized by selective motor neurons degeneration, which in its familial form is associated with several mutations of the SOD1 gene; a role for copper-mediated neurodegeneration in this pathology relies on aberrant reactivity of the metal of the mutated protein (see section 2).

Alzheimer's disease (AD), which occurs in a sporadic and an inherited form, is characterized by progressive neuronal dysfunction and the formation of copper- and iron-containing amyloid plaques in the brain. Several studies have indicated that Zn^{2+}, Fe^{3+} and Cu^{2+} are significantly elevated in AD patients. Those metals participate in the deposition of Aβ from a precursor (APP) within amyloid plaques [77]. It has also been suggested that APP may possibly be involved in intracellular copper transport, since it shows Cu^{+1} binding domains. Bound reduced copper can be re-oxidised by H_2O_2, leading to oxidative fragmentation of APP, and can favour oxygen radicals-mediated aggregation and deposition of Aβ [100]. The role of copper in AD is further indicated by the observation that copper levels are increased in the cerebral cortex and liver of mice made knockout for the APP-like proteins [101]. Evidence for the role of oxidative stress in AD includes an increase of brain levels of damaged DNA, oxidised proteins, and a decline in polyunsaturated fatty acids. Furthermore, serum copper levels and total peroxides, as well as red blood cells SOD1, were found to be elevated in AD patients [102, 103], indicating a dysbalance in copper metabolism and redox status. Therefore, treatment of AD patients with copper chelators has been proposed in order to control copper reactivity [102-104]: in particular, clioquinol, a copper chelator that can cross the blood-brain barrier, significantly decreased Aβ deposition in brain and improved general behaviour in transgenic mouse model of AD [104].

The human form of the prion diseases, the Kreutzfeld-Jacob disease, is characterized by a rapidly progressing dementia and cerebellar ataxia, resulting from neuronal spongiform degeneration and astrocytic glyosis. Prion diseases are widely believed to arise when a membrane prion protein (PrP) undergoes conformational changes to a pathogenic isoform (PrP^{Sc}). It has been shown that PrP binds copper to an octapeptide region [105]: this may give it an antioxidant (superoxide dismutating) activity, though this hypothesis has been recently questioned [106]. It has also been suggested that PrP plays a physiological role in the synaptic uptake of copper ions [107]. Actually, cerebellar cells from mice deficient in PrP reveal increased sensitivity to the toxicity of copper salts and marked decrease in membrane copper content and decreased SOD1 activity. On the other hand, copper may also play a pathogenetic role in the onset of prion diseases: it can induce conformational changes of PrP and may generate PrP^{Sc}-like species [108]. It has recently been shown that copper chelation can delay the onset of prion disease in mice, confirming that the levels of this metal can influence the infectivity of PrP [109].

Some evidence for the involvement of copper in the mechanism underlying the onset of Parkinson's disease (PD) has also emerged. Established aetiology of this disease involves environmental factors (exposure to pesticides, herbicides, industrial chemicals) and genetic factors (approximately 5-10% of PD patients have a familial form of parkinsonism with an autosomal-dominant pattern of inheritance) [110]. On the basis of epidemiological studies, it has been suggested that occupational exposure to specific metals, including copper, appears to be a risk factor for PD. Unbalance of copper homeostasis in PD patients is suggested by defects of Cytox in nigral neurones as well as by lower SOD1 activity in blood [77]. The pathogenesis of PD may involve oxidative stress, since oxidised marker molecules have been detected in the brains of PD patients. Familial PD was linked to mutations in the gene coding for the protein α-synuclein [111]. While α-synuclein physiological role is still largely unknown, in the familial cases of PD mutations of this protein might favour accumulation and aggregation that are crucial events in the development of the disease. A role for copper in the aetiology of PD is suggested by the finding that Cu^{2+} induces α-synuclein to form self-oligomers [112, 113].

3.3 Copper deficiency in neuronal cells: a genetic and an in vitro model of neurodegeneration

The mechanisms underlying the involvement of copper in WD or conformational neurodegeneration are supposedly based on uncontrolled redox activity, due to excess of the metal in brain or to its aberrant binding to brain proteins, which may play a physiological role in copper homeostasis. The death of neuronal cells is mediated by oxidative stress, protein aggregation and mitochondrial damage (Figure 5). Then, how can copper deficiency induce oxidative stress and neuronal cell death like in MD?

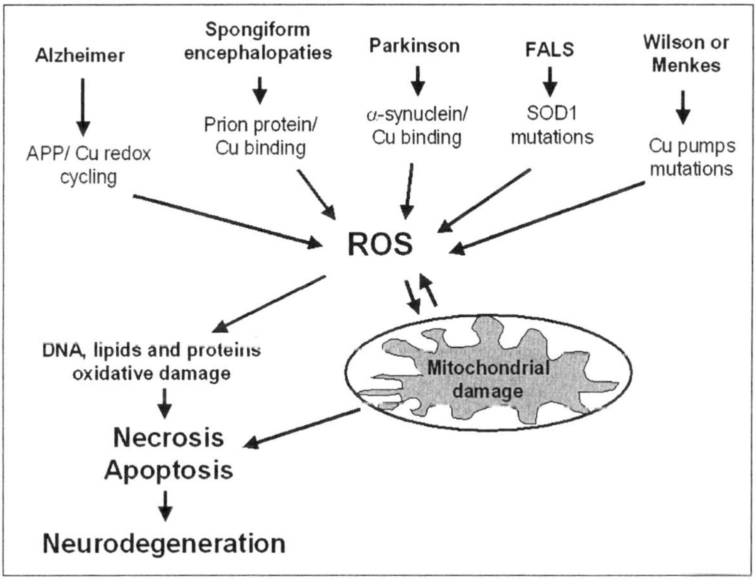

Figure 5. Oxidative stress in neurodegeneration associated with alteration of copper homeostasis

MD is usually lethal by the age of 3 years, but there are two milder allelic variants of this disorder, called occipital horn syndrome and mild MD [114, 115]. Due to impairment of

ATP7A function, nutritional copper is not released by the enterocytes and accumulates in the intestine whilst brain and liver become copper-deficient. Systemic depletion of copper-dependent enzymes may justify the phenotype and the symptoms of MD patients. The most striking feature of this disease is the coarse and hypopigmented hair: therefore, it is also called "kinky or steely hair disease". Menkes children also show impaired synthesis of collagen and elastin. However, the most relevant damage occurs to CNS: they are severely mental retarded and altered brain development and neurodegeneration have been detected by post-mortem histological assay [116]. In particular, diffuse atrophy, focal degeneration of grey matter and prominent neuronal loss has been detected in the cerebellum. Purkinje cells show abnormal dendridic arborisation and focal axonal swelling. These features are present at birth, strongly suggesting that copper is essential for prenatal growth and development of the CNS. Copper content is particularly low in the brain with respect to other organs: indeed, it has been reported that ATP7A is particularly expressed at the choroid plexes of the brain and transports copper across the blood-brain barrier in embryonic mice [117]. Therefore, mutations of this copper pump result in accumulation of copper in brain blood vessels and in astrocytes, without reaching neurons: the consequent lower activities of copper-dependent enzymes in these cells may strongly contribute to the altered development of the CNS.

The mechanisms underlying prenatal cerebral and cerebellar degeneration seem to imply programmed cell death, possibly mediated by a copper-dependent factor, very likely Cytox, indicating that mitochondrial function plays an essential role in neuronal growth and differentiation. This hypothesis is supported by the results of studies on the mechanisms of neurodegeneration in the closest animal model of MD, the mottled/brindled ($Mo^{br/Y}$) mouse, which carries a spontaneous mutation of the X-linked mottled locus, homologous to the ATP7A locus [118]. In the brain of these animals copper deficiency leads to specific decrease of Cytox and SOD1 activities (Figure 6) [119]. In addition dramatic changes of some markers for apoptosis, all related to mitochondria, occur: loss of the antioxidant Bcl-2 protein, release of cytochrome c from the mitochondria and depletion of ATP. Bcl-2 is a crucial protein in protecting neurons from naturally occurring degeneration or from pathological insults, in that its deficiency in brain is associated with impaired brain development and neurodegeneration [120]. Indeed, histological analysis of $Mo^{br/Y}$ brain revealed a high percentage of apoptotic cells in the neocortex and the hippocampus (Figure 6). This evidence allows to hypothesize that copper deficit in brain may cause mitochondrial damage consequent to inactivation of Cytox. In turn, this event may trigger leakage of oxygen radicals out of damaged mitochondria, leading to neurodegeneration via oxidative stress-mediated apoptosis. Tentative treatment of MD consists in intravenous administration of copper-histidine complex, but this therapy can only delay the progression of the disease. The crucial role of Cytox alteration in neurodegeneration is demonstrated by studies on the timing of treatment of $Mo^{br/Y}$ with copper, showing that delayed administration results in irreversible changes of Cytox of the brain leading to irresponsiveness to the treatment [121]. On the other hand, once the blood-brain barrier is fully developed, the impairment of ATP7A at this site makes impossible brain copper uptake, even when circulating copper levels are normalized by parenteral copper therapy. The idea that Cytox failure seems likely to cause severe brain damage associated with MD is strengthened by the observation that symptoms at CNS in MD are similar to those found in Leigh disease, caused by a deficient mitochondrial complex IV [122].

Studies on copper deficiency in neuroblastoma cells confirm the molecular mechanisms that link copper-imbalance to neurodegeneration. In SH-SY5Y neuroblastoma cells growing in the presence of the copper chelator Triethylene tetramine tetrahydrochloride (Trien) [123, 124] copper content decreases to about 40% in few days. This is a situation that resembles the effects of MD on *in vivo* brain cells. Unavailability of copper is confirmed by the decreased activity of the cuproenzymes SOD1 and Cytox. Interestingly, no changes were observed in the expression or the activities of other components of the mitochondrial transport chain, such as complex I or complex II.

Copper-depleted neuroblastoma cells are more vulnerable than copper-adequate control cells to oxidative stress, like that elicited by paraquat. This is a pro-oxidant agent: it can undergo the so called redox-cycling in cells, being activated by cellular reductases to free radical and then re-oxidised by molecular oxygen, with the production of $O_2^{\cdot-}$. It is of relevance for the CNS, because it is chemically analogous to 1-methyl-4-phenyl-piridinium ion (MPP^+), the active metabolite of a dopaminergic neurotoxin, and it has been proposed as a possible environmental aetiological agent of Parkinson's disease. In copper-depleted cells it provokes the formation of oxidized glutathione, as a sign of oxidative stress, and apoptosis [123]. This increased sensitivity to paraquat-elicited $O_2^{\cdot-}$ production is likely due to the decreased activity of SOD1, thus confirming the critical role played by this enzyme in counteracting oxygen free radicals.

Prolonging copper-deficiency in neuroblastoma cells by chelator-treatment for several days leads to a progressive decrease of Cytox and SOD1. This phenomenon suggests that the residual copper pool is unavailable for binding to the chaperones that mediate the delivery of the metal to these cuproenzymes. In particular, Cytox activity decrement shows a higher rate than that of SOD1 and this is consistent with the existence of a stable pool of apo-SOD1 that accumulates during copper deficiency and may be ready to catch any available copper ion [125]. The effect of copper deficiency severely affects also the protein content of the subunit II of Cytox and this is in line with the fact that this metal is required for the maturation and the assembly of Cytox subunits and no apo-Cytox exists under condition of copper deficiency. As a consequence of the dysfunction of electron transport chain and oxidative phosphorylation, ATP level in these copper-deficient cells drops to about 40 % (Figure 6).

Copper depletion induces in SH-SY5Y cells an increment in ROS production. This may be due to the loss of Cytox activity followed by mitochondrial electron transport chain failure. It has been reported that electrons accumulated upstream of Cytox can leak from complex I and III and react with molecular oxygen to give ROS [126]. The concomitant decrement in SOD1 activity may allow ROS to accumulate in the IMS, thus enhancing their noxious effects. However, in this experimental model no significant variation in oxidized and reduced glutathione or any increment of carbonylated proteins occurs: therefore, it is conceivable that under copper deficiency mitochondria produce a low but continuous flow of ROS, somewhat acting as redox signals. Among the intracellular targets of redox signalling manganese-dependent superoxide dismutase (SOD2), Bcl-2, and p53 are strongly upregulated. Bcl-2 and SOD2 are part of the mitochondrial antioxidative defence, and have been reported to be induced by oxidative stress [127]. The increase of SOD2 appears to be a common mechanism of defence against copper-deficiency elicited oxidative stress: in fact, it has been demonstrated that its mRNA, activity and protein levels were increased in copper deficient rats [128]. Besides, increased SOD2 immunoreactivity has been observed in the cerebella of patients affected by MD [129]. Bcl-2 protein exerts a protective anti-apoptotic action on mitochondria by a not well-elucidated mechanism(s), being able to block pro-apoptotic proteins and enhancing SOD1 activity *via* an unknown mechanism [130]. In neuroblastoma undergoing prolonged shortness of copper, the increase of Bcl-2 seems to compensate the low activity of

SOD1; that phenomenon could be a response to higher level of mitochondrial oxidative stress. These findings suggest a link between the two proteins and mitochondrial protection.

Another target of ROS signalling is the tumour suppressor protein p53, a transcription factor, exerting multiple, antiproliferative effects in response to genotoxic exposure. p53 can be an early sensor of intracellular redox unbalance [50], controlling the cell cycle progression and apoptosis. It has been demonstrated that ROS are involved at several levels in the p53 signalling pathways [131]. In reality, in copper-deficient cells, the activated form of p53 increases in the early stage of the treatment with the copper chelator, together with the increase of the expression of the product of one of its target genes, p21.

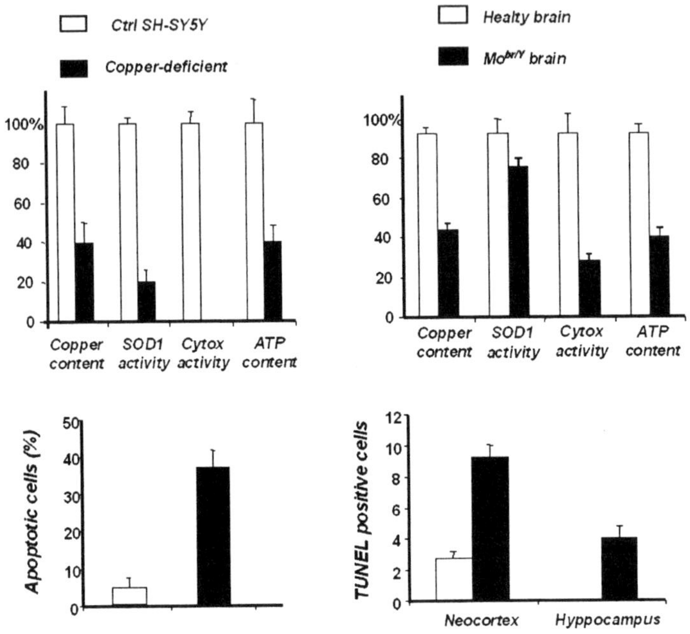

Figure 6. Changes in copper-dependent enzymes and ATP levels, and occurrence of apoptosis upon copper deficiency: a comparison between an *in vivo* and *in vitro* model (for details see refs. 119, 124)

Consistently with the idea that low and continuative levels of oxidative insult can induce apoptosis, while higher acute levels can induce necrosis [94], prolonged copper deficiency is eventually able to induce in SH-SY5Y cells both morphological changes occurring to the chromatin in the nuclei and cell cycle plot modifications typical of apoptosis (Figure 6). The role of ROS produced in mitochondria by impairment of the transport chain is a likely event triggering apoptosis: it has been found, in fact, that inhibitors of mitochondrial electron transport chain complexes induce ROS production and apoptosis in several types of cultured cells [132].

Another biochemical event related to the progress of the apoptotic pathway is the activation of the proteases belonging to the caspases family; they are useful tools to understand which one of the several pathways of apoptosis is active. As said, apoptosis triggered by stimuli at the surface receptors proceeds *via* caspase-8 activation, while apoptosis triggered by mitochondrial factors proceeds via caspase-9. In prolonged copper deficiency in SH-SY5Y neuroblastoma the activation of caspase-9 rather than that of caspase-8 occurs, demonstrating that apoptosis proceeds through a mitochondrial-driven pathway. Caspase-3 activation then takes place.

These findings strongly suggest that copper depletion stimulates the production of low levels of ROS in the mitochondria by both Cytox impairment and decrease of SOD1 activity. To cope with this challenge, cell upregulates SOD2 and Bcl-2; however, since ROS act simultaneously as inducers of antioxidants and pro-apoptotic stimuli, this may counteract antioxidants prevention of cell death. Then apoptosis proceeds through p53 activation. Caspase-9 and -3 carry out the cell death program confirming the involvement of mitochondrial effectors (Figure 7).

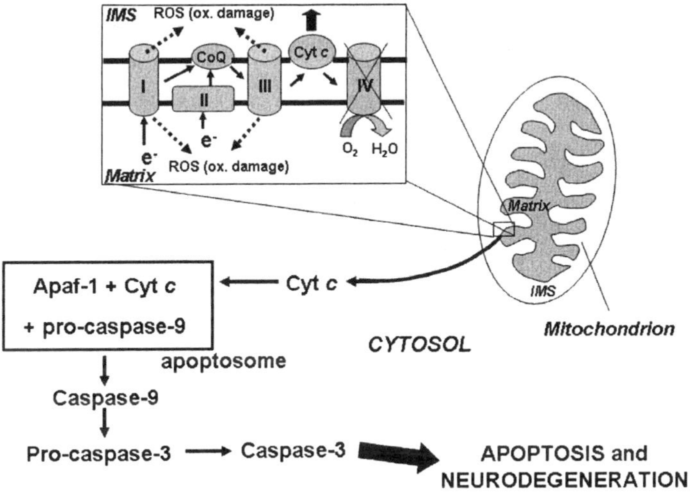

Figure 7. Hypothetical mechanism for apoptosis induced by copper deficiency

The described *in vitro* model of copper-depleted SH-SY5Y cells shows some similarities with MD and its animal model: i) the decrement in intracellular copper content of neuroblastoma cells is similar to those of the $Mo^{br/Y}$ brain [119, 123, 124]; ii) SOD2 increment has also been reported in the cerebella of MD patients [129]; iii) a comparable decrement of ATP content is observed in copper-depleted neuroblastoma cells and in the $Mo^{br/Y}$ brain; iv) in brain of $Mo^{br/Y}$ mouse neurodegeneration occurs via apoptosis [119]. Furthermore, another parallelism consists in the response of the two models to copper supplementation. In fact, parenteral administration of copper-histidine prevents the neurological disturbances present in the $Mo^{br/Y}$ mouse [121] as well as it is a useful, though not resolutive, therapy for MD patients [114]. Likewise, copper addition was able to restore Cytox and SOD1 levels and to ameliorate cell viability in copper-deficient neuroblastoma cells.

These findings demonstrate that Trien-treated neuroblastoma cells are a good model to study the effects of copper depletion on neuronal cells. However, models, thought similar, are not always fully super imposable. In fact, at least an important difference exists between copper-depleted SH-SY5Y cells and neonatal $Mo^{br/Y}$ brain. In the latter case low levels of Bcl-2 accompanied apoptosis. The reason of this discrepancy may reside in the intrinsic differences of the two experimental models (*in vitro* tumour cells versus *in vivo* neurons). It is conceivable that tumour cells are more prone to activate mechanisms of resistance to death stimuli than normal neurons in a developing brain. As a matter of fact, apoptosis is a physiological process in the remodelling of the growing neuronal tissue [133].

In conclusion, copper deficiency represents a potential harmful condition to neuronal cells because it induces a constant, low ROS production, probably arising in mitochondria, due to inhibition of Cytox. Thus, copper-depleted neuronal cells become very sensitive to any oxidizing agent. Furthermore, copper depletion affects cellular antioxidants defence. This pro-oxidant situation alerts biochemical factors involved in apoptosis, thus leading to neurodegeneration.

4. Intracellular redox state as modulator of cell signalling and death response

Filomeni, G. and Ciriolo, M.R.

4.1 Intracellular redox state

The energy required to maintain the ordered state of a single cell or a more structured organism comes from electron flow, which starts from oxidisable organic molecules (carbohydrates and lipids) and culminates at oxygen, the final acceptor of reducing equivalents. The mediators of this electron flow are molecules able to cycle from reduced into oxidized form, in a sequence-dependent on their electro-chemical potential. Furthermore, redox couples [nicotinamide adenine dinucleotide phosphate ($NADP^+$/NADPH), glutathione (GSSG/GSH), and thioredoxin ($TrxSS/Trx(SH)_2$) systems] are the most important systems in maintaining the intracellular redox environment. These *redox couples* are often linked each other to form a set of related couples responsive to electron flow. The redox state of each couple can be considered the sum of the *reduction potential*, which is a measure of the electric gradient for the two inter-convertible forms of a specific redox couple and of the *reducing capacity* which, by defining the number of electrons available, simply depends on the concentration of the reducing form of the redox couple [134].

NADPH is the major source of electrons for bio-reductive biosynthesis; furthermore, it limits the action of freely diffusing oxidizing radicals, which alter redox environment, by scavenging them or re-reducing the oxidized biomolecules directly operating as an antioxidant. In this context, NADPH acts as hydrogen anion donor in several enzymatic processes such as the reduction of glutathione, catalyzed by the NADPH-dependent glutathione disulfide reductase (GSSG-Red). Besides such co-factor role, recently, a direct action on reduction reactions has been suggested for NADPH, especially in the mitochondrial compartment where it can scavenge toxic free radicals and repair biomolecule-derived radicals [135].

Glutathione represents the most prevalent low molecular weight thiol with several fundamental functions ranging from detoxification to messenger molecule. It exists as a reduced predominant form (GSH), as a disulfide oxidised form (GSSG), or as mixed disulfide with protein thiols (GS-R). GSH can represent a cofactor for antioxidant enzymes such as GSH-peroxidase, a selenium containing enzyme involved in the reduction of many peroxides, especially membrane lipids peroxides formed upon oxidative insults. A further role for GSH has been suggested in intracellular copper transport and detoxification [136]. Therefore, GSH decreases the dangerous effect of free intracellular copper by impeding potentially toxic redox reactions among the metal and ROS (Fenton reaction). Finally, GSH may represent a storage for cysteine, which can be toxic when present at high concentration.

Mammalian and prokaryotic Trx are proteins with oxido-reductase activity. They contain a highly conserved -Cys-Gly-Pro-Cys- active site, essential for the function as a general and potent protein disulfide oxido-reductase. Specific protein disulfide targets for reduction by Trx are ribonucleotide reductase, protein disulfide isomerase and several transcription factors including p53, NF-κB and AP-1 [137].

Since GSH concentration is 100-1000 fold higher than the reduced form of the other couples, glutathione redox state usually reflects the status of intracellular redox environment. Moreover, the other redox couples are strictly related by chemical reactions in maintaining GSH/GSSG proper ratio: in fact, both Trx and NADPH are necessary to allow the re-reduction of the two oxidized species of glutathione. In particular, GSSG-Red catalyzes the reduction of GSSG by using the NADPH-supplied reducing equivalents, while Trx participates as electron donor for the reduction of mixed disulfide between GSH and protein thiols (GS-R).

4.2 Thiol/disulfide exchange: a redox switch for cell signalling and survival

Processes that involve oxidative changes and intracellular thiols modification have been recently associated with the modulation of several protein functions. The primary target of redox regulation can be the sulfhydryl group of specific cysteine residues, named "reactive" cysteines. Owing to their low pKa, which is a function of neighbouring residues, these cysteines can be easily oxidized to form a disulfide bond, sulfenic (R-SOH), sulfinic ($R-SO_2H$), or sulfonic ($R-SO_3H$) acid [138], the last two oxidative modifications being irreversible. Proteins possessing reactive cysteines should be more sensitive to oxidative alteration that could eventually lead to irreversible modifications in their structure and function. Sulfenic acid can be either re-reduced to a thiol form or transformed in thiol derivatives, such as nitrosylated (by reaction with NO) and glutathiolated thiols or disulfide bridges. These chemical species can be reduced back through the reaction catalysed by Trx and glutaredoxin (GRX) (Figure 8).

4.2.1 Thiol oxidation: "gain" or "loss" of function

Cysteine redox state influences structure of sensitive proteins leading to "gain" or "loss" of function. In particular, it has been suggested that, while intra-molecular disulfide bond formation results in alteration of protein three-dimensional conformation, the inter-molecular disulfide bridge formation could lead to protein arrangement in dimers and/or multimers. The latter process could influence the association between different cellular proteins and be implicated in regulatory pathways [139].

γ-glutamyl-cysteinil synthetase (γ-GCS) is the rate-limiting enzyme involved in the two-step synthesis of GSH. It belongs to the class of proteins that "sense" oxidizing conditions as a regulatory mechanism because, through reversible disulfide bonds formation, the enzyme undergoes a gain of function [140]. The holoenzyme is formed by a 70 kDa catalytic subunit (γ-GCSc) and a 27 kDa regulatory subunit (γ-GCSr). Although both subunits present several cysteine residues, only two disulfide bonds and a thiol cysteine residue at the active site are

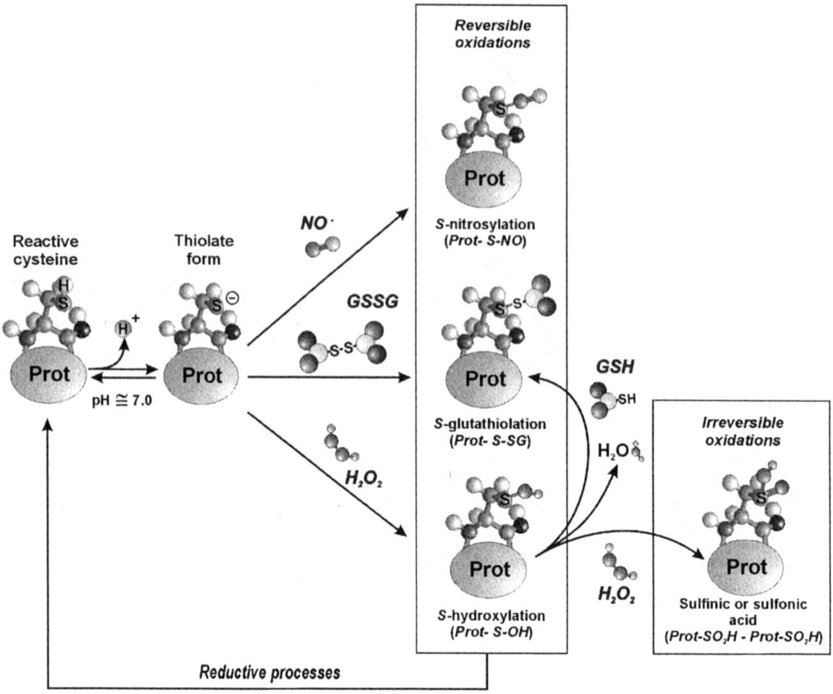

Figure 8. Oxidised species of reactive cysteines

required for optimal enzyme activity. One disulfide bond is inter-molecular and it is necessary to link the two subunits; the other is intra-molecular and does not affect the active site [141]. Oxidizing conditions that result in GSH depletion promote formation of the inter-molecular disulfide. This produces a conformational change that increases the affinity and the specificity of the glutamate binding site. On the other hand, physiological GSH concentration reduces the inter-molecular disulfide, thus producing changes in conformation that favours GSH feedback inhibition [140].

Differently from γ-GCS, protein tyrosin phosphatases (PTPs) are well-characterized examples of negatively redox-regulated proteins by disulfide bridge formation. PTPs activity seems to be modulated by oxidation/reduction reactions involving the cysteine residue required for catalysis [142]. PTPs share a conserved 230-amino acid domain containing the cysteine residue that catalyses the hydrolysis of phosphate from phospho-tyrosine residues by the formation of a cysteinyl-phosphate intermediate [143]. PTPs are involved in the regulation of reversible tyrosine phosphorylation in the pathway induced by insulin. Recently, it has been established that insulin stimulation generates a burst of intracellular H_2O_2 in insulin-sensitive cells, which is associated with reversible oxidative inhibition of overall cellular PTPase activity, especially the PTP-1B family member [144].

On the basis of these findings, the question to which researchers are trying to answer is whether protein thiols redox state may represent a "molecular switch" able to reversibly activate/deactivate protein function, comparable to the well-established phosphorylative regulation where the addition of a phosphate group dramatically changes protein activity.

4.2.2 Trx/ASK-1 and GST-πl/JNK complexes: transformation of disulfide into phosphorylative potential

Among proteins that are responsive to the alteration of the redox state, Trx and glutathione-*S*-transferase-π1 (GST-π1) represent other well-established examples. Studies, performed using the yeast two-hybrid system, led to identify Trx as a regulatory protein interacting with apoptosis signal-regulating kinase (ASK-1) [145]. The Trx/ASK-1 association gives rise to the inactivation of kinase activity of ASK-1; moreover, this interaction is found only in non-stressed cells and seems to be modulated by intracellular ROS levels. In particular, increase in ROS concentration causes disulfide bridge formation between or within Trx molecules and, as a result, ASK-1 can undergo multimerization, which correspond to the active form of the enzyme [146]. ASK-1 has been suggested to activate MKK 3/6 and MKK4/7, upstream kinases of p38 mitogen activated protein (MAP) kinase and c-Jun NH_2-terminal kinase (JNK) respectively [147]. Signal transduction mediated by the phosphorylation cascade has to be tightly regulated because, once induced, it leads to the activation of different substrates, including several transcription factors involved in cell response to stress and damage (such as ATF-2, c-Jun and p53).

One example of such regulation could be represented by JNK, the activity of which is maintained at low levels within the cell, even in the presence of high concentrations of growth factors. As described for ASK-1, JNK activity seems to be inhibited in unstressed cells. Adler and co-workers purified the inhibitory component of JNK and identified it as GST-π1 [148]. Under resting conditions, JNK phosphorylation is inhibited upon its association with GST-π1, while under H_2O_2 or UV treatment, the GST-π1/JNK complex dissociates leading to GST-π1 dimer and/or multimer structures formation and JNK activation [139]. The identification of Trx and GST-π1 proteins as modulators of JNK and ASK-1 activities provides a potential molecular mechanism through which redox-mediated signalling events could be strictly related to downstream processes mediated by stress kinases activation. Upon oxidative unbalance, intracellular free thiols are oxidized to disulfides; as a result, the increase of disulfide potential indirectly leads to protein kinases activation and, in some cases, induction of apoptosis. This redox regulation of apoptotic process has been recently suggested to occur upon cell treatment with different pro-oxidizing compounds. It has been demonstrated that exogenous GSSG, a non-permeable compound, or diallyl disulfide (DADS), a cell permeable molecule extracted from garlic, are able to specifically activate different protein kinase-mediated apoptotic pathways in response to oxidative stress. In particular, treatment of a promonocytic cell line U937 with GSSG results in a significant decrease of exofacial cell membrane thiol groups and decrement of intracellular GSH content, owing to its engagement in the formation of mixed disulfides with protein thiols [149]. Concomitantly, redox changes in Trx thiol state and activation of p38 MAP kinase pathway are observed. Under these conditions cells are committed to apoptosis along the mitochondrial apoptotic pathway, characterized by Bcl-2 down-regulation, cytochrome *c* release, caspase-9 cleavage and caspase-3 activation. GSSG-mediated apoptosis is efficiently inhibited by counteracting the intracellular mixed disulfides formation, or by increasing the stability of Trx/ASK-1 complex [149].

Also treatment of the neuroblastoma cell line SH-SY5Y with DADS results in arrest of cell cycle in G2/M phase and commitment to apoptosis through the activation of the mitochondrial pathway. The earliest oxidative event observed following DADS addition was an increase in ROS production that gave rise to protein and phospholipids damage and to the activation of the redox-sensitive JNK/c-Jun pathway. In particular, it has been demonstrated that DADS treatment induces JNK dissociation from GST-π1 and its activation by phosphorylation [150].

4.2.3 Sulfhydryls oxidation modulates redox sensitive transcription factors activity

The regulation of several transcription factors seems to be dependent on the redox state of specific cysteine residues. Although the understanding of redox regulation of mammalian transcription factors is still rudimentary, a huge amount of information is available from bacteria. To survive in adverse environments, bacteria have evolved different and sophisticated mechanisms able to rapidly modulate gene transcription. These genes encode enzymes involved in detoxification of reactive molecules, export, repair and other homeostatic functions. A number of different classes of transcription factors are implicated in such control of gene expression, among which the OxyR system is the most deeply understood. OxyR activity depends on modification of specific cysteine residues in response to H_2O_2, GSH reactive compounds and RNS [151]. Pioneering studies by Storz and co-workers showed that one mechanism responsible for the activation of OxyR upon exposure to H_2O_2 involves the formation of a disulfide bond between Cys 199 and Cys 208, two residues that are separated by 17 Å in the reduced – and inactive – form of the protein [152]. The result of this reaction is a change in DNA binding specificity, which occurs under a tetrameric conformation, and the recruitment of RNA polymerase. Recent findings from Stamler's laboratory demonstrate that, besides this "on-off" modulation, a finer regulation for OxyR binding to DNA can also occur. In fact, they suggest that different redox stimuli result in a different strength of binding of OxyR to DNA, which occurs through the modulation of cooperative effect among its subunits [153]. This new theory not only suggests that OxyR (and maybe other proteins) can discriminate among redox-related signalling, but also that different thiol modification can have unique functional effects. It predicts that cysteine modification by *S*-nitrosylation (S-NO), oxidation to form a mixed disulfide with glutathione (S-SG, *S*-glutathiolation), intramolecular disulfide (S-S), or by sulfenic acid (S-OH, *S*-hydroxylation), may be alternatively exploited to control gene expression [153] (Figure 9).

In yeast, elevated concentrations of H_2O_2 stimulate the synthesis of at least 115 proteins, including the transcriptional regulator Yap1, a functional homologue of the bacterial OxyR protein. Its deletion results in hypersensitivity not only to H_2O_2, but also to GSH depletors, several electrophiles and metals. Yap1 contains a non-canonical leucine-rich export signal (NES) embedded within the C-terminal cysteine-rich domain including the residues Cys 598, Cys 620 and Cys 629. Oxidative stress results in conformational changes, due to an internal disulfide bond formation between Cys 598 and Cys 303 that inhibit export of Yap1 from the nucleus [154]. Differently from its homologue OxyR, Yap1 is insensitive to stress associated with increased intracellular levels of GSSG due to the presence of only a reactive cysteine [154] (Figure 9).

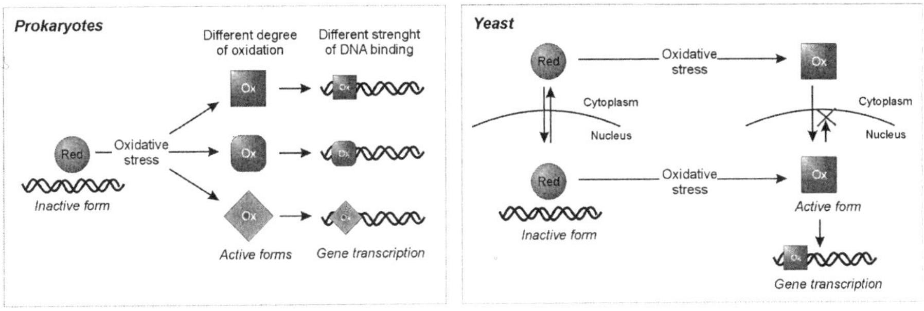

Figure 9. Regulation of transcription factors activity and localization by oxidative stress

In multicellular eukaryotes, the activity of several transcription factors has been suggested to be modulated by redox changes of specific cysteines (Figure 10); however the molecular mechanisms through which this modulation occur has not been elucidated yet. Some of these redox-sensitive factors are involved in the control of gene expression associated with cell cycle regulation and apoptosis.

NF-κB

NF-κB is a heterodimer of p50/p65 subunits that is bound to the inhibitory protein IκB within the cytoplasm. Under appropriate stimuli, NF-κB translocates into the nucleus and activates gene transcription [155]. This event relies on the dissociation from IκB, which in turn is phosphorylated by IκB kinase (IKK) and targeted for the ubiquitination/degradation pathway. NF-κB regulates a wide array of genes involved in the inflammatory response. It is now established that reducing conditions are required into the nucleus for NF-κB DNA binding [156], whereas oxidizing conditions in the cytoplasm promote NF-κB activation [157] (Figure 10). Such pro-oxidant-dependent activation relies on the evidence that H_2O_2, $O_2^{\cdot-}$, or mitochondrial-derived ROS induce cytosolic redox changes that allow NF-κB activation [158]. On the other hand, pre-treatment of cells with antioxidant compounds, such as N-acetyl cysteine or pyrrolidine dithiocarbamate prevents cytokine-induced NF-κB activation [159]. Although, a cysteine residue in the DNA binding region of the p50 subunit (Cys 62) of NF-κB must be in the reduced state [160], in order to allow DNA binding, the redox-sensitive step or the "switch-on" for NF-κB in the cytoplasm has still to be elucidated. In particular, the type of post-translational modifications that mediates the cellular control mechanisms, and the components of NF-κB system that undergo redox modifications (i.e., p50, p65, IκB proteins, IKK), have not been clearly identified. It has been suggested that one potential redox-mediated inducer of NF-κB could be the cyclin dependent kinase inhibitor p21, which is able to activate the MAP kinase cascade [161]. This process results in both IκB dissociation and phosphorylation of the p65 subunit.

AP-1

AP-1 is a transcription factor that belongs to the basic leucine zipper (bZip) family. It is a heterodimeric protein consisting of c-Fos and Jun subunit (c-Jun, JunB, JunD), with the primary activating form being c-Fos/c-Jun. However, Jun-Jun homodimers can also activate transcription with less efficiency. AP-1 activation has an important role in the control of cell proliferation and differentiation. Several different growth factors (e.g. βFGF, EGF), cytokines (e.g. TNF-α, TGFβ), and tumour promoters (e.g. phorbol esters, asbestos fibers) increase cellular AP-1 activity *in vitro* [162]. Regulation of AP-1 activity occurs through an increase in the transcription of *c-fos* and *c-jun* and phosphorylation of c-Fos and c-Jun proteins. JNK1/2 (c-Jun NH_2-terminal kinase), ERK1/2 (extracellular stimulus responsive kinase), and other members of the MAP kinase family participate in phosphorylation of the c-Jun and c-Fos proteins [163]. Moreover, oxidative stress by H_2O_2 and $O_2^{\cdot-}$-generating systems induces AP-1 by increasing the transcription of *c-fos* and *c-jun* [164]. The stimulation of AP-1 activity by cytokines and growth factors also appears to be dependent on $O_2^{\cdot-}$ production. On the contrary, increased cellular GSH levels inhibit the expression of c-Fos and Jun proteins as well as the activation of AP-1 [165]. This redox sensitivity is likely transduced through the JNK and ERK pathways.

Similarly to NF-κB, AP-1 binding to DNA is favoured under reducing conditions (Figure 10). A single cysteine residue in the basic region (i.e. DNA binding domain) of the c-Fos and c-Jun proteins confers this redox sensitivity [166]. Redox factor 1 (Ref-1) appears to be the principal regulator of the redox status of AP-1. The reducing capability of Ref-1 relies on a cysteine residue located at the N-terminal end of the protein [167]. Ref-1, in turn, is modulated by Trx, which translocates into the nucleus upon cell stimulation [168]. Recent studies demonstrate that a decrease in the GSH/GSSG ratio induces *S*-glutathiolation of the redox-sensitive cysteine in the basic region of c-Jun thus preventing DNA binding *in vitro* [169]. Therefore, oxidative modifications of a single cysteine seem to be the key factor in the modulation of AP-1 activity *in vitro*.

p53

The tumour suppressor protein p53 binds to its specific DNA sites more favourably in a reducing environment [170] (Figure 10), and mutation or oxidation of cysteine residues in the p53 core binding domain prevents DNA binding and p53-induced transcription [171]. Moreover, some of the cysteine residues are involved in the coordination of zinc ions, which are essential for protein structure and function. It also appears that Ref-1 regulates p53 DNA binding and gene transactivation like it regulates NF-κB and AP-1 [172]. As far as the redox regulation of p53 is concerned, it has been demonstrated that *in vitro* oxidation of Cys 182 may occur and it involves the formation of a mixed disulfide with glutathione. The glutathione adduct may prevent proper helix-helix interaction within the DNA binding domain and contribute to tetramer dissociation.

HSF1

HSF1 belongs to a family of heat shock factors whose activation and DNA binding is mediated by stress that alters thiols homeostasis. The activation of HSF1 is characterized by its conversion from the monomeric to trimeric form and it is induced by heat shock and by a wide variety of chemical and physical stresses that generate misfolded proteins. HSF1 activation results in heat shock proteins (Hsps) expression, such as the inducible isoforms of Hsp70 and Hsp27. Conditions that triggers GSH oxidation leading to GSSG, mixed disulfides (GS-R) or protein-protein disulfides formation, are able to induce HSF1 trimerization and DNA binding. These observations, together with the fact that HSF1 binding activity is attenuated under anoxic condition, suggest the involvement of a redox-dependent step during HSF1 activation. A pro-oxidant environment favours the nuclear translocation of HSF1, while HSF1 binding activity is increased by the reduction of critical cysteine residues. It has been demonstrated that H_2O_2 up-regulates Trx before HSF1 activation indicating that Trx reduces HSF1 allowing its DNA binding during oxidative stress [173].

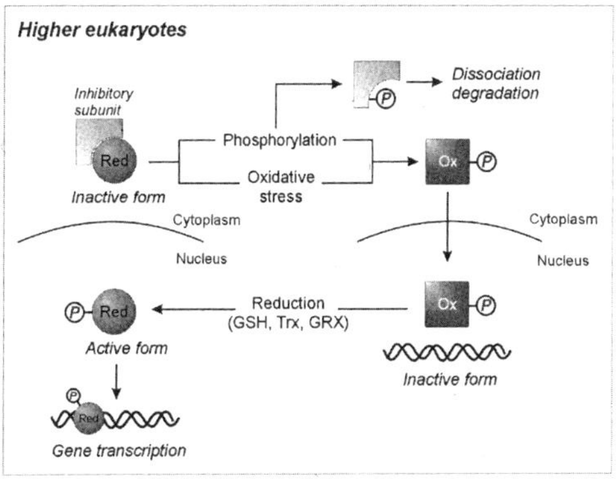

Figure 10. Phosphorylative and oxidative processes in the regulation of transcription factors in higher eukaryotes

4.2.4 Gene transcription can modulate cellular redox state: a novel hypothesis

As outlined above, the redox state of cysteines can finally result in cell proliferation or death by directly modulating transcription factors or indirectly inducing phosphorylative cascades implicated in cell cycle regulation. The choice between death and proliferation is often cell-type dependent: phosphorylative pathway mediated by JNK represents a good example, as it is able to induce cell proliferation [174], or apoptosis [150] under appropriate stimuli. Indeed, redox changes seem to represent the *primum movens* in the cascade of events that leads to the activation of these divergent cellular processes. On the other hand, we demonstrate that gene expression can in turn control the redox state. In fact, recently we identified c-Myc as a transcription factor that has the potentiality to play this role. c-Myc has a central and necessary role in the proliferation of normal cells; following mitogenic stimulations, c-Myc is rapidly induced in quiescent cells [175], suggesting that it is required for continuous cell growth, while inhibition of c-Myc can block mitogenic signals and facilitate cell differentiation [176, 177]. Conversely, c-Myc can also activate apoptosis [178], and this death-dealing aspect has gained attention because of its potential therapeutic approach in advanced malignancy. Since c-Myc is frequently deregulated in tumour cells, an effort has been made in characterizing target genes, which may mediate its apoptotic properties. Recent data have suggested that c-Myc is involved in the CD95/Fas and TNF apoptotic pathways and in p53 activity modulation. Besides c-Myc function as an upstream regulator of apoptosis, we demonstrated that its downregulation induces cell death through the activation of the mitochondrial pathway in melanoma cells [179]. Moreover, under c-Myc downregulation, a dramatic alteration in the GSH/GSSG ratio occurs early before the appearance of apoptotic features. c-Myc downregulation is associated with a general dysfunction of glutathione homeostasis: the activities of GSSG-Red and γ-GCS as well as the expression level of the latter enzyme, are decreased in *c-myc* antisense clones. Furthermore, the extrusion of GSSG is activated in order to maintain a high GSH/GSSG ratio. The impairment in both the GSSG reduction and the GSH neo-synthesis has been suggested to be causative of cell death, as N-acetyl cysteine, a well-known reducing compound, completely inhibits apoptosis by recovering the proper cellular reducing power [179]. This evidence outlines a new concept of redox-mediated signalling, in which proper gene expression of transcription factors functions in keeping the correct redox milieu.

4.3 Relationship between cellular thiols and function of apoptotic mitochondrial factors

Oxidative stress-induced apoptosis takes place preferentially through the activation of the mitochondrial pathway, because these organelles are both the target in the induction phase of apoptosis and the main source of ROS that, in turn, represent the effectors of apoptosis execution. In particular, caspases-mediated proteolysis of complex II causes an impairment of the electron transport chain and a massive production of oxyradicals, a phenomenon that represents an amplifying process for the establishment of degenerative conditions. Besides this novel function hypothesized for caspases, several mitochondria-sited proteins involved in the apoptotic process seem to be affected by the cytosolic redox state, such as cytochrome *c*, Bcl-2, caspases and the MPTP.

We demonstrated that GSH plays a fundamental role in the release of cytochrome *c* from mitochondria and subsequent commitment to apoptosis [180-182]. A massive extrusion of GSH through specific membrane translocators [181] has been identified as a primary event in the process leading to cell death and it is paralleled by the release of cytochrome *c* into the cytosol [182]. GSH-dependent cytochrome *c* release is also observed upon treatment with buthionine sulfoximine, a specific inhibitor of glutathione synthesis, without commitment of cell death. Moreover, neither GSH extrusion nor cytochrome *c* release from mitochondria is observed by inducing apoptosis through a thiol-reducing compound, such as dithiothreitol. This allows hypothesizing that the process of cytochrome *c* release is strictly redox-dependent and not a mere consequence of mitochondrial membrane alteration.

Bcl-2

Bcl-2, in addition to its role in the regulation of the permeability of the outer mitochondrial membrane, might function as an antioxidant partner to modulate ROS concentration. For example, during TNF-α-induced apoptosis, which involves ROS signalling [183], Bcl-2 prevents ROS accumulation and therefore mitochondrial membrane depolarization, Bax relocalization, cytochrome *c* release, executer caspases activation and nuclear fragmentation. However, even if the molecular mechanisms that underline Bcl-2 mediated protection remain unclear, its antioxidant properties are based on the evidence that: i) Bcl-2, or the homologue anti-apoptotic Bcl-X_L, influences the generation of ROS [184]; ii) it prevents oxidative damage to cellular compartments [185]; iii) it functions as a pro-oxidant, by inducing cellular antioxidant systems [186]. Cells overexpressing Bcl-2 show unaltered antioxidant enzyme activities and an increase in GSH content [187]. These results indicate that Bcl-2 is able to induce a shift in the cellular redox potential towards a more reduced state. Therefore, a cross talk between Bcl-2 and GSH can occur, deeply influencing virus infection and replication [188]. Low or undetectable levels of Bcl-2 are associated with low levels of GSH and these are permissive conditions to viral infection, whereas high levels of Bcl-2 correlate with higher GSH content and, at the same time, induce cell resistance to viral infection [189].

Caspases

Caspases exist as inactive monomeric zymogens (procaspases) that are converted in the active form upon proteolysis and subsequent assembly into two identical heterodimers. Their action on target proteins finally leads to the characteristic features of apoptosis and organized disassembly of the cell. Caspases are cysteine-dependent enzymes and, as such, may be expected to be sensitive to the redox status of the cell. It has been demonstrated that low levels of hydrogen peroxide could temporary inactivate caspases during Fas-mediated apoptosis [190], while under higher flux of hydrogen peroxide caspases remain inactive and cell dies by necrosis. This process seems to be common during cell treatment with oxidants or redox-active compounds [191], where extensive oxidative inactivation of caspases occurs preventing the apoptotic pathway, allowing induction of necrosis. NO has also been reported to inhibit apoptosis, *via* caspase inactivation, and direct *S*-nitrosylation of the thiol group at the active site is implicated (see section 2). In addition to ROS and RNS, intracellular GSH seems to have an important role in ensuring caspase activity by maintaining a reducing environment and preserving critical cysteine residues oxidation. Moreover, an additional role for GSH as *upstream* redox-modulator of caspase-8 activity has been recently proposed [192]. In lymphoblastoid B cells, glutathione depletion prevents Fas-mediated apoptosis upstream of caspase-8 activation. Immunoprecipitation of the death-inducing signalling complex (DISC) revealed that DISC was still formed under glutathione depletion, while the first cleavage step of procaspase-8 was inhibited. Accordingly, under cell-free conditions, radiolabeled procaspase-8 was processed at the immunoprecipitated DISC only after the addition of exogenous dithiothreitol or reduced glutathione. GSH appears to be a prerequisite for death receptor-mediated apoptosis and this might be due to the redox sensitivity of either caspases or the DISC, because death domain-containing receptors and procaspase-8 have a number of reactive cysteine residues. Overall, this evidence indicates that the activation of caspase-8 at the DISC and, hence Fas-mediated apoptosis induction, shows a cell-specific requirement for glutathione.

Mitochondrial Permeability Transition Pore (MPTP)

The capability of mitochondrion to integrate death signals is firstly related to changes in transmembrane potential. This phenomenon is associated with the mitochondrial permeability transition (PT), initially described as general swelling due to a non-specific damage at the level of external mitochondrial membrane. Several proteins are associated with the nucleus of MPTP, but only a few numbers have been still identified; among those benzodiazepine receptor, creatin kinase and hexokinase II are the most important [193]. Furthermore, co-immunoprecipitation analyses indicate that a protein/protein interaction with the regulatory proteins Bcl-2 and Bax also occurs [193, 194], although it has to be established whether these are able to independently induce membrane permeabilization. The capability of cyclosporin A to inhibit MPTP opening through the binding with the mitochondrial protein cyclophilin-D has contributed to the finding of the molecular mechanism governing this phenomenon. Cyclophilin-D has a peptidilprolil cis-trans isomerase activity; therefore, it is able to catalyze the rotation of peptide bound neighbouring proline residues. Halestrap and coworkers that also proposed the formation of an intramolecular disulfide bridge in the ANT structure upon oxidative stress suggested a putative interaction of cyclophilin-D with ANT. The resulting conformational change seems to involve a cis-trans isomerization, which plays a pivotal role for the opening of the pore [7]. Moreover, Chernyak and Bernardi have provided data suggesting that two distinct thiol groups are implicated in modulating the activity of MPTP [195]. One is sensitive to glutathione oxidation, while the other is sensitive to the redox state of the mitochondrial matrix NAD(P)H. The latter cysteine accounts for the well-documented stimulatory effect of the matrix NADH on MPT, perhaps through the mediation of Trx. ANT is known to have three cysteine residues that show differential reactivity towards various thiol reagents and oxidizing agents. These cysteines may represent the thiol groups that regulate both cyclophilin-D binding and the inhibitory effects of ADP on the MPTP [196]. Recent data suggest that oxidative cross-linking of the two matrix facing cysteine residues on the ANT (Cys 56 and Cys 159) plays the key role in regulating the MPTP. Adenine nucleotide binding to the ANT is inhibited by Cys 159 modification whilst oxidation of Cys 56 increases Cyclophilin-D binding to the ANT, probably at Pro 61.

4.4 Extracellular oxidative environment and intracellular redox response

The extracellular environment can dialogue with the intracellular compartments in a wide range of modalities. External molecules such as lipophylic hormones or esterified compounds can freely cross the plasma membrane owing to their chemical nature and act inside the cell without restrictions. On the other hand, hydrophylic molecules can enter the cell only through the action of specific channels or ATP-dependent pumps. There are also compounds that are totally membrane-impermeable but can stimulate a cell response by their binding to specific receptors that transduce the signal into the cytosol. Each molecule could then represent a specific marker of the extracellular environment and induce a stimulus to which cell responds.

Reducing or oxidizing molecules, such as Trx and/or H_2O_2, can be present outside the cell thus changing extracellular redox milieu. Furthermore, H_2O_2 can cross the plasma membrane and enter the cell leading to changes in the intracellular redox environment. Many membrane proteins can produce H_2O_2 upon different stimuli. These include the NADPH oxidase expressed on neutrophil membrane generating high levels of H_2O_2 as a defence mechanism in response to bacterial attack. Besides this "non-futile" generation of oxidant species, during an inflammatory response, cells produce low amount of H_2O_2 at plasma membrane level, by non phagocyte NADPH-oxidase protein homologue, during binding of hormones to their receptors (e.g. insulin), or as by-product of enzyme reactions, such as that catalysed by the membrane-associated enzyme γ-glutamyl transpeptidase (γ-GT) [197]. As a consequence of H_2O_2 generation, intracellular redox environment shifts towards oxidative conditions leading to activation of several transcription factors (see above). It is interesting to remind that several ligands such as those belonging to TNF superfamily can produce H_2O_2 upon binding to their receptors. Moreover, protein *S*-glutathiolation [198] and protein/protein disulfide bond formation [139] have also been suggested to be formed during the TNF receptor-mediated signals. Taking into account that oxidative alteration can function either as activator of upstream protein kinases (such as stress activated protein kinase (SAPK), extracellular signal regulated kinase (ERK) 1, 2, JNK and p38 [199]) or as inhibitor of downstream transcription factors (such as AP-1 and NF-κB), the decision between life and death depends on the relative strength of the oxidative stress and on the type of cell involved.

While the mechanisms by which redox-active permeable molecules, such as dithiothreitol, diamide and H_2O_2 alter the intracellular environment are well established, we tested if impermeable redox-active molecules were also able to change intracellular redox environment. Pioneering work performed with isolated erythrocytes demonstrated that intracellular GSH content could be modulated by external oxidants. In fact, Reglinski and co-workers demonstrated that by adding increasing concentrations of the non-permeable Ellmann's reagent to red blood cells, intracellular GSH levels decreased in a dose dependent manner [200] due to the formation of intracellular mixed disulfides. Moreover, by adding GSH, a membrane non-permeable compound, to red blood cells, an increase in the intracellular glutathione content previously engaged with protein thiols was envisaged [201]. The mechanism underlining these phenomena was explained in terms of a thiol/disulfide exchange among cysteine residues of proteins spanning across the plasma membrane. This process could represent another mode for transducing signals from extracellular milieu to intracellular environment (figure 11).

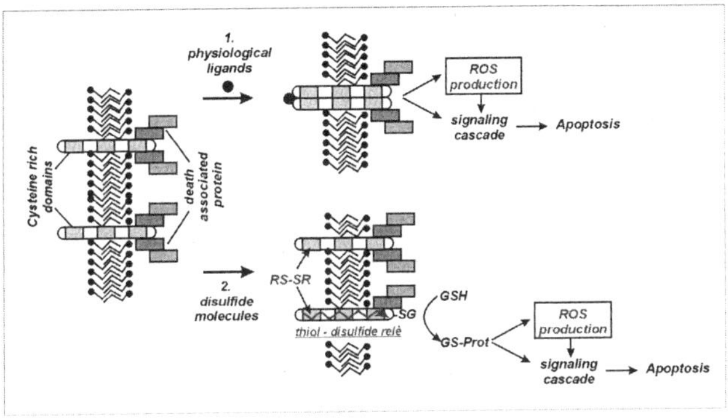

Figure 11. Schematic model of redox signalling mediated by non-permeable oxidants

This hypothesis was also strengthened by the results obtained with GSSG on tumour cells, where this compound was able to induce apoptosis *via* the mitochondrial pathway. In this experimental model a disulfide/thiol exchange along a chain of cysteine residues of transmembrane proteins was evidenced. Putative protein targets of GSSG-mediated oxidation could be represented by the cysteine-rich TNF receptors that are particularly concentrated on the plasma membrane of tumour cells. Even if interactions between redox-active molecules and these receptors are probably not so efficient as well as those mediated by binding of physiological effectors, the structure and the function of membrane receptors may be modified by reaction with these compounds in such a way as to start a signalling pathway. These results highlight a novel modality for the extracellular redox milieu in cell signalling and viability without the intervention of ROS. This is particularly evident in the mechanisms of signalling mediated by specialized cells: antigen-presenting cells increase extracellular cysteine levels in order to stimulate the proliferation of activated T cells [202]. Under physiological conditions extracellular cysteine equivalents exist as the oxidized form, cystine, which T cells are unable to internalize; during immune response, antigen-presenting cells take up cystine and extrude cysteine into the extracellular space where it becomes available for T cells [203].

Acknowledgements

This work was partially supported by grants from MIUR, FIRB, CNR and Ministero della Sanità.

References

[1] Strasser, A., O'Connor, L. and Dixit, V.M. (2000) Apoptosis signaling. Annu. Rev. Biochem. 69: 217-245
[2] Thornberry, N.A. and Lazebnik, Y. (1998) Caspases: enemies within. Science 281: 1312-1316
[3] Levine, A.J. (1997) p53, the cellular gatekeeper for growth and division. Cell 88: 323-331
[4] Chen, M., and Wang, J. (2002) Initiator caspases in apoptosis signaling pathways. Apoptosis 7: 313-319
[5] Cain, K., Bratton, S.B. and Cohen, G.M. (2002) The Apaf-1 apoptosome: a large caspase-activating complex. Biochimie 84: 203-214
[6] Martinou, J.C. and Green, D.R. (2001) Breaking the mitochondrial barrier. Nat. Rev. Mol. Cell. Biol. 2: 63-67
[7] Halestrap, A.P., McStay, G.P and Clarke, S.J. (2001) The permeability transition pore complex: another view. Biochimie 84: 153-166
[8] Mattson, M.P. and Kroemer, G. (2003) Mitochondria in cell death: novel targets for neuroprotection and cardioprotection. Trends Mol. Med. 9: 196-205
[9] Van Gurp, M., Festjens, N., Van Loo, G., Saelens, X. and Vandenabeele, P. (2003) Mitochondrial intermembrane proteins in cell death. Biochem. Biophys. Res. Commun. 304: 487-497
[10] Adrain, C. and Martin, S.J. (2001) The mitochondrial apoptosome: a killer unleashed by the cytochrome seas. Trends Biochem. Sci. 26: 390-397
[11] Saleh, A., Srinivasula, S.M., Balkir, L., Robbins, P.D. and Alnemri, E.S. (2000) Negative regulation of the Apaf-1 apoptosome by Hsp70. Nat. Cell Biol. 2: 476-483
[12] Bruey, J.M., Ducasse, C., Bonniaud, P., Ravagnan, L., Susin, S.A., Diaz-Latoud, C., Gurbuxani, S., Arrigo, A.P., Kroemer, G., Solary, E. and Garrido, C. (2000) Hsp27 negatively regulates cell death by interacting with cytochrome c. Nat. Cell Biol. 2: 645-652
[13] Crompton, M. (2000) Bax, Bid and the permeabilization of the mitochondrial outer membrane in apoptosis. Curr. Opin. Cell Biol. 12: 414-419
[14] Penninger, J.M. and Kroemer, G. (2003) Mitochondria, AIF and caspases--rivaling for cell death execution. Nat. Cell Biol. 5: 97-99
[15] Moncada, S., Palmer, R.M. and Higgs, E.A. (1988) The discovery of nitric oxide as the endogenous nitrovasodilator. Hypertension 12: 365-372
[16] Stamler, J.S. (1994) Redox signaling: nitrosylation and related target interactions of nitric oxide. Cell 78, 931-936
[17] Kuo, R.C., Baxter, G.T., Thompson, S.H., Stricker, S.A., Patton, C., Bonaventura, J. and Epel D. (2000) NO is necessary and sufficient for egg activation at fertilization. Nature 406: 633-636
[18] Wingrove, J.A. and O'Farrell, P.H. (1999) Nitric oxide contributes to behavioral, cellular, and developmental responses to low oxygen in Drosophila. Cell 98: 105-114
[19] Dawson, T.M. and Dawson, V.L. (1996) Nitric oxide synthase: role as a transmitter/mediator in the brain and endocrine system. Annu. Rev. Med. 47: 219-27
[20] Moncada, S., Palmer, R.M. and Higgs, E.A. (1991) Nitric oxide: physiology, pathophysiology, and pharmacology. Pharmacol Rev. 43: 109-142
[21] Albina, J.E., Abate, J.A. and Henry, W.L. Jr. (1991) Nitric oxide production is required for murine resident peritoneal macrophages to suppress mitogen-stimulated T cell proliferation. Role of IFN-gamma in the induction of the nitric oxide-synthesizing pathway. J. Immunol. 147: 144-148
[22] Liu, L. and Stamler J.S. (1999) NO: an inhibitor of cell death. Cell Death Differ. 6: 937-942
[23] Beyer, R.E. (1992) An analysis of the role of coenzyme Q in free radical generation and as an antioxidant. Biochem. Cell. Biol. 70: 390-403
[24] Vignais, P.V. (2002) The superoxide-generating NADPH oxidase: structural aspects and activation mechanism. Cell. Mol. Life Sci. 59: 1428-1459
[25] Li, J.M. and Shah, A.M. (2003) ROS generation by nonphagocytic NADPH oxidase: potential relevance in diabetic nephropathy. J. Am. Soc. Nephrol. 14: S221-S226
[26] Curtin, J.F., Donovan, M. and Cotter, T.G. (2002) Regulation and measurement of oxidative stress in apoptosis. J. Immunol. Methods. 265: 49-72

[27] Alderton, W.K., Cooper, C.E. and Knowles, R.G. (2001) Nitric oxide synthases: structure, function and inhibition. Biochem J. 357: 593-615

[28] Stamler, J.S., Singel, D.J. and Loscalzo, J. (1992) Biochemistry of nitric oxide and its redox-activated forms. Science 258: 1898-1902

[29] Ames, B.N. (1989) Endogenous oxidative DNA damage, aging, and cancer. Free Radic. Res. Commun. 7: 121-128

[30] Demple, B. and Harrison, L. (1994) Repair of oxidative damage to DNA: enzymology and biology. Annu. Rev. Biochem. 63: 915-948

[31] Vogt, W. (1995) Oxidation of methionyl residues in proteins: tools, targets, and reversal Free Rad Biol. Med. 18: 93-105

[32] Filomeni, G., Rotilio, G. and Ciriolo, M.R. (2002) Cell signalling and the glutathione redox system. Biochem. Pharmacol. 64: 1057-1064

[33] Wolff, S.P. and Dean, R.T. (1986) Fragmentation of proteins by free radicals and its effect on their susceptibility to enzymic hydrolysis. Biochem. J. 234: 399-403

[34] Davies, K.J.A. (1987) Protein damage and degradation by oxygen radicals. General aspects. J. Biol. Chem. 262: 9895-9901

[35] Squier, T.C. (2001) Oxidative stress and protein aggregation during biological aging. Exp. Gerontol. 36: 1539-1550

[36] Van der Vliet, A., Eiserich, J.P. et al. (1996) Nitrotyrosine as biomarker for reactive nitrogen species. Methods Enzymol. 269: 175-184

[37] Stamler, J.S., lamas, S. and Fang, F.C. (2001) Nitrosylation: the prototypic redox-based signaling mechanism. Cell 106: 675–683

[38] Davies, K.J. (2001) Degradation of oxidized proteins by the 20S proteasome. Biochimie 83: 301-310

[39] Esterbauer, H. (1993) Cytotoxicity and genotoxicity of lipid-oxidation products. Am. J. Clin. Nutr. 57: 779S-785S

[40] Scandalios, J.G. (1997) Oxidative stress and the molecular biology of antioxidant defences. Monograph 34. Cold Spring Harbor Laboratory Press, New York

[41] Marklund, S. L. (1982) Human copper-containing superoxide dismutase of high molecular weight. Proc. Natl. Acad. Sci. 79: 7634-7638

[42] Barra, D., Schininà, M.E., Simmaco, M., Bannister, J.V., Bannister, W.H., Rotilio, G. and Bossa, F. (1984) The primary structure of human liver manganese superoxide dismutase. J. Biol. Chem. 259: 12595–12601

[43] Weisiger, R.A. and Fridovich, I. (1973) Mitochondrial superoxide dismutase: site of synthesis and intramitochondrial localization. J. Biol. Chem. 248: 4793–4796

[44] St. Clair, D.K., Oberley, T.D., Muse, K.E. and St. Clair, W.H. (1994) Expression of manganese superoxide dismutase promotes cellular differentiation. Free Rad. Biol. Med. 16: 275-282

[45] Wispe, J.R., Warner, B.B., Clark, J.C., Day, C.R., Neuman, J., Glasser, S.W., Crapo, J.D., Chang, L.Y. and Whitsett, J.A. (1992) Human Mn-superoxide dismutase in pulmonary epithelial cells of transgenic mice confers protection from oxygen injury. J. Biol. Chem. 267: 23937–23941

[46] Rotilio, G., Aquilano, K. and Ciriolo, M.R. (2003) Interplay of Cu,Zn superoxide dismutase and nitric oxide synthase in neurodegenerative processes. IUBMB Life, in press

[47] Zelko, I.N., Mariani, T.J. and Folz, R.J. (2002) Superoxide dismutase multigene family: a comparison of the CuZn-SOD (SOD1), Mn SOD (SOD2), and EC-SOD (SOD3) gene structures, evolution, and expression. Free Rad. Biol. Med. 33: 337-349

[48] Yoo, H.Y., Chang, M.S. and Rho, H.M. (1999) Heavy metal-mediated activation of the rat Cu/Zn superoxide dismutase gene via a metal-responsive element. Mol. Gen. Genet. 262: 310-313

[49] Frank, S., Kampfer, H., Podda, M., Kaufmann, R. and Pfeilschifter, J. (2000) Identification of copper/zinc superoxide dismutase as a nitric oxide-regulated gene in human (HaCaT) keratinocytes: implications for keratinocyte proliferation. Biochem J. 346: 719-728

[50] Ciriolo, M.R., De Martino, A., Lafavia, E., Rossi, L., Carrì, M.T. and Rotilio, G. (2000) Cu,Zn-superoxide dismutase-dependent apoptosis induced by nitric oxide in neuronal cells. J. Biol. Chem. 275: 5065-5072

[51] Okado-Matsumoto, A. and Fridovich, I. (2001) Subcellular distribution of superoxide dismutases (SOD) in rat liver: Cu,Zn-SOD in mitochondria. J. Biol. Chem. 276: 38388-38393

[52] Larrick, J.W. and Wright, S.C. (1990) Cytotoxic mechanism of tumor necrosis factor-alpha. FASEB J. 4: 3215-3223

[53] Kim, Y.M., Bombeck, C.A. and Billiar, T.R. (1999) Nitric oxide as a bifunctional regulator of apoptosis. Circ. Res. 84: 253-256

[54] Szabo, C. (2003) Multiple pathways of peroxynitrite cytotoxicity. Toxicol. Lett. 140-141: 105-112

[55] Inoue, K., Akaike, T., Miyamoto, Y., Okamoto, T., Sawa, T., Otagiri, M., Suzuki, S., Yoshimura, T. and Maeda, H. (1999) Nitrosothiol formation catalyzed by ceruloplasmin. Implication for cytoprotective mechanism in vivo. J. Biol. Chem. 274: 27069-27075

[56] Ciriolo, M.R., Aquilano, K., De Martino, A., Carrì, M.T. and Rotilio G. (2001) Differential role of superoxide and glutathione in S-nitrosoglutathione-mediated apoptosis: a rationale for mild forms of familial amyotrophic lateral sclerosis associated with less active Cu,Zn superoxide dismutase mutants. J Neurochem. 77: 1433-1443

[57] Brown, G.C. and Borutaite, V. (2002) Nitric oxide inhibition of mitochondrial respiration and its role in cell death. Free Rad. Biol. Med. 33: 1440-1450

[58] Schonhoff, C.M., Gaston, B. and Mannick, J.B. (2003) Nitrosylation of cytochrome c during apoptosis. J. Biol. Chem. 278: 18265-18270

[59] Jemmerson, R., Liu, J., Hausauer, D., Lam, K.P., Mondino, A. and Nelson, R.D. (1999) A conformational change in cytochrome c of apoptotic and necrotic cells is detected by monoclonal antibody binding and mimicked by association of the native antigen with synthetic phospholipid vesicles. Biochemistry 38: 3599-3609

[60] Yu, T., Wang, X., Purring-Koch, C., Wei, Y. and McLendon, G. L. (2001) A mutational epitope for cytochrome C binding to the apoptosis protease activation factor-1. J. Biol. Chem. 276: 13034–13038

[61] Mannick, J.B., Schonhoff, C., Papeta, N., Ghafourifar, P., Szibor, M., Fang, K. and Gaston, B.S. (2001) Nitrosylation of mitochondrial caspases. J. Cell. Biol. 154: 1111-1116

[62] Kim, Y.M., Kim, T.H., Chung, H.T., Talanian, R.V., Yin, X.M. and Billiar, T.R. (2000) Nitric oxide prevents tumor necrosis factor alpha-induced rat hepatocyte apoptosis by the interruption of mitochondrial apoptotic signaling through S-nitrosylation of caspase-8. Hepatology 32: 770-778

[63] Torok, N.J., Higuchi, H., Bronk, S. and Gores G.J. (2002) Nitric oxide inhibits apoptosis downstream of cytochrome C release by nitrosylating caspase 9. Cancer Res. 62: 1648-1653

[64] Levanon, D., Lieman-Hurwitz, J., Dafni, N., Wigderson, M., Sherman, L., Bernstein, Y., Laver-Rudich, Z., Danciger, E., Stein, O. and Groner, Y. (1985) Architecture and anatomy of the chromosomal locus in human chromosome 21 encoding the Cu/Zn superoxide dismutase. EMBO J. 4: 77-84

[65] Avraham, K.B., Schickler, M., Sapoznikov, D., Yarom, R. and Groner, Y. (1988) Down's syndrome: abnormal neuromuscular junction in tongue of transgenic mice with elevated levels of human Cu/Zn-superoxide dismutase. Cell 54: 823–829

[66] Rosen, D.R., Siddique, T. et al. (1993) Mutations in Cu/Zn superoxide dismutase gene are associated with familial amyotrophic lateral sclerosis. Nature 362: 59-62

[67] Gurney, M.E., Pu, H. et al. (1994) Motor neuron degeneration in mice that express a human Cu,Zn superoxide dismutase mutation. Science 264: 1772-1775

[68] Ho, Y.S., Gargano, M., Cao, J., Bronson, R.T., Heimler, I. and Hutz, R.J. (1998) Reduced fertility in female mice lacking copper-zinc superoxide dismutase. J. Biol. Chem. 273: 7765-7769

[69] Julien, J. (2001) Amyotrophic lateral sclerosis: unfolding the toxicity of the misfolded. Cell 104: 581-591

[70] Morrison, B.M. and Morrison, J.H. (1999) Amyotrophic lateral sclerosis associated with mutations in superoxide dismutase: a putative mechanism of degeneration. Brain Res. Brain Res. Rev. 29: 121-135

[71] Spooren, W.P. and Henger, B. (2000) DNA laddering and caspase 3-like activity in the spinal cord of a mouse model of familial amyotrophic lateral sclerosis. Cell Mol. Biol. 46: 63-69

[72] Boll, M.C., Alcaraz-Zubeldia, M., Montes, S., Murillo-Bonilla, L. and Rios, C. (2003) Raised nitrate concentration and low SOD activity in the CSF of sporadic ALS patients. Neurochem. Res. 28: 699-703

[73] Sasaki, S., Shibata, N., Komori, T. and Iwata, M. (2000) iNOS and nitrotyrosine immunoreactivity in amyotrophic lateral sclerosis. Neurosci. Lett. 291: 44-48

[74] Roe, J.A., Wiedau-Pazos, M., Moy, V.N., Goto, J.L., Gralla, E.B. and Valentine J. (2002) In vivo peroxidative activity of FALS-mutant human Cu,Zn SODs expressed yeast. Free Rad. Biol. Med. 32: 169-174

[75] Carrì, M.T., Ferri, A., Battistoni, A., Famhy, L., Gabbianelli, R., Poccia, F. and Rotilio G. (1997) Expression of a Cu,Zn superoxide dismutase typical of familial amyotrophic lateral sclerosis induces mitochondrial alteration and increase of cytosolic Ca2+ concentration in transfected neuroblastoma SH-SY5Y cells. FEBS Lett. 414: 365-368

[76] Aquilano, K., Rotilio, G. and Ciriolo, M.R. (2003) Proteasome activation and nNOS down-regulation in neuroblastoma cells expressing a Cu,Zn superoxide dismutase mutant involved in familial ALS. J Neurochem. 85: 1324-1335

[77] Rotilio, G., Ciriolo, M.R, Carrì, M.T. and Rossi, L. (2002) Disturbances of copper homeostasis and brain function. in: Handbook of Copper Pharmacology and Toxicology (Massaro, E.J. ed.), pp 277-296 Humana Press, Totowa, NJ.
[78] Puig, S. and Thiele, D.J. (2002) Molecular mechanisms of copper uptake and distribution. Curr. Op. Chem. Biol. 6: 171-180
[79] Huffman, D.L. and O'Halloran, T.V. (2001) Function, structure, and mechanism of intracellular copper trafficking proteins. Ann. Rev. Biochem. 70: 677-701
[80] Lee, J., Pena, M.M.O., Nose, J. and Thiele, D.J. (2002) Biochemical characterization of the human copper transporter Ctr1. J. Biol. Chem. 277: 4380-4387
[81] Lee, J., Prohaska, J.R. and Thiele, D.J. (2001) Essential role for mammalian copper transporter Ctr1 in copper homeostasis and embryonic development. Proc. Natl. Acad. Sci. 98: 6842-6847
[82] Punter, F.A. and Glerum, D.M. (2003) Mutagenesis reverses a specific role for Cox17p in copper transport to cytochrome oxidase. J. Biol. Chem. 278: 30875-30880
[83] Carr, H.S., George, G.N. and Winge, D.R. (2002) Yeast Cox11, a protein essential for cytochrome c oxidase assembly, is a Cu(I)-binding protein. J. Biol. Chem. 277: 31237-31242
[84] Jaksch, M., Paret, C. et al. (2001) Cytochrome c oxidase deficiency due to mutations in SCO2, encoding a mitochondrial copper-binding protein, is rescued by copper in human myoblast. Hum. Mol. Genet. 10: 3025-3035
[85] Torres, A.S., Petri, V., Rae, T.D. and O'Halloran, T.V. (2001) Copper stabilizes a heterodimer of the yCCS metallochaperone and its target superoxide dismutase. J. Biol. Chem. 276: 38410-416
[86] Prohaska, J.R., Broderius M. and Brokate B. (2003) Metallochaperone for Cu,Zn-superoxide dismutase (CCS) protein but not mRNA is higher in organs from copper-deficient mice and rats. Arch Biochem Biophys. 417: 227-34
[87] Field, L.S., Furukawa, Y., O'Halloran, T.V. and Culotta, V.C. (2003) Factors controlling the uptake of yeast Cu/Zn superoxide dismutase into mitochondria. J. Biol. Chem. 27: 28052-28059
[88] Wernimont, A.K., Huffman, D.L., Lamb, A.L. and O'Halloran, T.V. (2000) Structural basis or copper transfer by the metallochaperone for the Menkes/Wilson disease proteins. Nat. Struct. Biol. 7: 766-771
[89] Hamza, I., Faisst, A., Prohaska, J.R., Chen, J., Grus, P. and Gitlin, J.D. (2001) The metallochaperone Atox1 plays a critical role in perinatal copper homeostasis. Proc. Natl. Acad. Sci. 98: 6848-6852
[90] Harris, E.D. (2000) Cellular copper transport and metabolism. Annu. Rev. Nutr. 20: 291-310
[91] Petris, M.J., Mercer, J.F., Culvenor, J.G., Lockart, P. and Gleeson, P.A. (1996) Ligand-regulated transport of the Menkes copper P-type ATPase efflux pump from the Golgi apparatus to the plasma membrane: a novel mechanism of regulated trafficking EMBO J. 15: 6084-6095
[92] Mercer, J.F.B., Livingston, J., Hall, B., Paynter, J.A., Begy, C., Chandrasekharappa, S., Lockhart, P., Grimes, A., Bhave, M., Siemieeniak, D. and Glomer, T. (1993) Isolation of a partial candidate gene for Menkes disease by positional cloning. Nat. Genet. 3: 20-25
[93] Tanzi, R.E., Petrukhin, K. et al. (1993) The Wilson disease gene is a copper transporting ATPase with homology to the Menkes disease gene. Nat. Genet. 5: 344-350
[94] Leist, M. and Nicotera, P. (1998). Apoptosis, excitotoxicity, and neuropathology. Exp. Cell Res. 239: 183-201
[95] Rossi, L., Lombardo, M.F., Ciriolo, M.R. and Rotilio, G. (2004) Mitochondrial dysfunction in neurodegenerative diseases associated with copper imbalance. Neurochem. Res., in press.
[96] Dobyns, W.B., Goldstein, N.P. and Gordon, H. (1979) Clinical spectrum of Wilson's disease (hepatolenticular degeneration). Mayo Clin. Proc. 54: 35-42
[97] Kodama, H., Okabe, I., Yanagisawa, M., Nomiyama, H., Nomiyama, K., Nose,O. and Kamoshita, S. (1988) Does CSF copper level in Wilson disease reflect copper accumulation in the brain? Pediatr. Neurol. 4: 35-37
[98] Weisner, B., Hartad, C.and Dieu, C. (1987) CSF copper concentration: a new parameter for diagnosis and monitoring therapy of Wilson's disease with cerebral manifestation. J. Neurol. Sci. 79: 229-237
[99] Hashimoto, M., Rockenstein, E., Crews, L. and Masliah, E. (2003) Role of protein aggregation in mitochondrial dysfunction and neurodegeneration in Alzheimer's and Parkinson's diseases. Neuromolecular Med. 4: 21-36
[100] Multhaup, G., Ruppert, T., Schlicksupp, A., Hesse, L., Bill, E., Pipkorn, R., Masters, C.L. and Beyreuther, K. (1998) Copper binding amyloid precursor protein undergoes a site-specific fragmentation in the reduction of hydrogen peroxide. Biochemistry 37: 7224-7230

[101] White, A.R., Reyes, R., Mercer, J.F., Camakaris, J., Zheng, H., Bush, A.I., Multhaup, G., Beyreuther, K., Masters, C.L. and Cappai, R. (1999) Copper levels are increased in the cerebral cortex and liver of APP and APLP2 knockout mice. Brain Res. 842: 439-444

[102] Squitti, R., Rossini, P.M., Cassetta, E., Moffa, F., Pasqualetti, P., Cortesi, M., Colloca, A., Rossi, L. and Finazzi-Agrò, A. (2002) D-penicillamine reduces serum oxidative stress in Alzheimer's disease patients. Eur. J. Clin. Invest. 32: 51-59

[103] Rossi, L., Squitti, R., Pasqualetti, P., Marchese, E., Cassetta, E., Forestiere, E., Rotilio, G., Rossini, P. M. and Finazzi-Agrò, A. (2002) Red blood cell copper, zinc superoxide dismutase activity is higher in Alzheimer's disease and is decreased by D-penicillamine. Neurosci. Lett. 329: 137-40

[104] Cherny, R.A., Atwood, C.S. et al. (2001) Treatment with a copper-zinc chelator markedly and rapidly inhibits β-amyloid accumulation in Alzheimer's disease transgenic mice. Neuron 30: 665-676.

[105] Viles, J.H., Cohen, F.E., Prusiner, S.B., Goodin, D.B., Wright, P.E. and Dyson, H.J. (1999) Copper binding to the prion protein: structural implications of four identical coperative bindings sites. Proc. Natl. Acad. Sci. 96: 2042-2047

[106] Hutter, G., Heppner, F.L. and Aguzzi, A. (2003) No superoxide dismutase activity of cellular prion protein in vivo. Biol Chem. 384:1279-1285

[107] Brown, D.R. (2001) Prion and prejudice: normal protein at the synapse. Trends Neurosci. 24: 85-50

[108] Qin, K., Yang, D.S., Yang, Y., Chishti, M.A., Meng, L.J., Kretzschmar, H.A., Yip, C.M., Fraser, P.E. and Westaway, D. (2000) Copper(II)-induced conformational changes and protease resistance in recombinant and cellular PrP. Effect of protein age and deamidation. J. Biol. Chem. 275: 19121-19131

[109] Sigurdsson, E.M., Brown, D.R., Alim, M.A., Scholtzova, H., Carp, R., Meeker, H.C., Prelli, F., Frangione, B. and Wisniewski, T. (2003) Copper chelation delays the onset of prion disease. J Biol Chem. 278: 46199-46202

[110] Olanow, C.W. and Tatton, W.G. (1999) Etiology and pathogenesis of Parkinson's disease. Annu. Rev. Neurosci. 22: 123-144

[111] Kruger, R., Kuhn, W., Muller, T., Woitalla, D., Graeber, M., Kosel, S., Przunter, H., Epplen, J. T., Schols, L. and Riess, O. (1998) Ala30Pro mutation in the gene encoding α-synuclein in Parkinson's disease. Nat. Genet. 18: 106-108

[112] Paik, S.R., Shin, H.J., Lee, J.H., Chang C.S. and Kim, J. (1999) Copper (II)-induced self-oligomerization of α-synuclein. Biochem. J. 340: 821-828

[113] Uversky, V.N., Li, J. and Fink, A.L. (2001) Metal-triggered structural transformations, aggregation, and fibrillation of human α-synuclein. J. Biol. Chem. 276: 44284-44296.

[114] Tumer, Z. and Horn, N. (1997) Menkes disease: recent advances and new aspects. J. Med. Gen. 34: 265-274

[115] Mercer, J.F.B. (1998) Menkes syndrome and animal models. Am. J. Clin. Nutr. 67: 1022S-1028S

[116] Menkes, J.H., Alter, M., Stegleder, G., Weakley, D.R. and Sung, J.H. (1962) A sex-linked recessive disorder with retardation of growth, peculiar hair and focal cerebral and cerebellar degeneration. Pediatrics 29: 764-779

[117] Quian, Y., Tiffany-Castiglioni E. and Harris E.D. (1998) Copper efflux from murine microvascular cells requires expression of the Menkes disease Cu ATPase. J. Nutr. 128: 1276-1282

[118] Grimes, A., Hearn, C.J., Lockhart, P., Newgreen, D.F. and Mercer, J.F. (1997) Molecular basis of the brindled mouse mutant (Mo(br)): a murine model of Menkes disease. Hum. Mol. Gen. 6: 1037-1042

[119] Rossi, L., De Martino, A., Marchese, E., Piccirilli, S., Rotilio, G. and Ciriolo, M.R. (2001) Neurodegeneration in the animal model of Menkes' disease involves Bcl-2 linked apoptosis. Neuroscience 103: 181-188

[120] Sadoul, R. (1998) Bcl-2 family members in the development and degenerative pathologies of the nervous system. Cell Death Differ. 5: 805-815

[121] Fuji, T., Ito, M., Tsuda, H. and Mikawa, H. (1990) Biochemical study on the critical period for treatment of the mottled brindled mouse. J. Neurochem. 55: 885-889

[122] DiMauro, S., Bonilla, E., Lombes, A., Shanske, S., Minetti, C. and Moares, C. (1990) Mitochondrial encephalomyophaties. Neurol. Clin. 8: 483-506

[123] Rossi, L., Marchese, E., Lombardo, M.F., Rotilio, G. and Ciriolo, M.R. (2001) Increased susceptibility of copper-deficient neuroblastoma cells to oxidative stress-mediated apoptosis. Free Rad. Biol. Med. 30: 1177-1187

[124] Lombardo, M.F., Ciriolo, M.R., Rotilio, G. and Rossi, L. (2003) Prolonged copper depletion induces expression of antioxidants and triggers apoptosis in SH-SY5Y neuroblastoma cells. Cell Mol. Life Sci. 60: 1733-1743

[125] Rossi, L., Ciriolo, M.R., Marchese, E., De Martino, A., Giorgi, M. and Rotilio, G. (1994) Differential decrease of copper content and of copper binding to superoxide dismutase in liver, heart and brain of copper-deficient rats. Biochem. Biophys. Res Commun. 203: 1028-1034
[126] Duranteau, J., Chandel, N.S., Kulisz, A., Shao, Z. and Schumacker, P.T. (1998) Intracellular signalling by reactive oxygen species during hypoxia in cardiomyocytes. J. Biol. Chem. 273: 11619-11624
[127] Robinson, B.H., Luo, X.P., Pitkanen, S., Bratinova, S., Bourgeois, J., Lehotay, D.C. and Raha, S. (1998) Diagnosis of mitochondrial energy metabolism defects in tissue culture. Induction of Mn SOD and Bcl-2 in mitochondria from patients with complex I deficiency. Biofactors 7: 229-230
[128] Lai, C-C., Huang, W., Klevay, L.M., Gunning, W.T. and Chiu, T.H. (1996) Antioxidant enzyme gene transcription in copper-deficient rat liver. Free Rad. Biol. Med. 21: 233-240
[129] Shibata, N., Hirano, A., Kobayashi, M., Umahara, T., Kawanami, T. and Asayama, K. (1995) Cerebellar superoxide dismutase expression in Menkes' kinky hair disease: an immunohistochemical investigation. Acta Neuropathol. 90: 198-202
[130] Lee, M.H., Hyun, D.H., Marshall, K.A., Ellerby, L. M., Bredesen, D.E., Jenne, P. and Halliwell, B. (2001) Effect of overexpression of Bcl-2 on cellular oxidative damage, nitric oxide production, antioxidant defences and the proteasome. Free Rad. Biol. Med. 31: 1550-1559
[131] Mèplan, C., Richard, M.J. and Hainaut, P. (2000) Redox signalling and transition metals in the control of the p53 pathway. Biochem. Pharmacol. 59: 25-33
[132] Wolvetang, E.J., Johnson, K.L., Krauer, K., Ralph, S.J. and Linnane, A.W. (1994) Mitochondrial respiratory chain inhibitors induce apoptosis. FEBS Lett. 339: 40-44
[133] Raff, M.C., Barres, B.A., Burne, J.F., Coles, H.S., Ishizaki, Y. and Jacobson, M.D. (1993) Programmed cell death and the control of cell survival: lessons from the nervous system. Science 262: 695-700
[134] Schafer, F.Q. and Buettner, G.R. (2001) Redox environment of the cell as viewed through the redox state of the glutathione disulfide/glutathione couple. Free Rad. Biol. Med. 30: 1191-1212
[135] Kirsgh, M. and De Groot, H. (2001) NAD(P)H, a directly operating antioxidant? FASEB J. 15: 1569-1574
[136] Ferreira, A.M., Ciriolo, M.R., Marcocci, L. and Rotilio G. (1993) Copper(I) transfer into metallothionein mediated by glutathione Biochem. J. 292: 673-676
[137] Nordberg, J. and Arner, S.J. (2001) Reactive oxygen species, antioxidants and mammalian thioredoxin system. Free Rad. Biol. Med. 31: 1287-1312
[138] Finkel, T. (2000) Redox-dependent signal transduction. FEBS Lett. 476: 52-54
[139] Adler, V., Yin, Z., Tew, K.D. and Ronai, Z. (1999) Role of redox potential and reactive oxygen species in stress signaling. Oncogene 18: 6104-6111
[140] Soltaninassab, S.R., Sekhar, K.R., Meredith, M.J. and Freeman, M.L. (2000) Multi-faceted regulation of γ-glutamylcysteine synthetase. J. Cell. Physiol. 182: 163-170
[141] Tu, Z. and Anders, M.W. (1998) Identification of an important cysteine in human glutamate-cysteine ligase catalytic subunit by sited direct mutagenesis. Biochem. J. 336: 675-680
[142] Barrett, W.C., DeGnore, J.P., Konig, S., Fales, H.M., Keng, Y.F., Zhang, Z.Y., Yim, M.B. and Chock, P.B. (1999) Regulation of PTP1B via glutathionylation of the active site cysteine 215. Biochemistry 38: 6699-6705
[143] Denu, J.M. and Dixon, J.E. (1998) Protein tyrosine phosphatases: mechanisms of catalysis and regulation. Curr. Opin. Chem. Biol. 2: 633-641
[144] Mahadev, K., Zilbering, A., Zhu, L. and Goldstein, B.J. (2001) Insulin-stimulated hydrogen peroxide reversibly inhibits protein-tyrosine phosphatase 1B *in vivo* and enhances the early insulin action cascade. J. Biol. Chem. 276: 21938-21942
[145] Saitoh, M., Nishitoh, H., Fujii, M., Takeda, K., Tobiume, K., Sawada, Y., Kawabata, M., Miyazono, K. and Ichijo, H. (1998) Mammalian thioredoxin is a direct inhibitor of apoptosis signal-regulating kinase (ASK) 1. EMBO J. 17: 2596 2606
[146] Gotoh, Y. and Cooper J.A. (1998) Reactive oxygen species- and dimerization-induced activation of apoptosis signal-regulating kinase 1 in tumor necrosis factor-alpha signal transduction. J. Biol. Chem. 273: 17477-17482
[147] Ichijo, H., Nishida, E., Irie, K., Dijke, P., Saitoh, M., Moriguchi, T., Takagi, M., Matsumoto, K., Miyzaono, K. and Gotoh, Y. (1997) Induction of apoptosis by ASK1, a mammalian MAPKKK that activates SAPK/JNK and p38 signaling pathways. Science 275: 90-94
[148] Adler, V., Yin, Z., Fuchs, S.Y., Benezra, M., Rosario, L., Tew, K.D., Pincus, M.R., Sardana, M., Henderson, C.J., Wolf, C.R., Davis, R.J. and Ronai, Z. (1999) Regulation of JNK signaling by GSTp. EMBO J. 18: 1321-1334

[149] Filomeni, G., Rotilio, G. and Ciriolo, M.R. (2003) Glutathione disulfide induces apoptosis in U937 cells by a redox-mediated p38 MAP kinase pathway. FASEB J. 17: 64-66

[150] Filomeni, G., Aquilano, K., Rotilio, G. and Ciriolo, M.R. (2003) Reactive oxygen species-dependent c-Jun NH_2-terminal kinase/c-Jun signaling cascade mediates neuroblastoma cell death induced by diallyl disulfide. Cancer Res. 63: 5940-5949

[151] Hausladen, A., Privalle, C.T., Keng, T., De Angelo, J. and Stamler, J.S. (1996) Nitrosative stress: activation of the transcription factor OxyR. Cell 86: 719-729

[152] Zheng, M., Aslund, F. and Storz, G. (1998) Activation of the OxyR transcription factor by reversible disulfide bond formation. Science 279: 1718-1721

[153] Kim, S.O., Merchant, K., Nudelman, R., Beyer, W.F. Jr., Keng, T., De Angelo, J., Hausladen, A. and Stamler, J.S. (2002) OxyR: a molecular code for redox-related signaling. Cell 109: 383-396

[154] Georgeou, G. (2002) How to flip the (redox) switch. Cell 111: 607-610

[155] Siebenlist, U., Franzoso, G. and Brown, K. (1994) Structure, regulation, and function of NF-kappa B. Annu. Rev. Cell Biol. 10: 405-455

[156] Mitomo, K., Nakayama, K., Fujimoto, K., Sun, X., Seki, S. and Yamamoto, K. (1994) Two different cellular redox systems regulate the DNA-binding activity of the p50 subunit of NF-kappa B in vitro. Gene 145:197-203

[157] Satriano, J. and Schlondorff, D. (1994) Activation and attenuation of transcription factor NF-kappa B in mouse glomerular mesangial cells in response to tumor necrosis factor-alpha, immunoglobulin G, and adenosine 3':5'-cyclic monophosphate. J. Clin. Invest. 94: 1629-1636

[158] Anderson, M.T., Staal, F.J., Gitler, C., Herzenberg, L.A. and Herzenberg, L.A. (1994) Separation of oxidant-initiated and redox-regulated steps in the NF-kappa B signal transduction pathway. Proc. Natl. Acad. Sci. 91: 11527-11531

[159] Staal, F.J., Roederer, M., Herzenberg, L.A. and Herzenberg, L.A. (1990) Intracellular thiols regulate activation of nuclear factor kappa B and transcription of human immunodeficiency virus. Proc. Natl. Acad. Sci. 87: 9943-9947

[160] Matthews, J.R., Kaszubska, W., Turcatti, G., Wells, T.N. and Hay, R.T. (1993) Role of cysteine 62 in DNA recognition by the P50 subunit of NF-kappa B. Nucleic Acids Res. 21: 1727-1734

[161] Lander, H.M., Ogiste, J.S., Teng, K.K. and Novogrodsky, A. (1995) p21ras as a common signaling target of reactive free radicals and cellular redox stress. J. Biol. Chem. 270: 21195-21198

[162] Janssen, Y.M.W., Heintz, N.H., Marsh, J.P., Borm, P.J.A. and Mossman, B.T. (1994) Induction of c-Fos and c-Jun proto-oncogenes in target cells of the lung and pleura by carcinogenic fibers. Am. J. Resp. Cell Mol. Biol. 11: 522-530

[163] Karin, M. (1995) The regulation of AP-1 activity by mitogen-activated protein kinases. J. Biol. Chem. 270: 16483-16486

[164] Wenk, J., Brenneisen, P., Wlaschek, M., Poswig, A., Briviba, K., Oberley, T.D. and Scharffetter-Kochanek, K. (1999) Stable overexpression of manganese superoxide dismutase in mitochondria identifies hydrogen peroxide as a major oxidant in the AP-1-mediated induction of matrix-degrading metalloprotease-1. J. Biol. Chem. 274: 25869-25876

[165] Janssen, Y.M.W., Heintz, N.H. and Mossman, B.T. (1995) Induction of c-fos and c-jun proto-oncogene expression by asbestos is ameliorated by N-acetyl-L-cysteine in mesothelial cells. Cancer Res. 55: 2085-2089

[166] Abate, C., Patel, L., Rauscher, F.J. and Curran, T. (1990) Redox regulation of fos and jun DNA-binding activity in vitro. Science 249: 1157-1161

[167] Walker, L.J., Robinson, C.N., Black, E., Gillespie, D. and Hickson, I.D. (1993) Identification of residues in the human DNA repair enzyme HAP1(Ref-1) that are essential for redox regulation of Jun DNA binding. Mol. Cell. Biol. 13: 5370-5376

[168] Hirota, K., Matsui, M., Iwata, S., Nishiyama, A., Mori, K. and Yodoi, J. (1997) AP-1 transcriptional activity is regulated by a direct association between thioredoxin and Ref-1. Proc. Natl. Acad. Sci. 94: 3633-3638

[169] Klatt, P., Molina, E.P., De Lacoba, M.G., Padilla, C.A., Martinez-Galisteo, E., Barcena, J.A. and Lamas, S. (1999) Redox regulation of c-Jun DNA binding by reversible S-glutathiolation. FASEB J. 13: 1481-1490

[170] Hainaut, P. and Milner, J. (1993) Redox modulation of p53 conformation and sequence-specific DNA binding in vitro. Cancer Res. 53: 4469-4473

[171] Rainwater, R., Parks, D., Anderson, M.E., Tegtmeyer, P. and Mann, K. (1995) Role of cysteine residues in regulation of p53 function. Mol. Cell Biol. 15: 3892-3903

[172] Jayaraman, L., Murthy, K.G., Zhu, C., Curran, T., Xanthoudakis, S. and Prives, C. (1997) Identification of redox/repair protein Ref-1 as a potent activator of p53. Genes Develop. 11: 558-570

[173] Jacquier-Sarlin, M.R. and Polla, B. (1996) Dual regulation of heat shock transcription factor (HSF) activation and DNA-binding activity by H2O2: role of thioredoxin. Biochem. J. 318: 187-193

[174] Liu, S.L., Lin, X., Shi, D.Y., Cheng, J., Wu, C.Q. and Zhang, Y.D. (2002) Reactive oxygen species stimulated human hepatoma cell proliferation via cross-talk between PI3-K/PKB and JNK signaling pathways. Arch. Biochem. Biophys. 406: 173-182

[175] Eilers, M., Picard, D., Yamamoto, K.R. and Bishop, J.M. (1989) Chimaeras of myc oncoprotein and steroid receptors cause hormone-dependent transformation of cells. Nature 340: 66-68

[176] Heikkila, R., Schwab, G., Wickstrom, E., Loke, S.L., Pluznik, D.H., Watt, R. and Neckers, L.M. (1987) A c-myc antisense oligodeoxynucleotide inhibits entry into S phase but not progress from G0 to G1. Nature 328: 445-448

[177] Hanson, K.D., Shichiri, M., Follansbee, M.R. and Sedivy, J.M. (1994) Effects of c-myc expression on cell cycle progression. Mol. Cell Biol. 14: 5748-5755

[178] Evan, G.I., Wyllie, A.H., Gilbert, C.S., Littlewood, T.D., Land, H., Brooks, M., Waters, C.M., Penn, L.Z. and Hancock, D.C. (1992) Induction of apoptosis in fibroblasts by c-myc protein. Cell 69: 119-128

[179] Biroccio, A., Benassi, B., Filomeni, G., Amodei, S., Marchini, S., Chiorino, G., Rotilio, G., Zupi, G. and Ciriolo, M.R. (2002) Glutathione influences c-Myc-induced apoptosis in M14 human melanoma cells. J. Biol. Chem. 277: 43763-43770

[180] Ghibelli, L., Coppola, S., Rotilio, G., Lafavia, E., Maresca, V. and Ciriolo, M.R. (1995) Non-oxidative loss of glutathione in apoptosis via GSH extrusion. Biochem. Biophys. Res. Commun. 216 : 313-320

[181] Ghibelli, L., Fanelli, C., Rotilio, G., Lafavia, E., Coppola, S., Colussi, C., Civitareale, P. and Ciriolo, M.R. (1998) Rescue of cells from apoptosis by inhibition of active GSH extrusion. FASEB J. 12: 479-486

[182] Ghibelli, L., Coppola, S., Fanelli, C., Rotilio, G., Civitareale, P., Scovassi, A.I. and Ciriolo, M.R. (1999) Glutathione depletion causes cytochrome c release even in the absence of cell commitment to apoptosis. FASEB J. 13: 2031-2036

[183] Chandel, N.S., Schumacker, P.T. and Arch, R.H. (2001) Reactive oxygen species are downstream products of TRAF-mediated signal transduction. J. Biol. Chem. 276: 42728-42736

[184] Hockenbery, D.M., Oltvai, Z.N., Yin, X.M., Milliman, C.L. and Korsmeyer, S.J. (1993) Bcl-2 functions in an antioxidant pathway to prevent apoptosis. Cell 75: 241-251

[185] Cory, S., Huang, D.C. and Adams, J.M. (2003) The Bcl-2 family: roles in cell survival and oncogenesis. Oncogene 22: 8590-8607

[186] Briehl, M.M., Baker, A.F., Siemankowski, L.M. and Morreale, J. (1997) Modulation of antioxidant defenses during apoptosis. Oncol. Res. 9: 281-285

[187] Voehringer, D.W. (1999) BCL-2 and glutathione: alterations in cellular redox state that regulate apoptosis sensitivity. Free Rad. Biol. Med. 27: 945-950

[188] Nencioni, L., Iuvara, A., Aquilano, K., Ciriolo, M.R., Cozzolino, F., Rotilio, G., Garaci, E. and Palamara, A.T. (2003) Influenza A virus replication is dependent on an antioxidant pathway that involves GSH and Bcl-2. FASEB J. 17: 758-760

[189] Ciriolo, M.R., Palamara, A.T., Incerpi, S., Lafavia, E., Bue, M.C., De Vito, P., Garaci, E. and Rotilio, G. (1997) Loss of GSH, oxidative stress, and decrease of intracellular pH as sequential steps in viral infection. J. Biol. Chem. 272: 2700-2708

[190] Hampton, M.B. and Orrenius, S. (1997) Dual regulation of caspase activity by hydrogen peroxide: implications for apoptosis. FEBS Lett. 414: 552-556

[191] Dypbukt, J.M., Ankarcrona, M., Burkitt, M., Sjoholm, A., Strom, K., Orrenius, S. and Nicotera, P. (1994) Different prooxidant levels stimulate growth, trigger apoptosis, or produce necrosis of insulin-secreting RINm5F cells. The role of intracellular polyamines. J. Biol. Chem. 269: 30553-30560

[192] Hentze, H., Schmitz, I., Latta, M., Krueger, A., Krammer, P.H. and Wendel, A. (2002) Glutathione dependence of caspase-8 activation at the death-inducing signaling complex. J. Biol. Chem. 277: 5588-5595

[193] Zamzami, N. and Kroemer, G. (2001) The mitochondrion in apoptosis: how Pandora's box opens. Nat. Rev. Mol. Cell Biol. 2: 67-71

[194] Marzo, I., Brenner, C., Zamzami, N., Jurgensmeier, J.M., Susin, S.A., Vieira, H.L., Prevost, M.C., Xie, Z., Matsuyama, S., Reed, J.C. and Kroemer G. (1998) Bax and adenine nucleotide translocator cooperate in the mitochondrial control of apoptosis. Science 281: 2027-2031

[195] Chernyak, B.V. and Bernardi, P. (1996) The mitochondrial permeability transition pore is modulated by oxidative agents through both pyridine nucleotides and glutathione at two separate sites. Eur. J. Biochem. 238: 623-630.
[196] McStay, G.P., Clarke, S.J. and Halestrap, A.P. (2002) Role of critical thiol groups on the matrix surface of the adenine nucleotide translocase in the mechanism of the mitochondrial permeability transition pore. Biochem. J. 367: 541-548
[197] Perego, P., Paolicchi, A., Tongiani, R., Pompella, A., Tonarelli, P., Carenini, N., Romanelli, S. and Zunino, F. (1997) The cell-specific anti-proliferative effect of reduced glutathione is mediated by gamma-glutamyl transpeptidase-dependent extracellular pro-oxidant reactions. Int. J. Cancer 71: 246-250
[198] Sullivan, D.M., Wehr, N.B., Fergusson, M.M., Levine, R.L. and Finkel, T. (2000) Identification of oxidant-sensitive proteins: TNF-alpha induces protein glutathiolation. Biochemistry 39: 11121-11128
[199] Nebreda, A.R. and Porrai, A. (2000) p38 MAP kinases: beyond the stress response. Trends Biochem. Sci. 25: 257-260
[200] Reglinski, J., Hoey, S., Smith, W.E. and Sturrock, R.D. (1988) Cellular response to oxidative stress at sulfhydryl group receptor sites on the erythrocyte membrane J. Biol. Chem. 263: 12360-12366
[201] Ciriolo, M.R., Paci, M., Sette, M., De Martino, A., Bozzi, A. and Rotilio, G. (1993) Transduction of reducing power across the plasma membrane by reduced glutathione. A 1H-NMR spin-echo study of intact human erythrocytes. Eur. J. Biochem. 215: 711-718
[202] Angelini, G., Gardella, S., Ardy, M., Ciriolo, M.R., Filomeni, G., Di Trapani, G., Clarke, F., Sitia, R. and Rubartelli, A. (2002) Antigen-presenting dendritic cells provide the reducing extracellular microenvironment required for T lymphocyte activation. Proc. Natl. Acad. Sci. 99: 1491-1496
[203] Edinger, A.L. and Thompson, C.B. (2002) Antigen-presenting cells control T cell proliferation by regulating amino acid availability. Proc. Natl. Acad. Sci. 99: 1107-1109

Frontiers in Neurodegenerative Disorders and Aging: Fundamental Aspects, Clinical Perspectives and New Insights
T. Özben and M. Chevion (Eds.)
IOS Press, 2004

Molecular Mechanism of HIV-1 Associated Neurodegeneration

M. Hakan Özdener*
Department of Neurology, School of Medicine, University of Pennsylvania, Philadelphia, Pennsylvania, USA

Abstract: Since the identification of Human Immunodeficiency Virus (HIV), all studies suggest that neurological impairments, and in particular dementia, are associated with acquired immunodeficiency syndrome (AIDS) with alarming occurrence worldwide. Approximately 60% of HIV infected people show some form of neurological impairment, and neuropathological changes are found in 90% of autopsied cases. The mechanism behind these pathological changes still is not well known. The mounting data obtained by *in-vivo* and *in vitro* experiments, suggest that neuronal apoptosis is a major feature of HIV associated dementia (HAD) and occurs in the absence of a direct infection. The major pathway to neuronal apoptosis occurs indirectly through release of neurotoxins by activated cells in the CNS involved in the induction of excitotoxicity and oxidative stress. A direct mechanism as induced by viral proteins in the pathogenesis of HAD may also play a role. In this review, we will focus on the molecular mechanisms of HIV associated dementia and possible therapeutic strategies.

1. Introduction

HIV-1 causative agent of AIDS is the cause of a worldwide health crisis. According to the World Health Organization (WHO), by 2002 more than 42 million people worldwide were infected by HIV, three times more than when surveyed in 1996 [1]. HIV-1 infection is a multi system infection. Transmission of HIV is dependent on biological and behavioral factors [2, 3]. HIV is transmitted by sexual relations, breast feeding, contaminated blood products, contaminated intravenous injectors, and through maternal-fetal circulation. Clinical features of HIV infection are dependent on the stage of HIV infection and vary from flu like symptoms to extreme multi system immunodeficiency symptoms and diseases. HIV enters into the bloodstream directly and is delivered to lymphoid tissues, spleen, lung and liver [4]. HIV-1 invades the central nervous system (CNS) at the early phase of infection and induces progressive multi symptoms of motor, cognitive dysfunction and behavioral changes. Major clinical symptoms include forgetfulness coupled with difficulty in mental concentration, leg weakness, slowness of hand movements and gait as well as depression [5]. The term of AIDS dementia complex or HIV-1 associated dementia (ADC, HAD respectively) is referred to describe these neurological and psychiatric symptoms caused by HIV infection [6, 7]. HIV-1 associated dementia affects 15-20% of the patients in the late stages of AIDS. HIV-1 induced

*Present Address: Monell Chemical Senses Center, 3500 Market Street, Philadelphia Pennsylvania USA
e-mail: hozdener@yahoo.com

neuropathology can be identified at autopsy in over 90% of cases. In the United States, HIV-1 infection is the most common cause of dementia in young adults [8, 9]

2. Biology of HIV-1 and cellular tropism

HIV-1 is the third retrovirus discovered after the adult T cell leukemia-associated viruses (HTLV-I and HTLV-II) [10, 11]. HIV-1 is an enveloped animal RNA virus with two positive strands, which is classified as a lentivirus within the retroviridae family. The HIV-1 genome is over 9200 base pairs long [12, 13]. The typical HIV genome includes the long terminal repeat (LTR) at both ends and has three major coding regions, which encode core (gag), polymerase (pol) and envelope (env) gene products. The HIV genome also encodes several "accessory" proteins such as Nef, Tat, Vpr, Vif, Rev and Vpu that may play key role in the pathogenesis of HIV infection [14].

CD4+ T cells and macrophages are major target for HIV infection [15]. HIV-1 infects CD4+ T cells by utilizing CD4 as receptor. HIV also needs certain chemokine receptors as co-receptors. The criteria for cellular tropism can be defined in terms of the ability of HIV to grow in cells *in vitro*. HIV isolates, which can infect and grow productively in macrophages and PBMC but less efficiently in T cell lines, are called macrophage or M tropic. Whereas HIV isolates which can grow productively in T cell lines and PBMC but not in macrophages are classified as T tropic [15]. HIV isolates that can grow both in T and macrophage cells called dual tropic. Most of M tropic viruses utilize the CCR5 chemokine receptor, whereas most T-tropic strains utilize CXR4 chemokine receptors [17]. HIV strains and cellular tropism may play a role in HAD [16]. The viral determinant of cellular and neurotropism is the gp120 envelope protein. In particular, the V3 region is the major co-determinant for co-receptor use. Nucleotide changes in the HIV sequence are distributed throughout the genome. However, the change in V3 region is crucial for determination of HIV binding and entry [18, 19, 20].

3. Pathological findings of HAD

Neurodegeneration is one of the characteristics of AIDS and is associated with neuronal apoptosis, brain atrophy and blood-derived monocytes infiltration into the brain [21 -25]. HIV associated neurodegeneration is clinically manifested after many years of seroconversion. Elevated viral RNA in the plasma and viral load in the CSF with low level of CD4+ T cells are indicators of greater risk to develop HAD [26, 27]. Neuronal apoptosis in the CNS is a common feature of HAD in the brains of adults and pediatric patients with HIV infection. Unlike other encephalopathies, HAD occurs without direct infection of neurons [28, 59]. Cortical neuronal loss has been often described post-mortem in the brain of patients with AIDS [22]. Typical pathological changes in patients with HAD is multinucleated giant cells (HIV-1 envelope mediated fusion of microglia or macrophages), diffuse white matter pallor, reactive gliosis and cerebral atrophy. The mechanisms of multinucleated giant cells formation are not well known, but the binding of HIV envelope protein to CD4+ cells may have a function in inducing this formation [29].

4. Viral entry into the CNS and development of cellular injury

How HIV-1 enters into the CNS remains obscure. It is generally accepted that HIV enters the CNS shortly after systemic infection via infiltration of infected CD4+ monocytes and perivascular macrophages (Trojan Horse hypothesis) [30, 31, 32]. The relative numbers of these infected cells are low, although they serve as a reservoir of HIV. Productive HIV infection has been shown in microglia, macrophages, and multinucleated giant cells in the CNS but not in neurons, oligodendrocytes and astrocytes [33]. Productive infection of HIV requires complex interaction between viral and host cell factors.

Infection of HIV in astrocytes is different from productive infection of HIV in microglia. Infection of astrocytes is restricted by post entry since early transcription products were detected [34, 35, 36, 37]. In contrast to HIV infection in microglia, which produces viral genomic RNA upon stimulation, astrocytes produce only multi spliced RNA even after stimulation [38]. HIV also can infect choroid plexus and blood brain barrier epithelial cells [39, 36]. Choroid plexus infection has been shown in experimental simian immunodeficiency virus and feline immunodeficiency virus infection [40, 41].

Chemokines have significantly diverse action mechanisms and cellular targets in the CNS. Chemokine receptors have important roles in the pathogenesis of HIV infection, since they are utilized as a co-receptor for HIV entry. There are more than a dozen chemokine receptors involved in HIV pathogenesis, however, three of them CXCR4, CCR5 and CCR3, are crucial for virus adhesion and entry into the target cells. HIV utilizing CXCR4 were found to be more cytopathic compared to CCR5 and CCR3. The envelope region of HIV may have major role in this process [48].

The presence of chemokine receptors on neurons suggests that chemokines may have roles in development of HAD [49, 50, 51]. A growing body of evidence suggests that the role of chemokines in the pathogenesis of HAD is not limited to virus entry but chemokine receptor signaling may also have role in modulating neuronal apoptosis and neurotoxicity via induction of glutamate release and through a G-protein-mediated modulation of L- and N-type calcium channel [45, 46, 47]. Additionally, some of chemokines are suppressive factors for HIV-1 infection. Antagonists of CXCR4 and CCR5 may inhibit HIV entry [42, 43, 44]. In particular, CXCR4 and its ligand, SDF-1 may play a crucial role in the inhibition of gp120 induced neuroapoptosis indicating that CXCR4 signaling plays a role in HIV induced dementia [52, 53, 54]. Another important chemokine receptor, CX3CR1, and its ligand, fractalkine (FKN) are expressed on the cell surface of microglia, neuron and macrophages [55, 56]. Increased level of CX3CR1 and FKN has been shown in pediatric patients with HIV-encephalitis [57]. In microglia and neurons, FKN signaling increases intracellular Ca^{+2} and induces Akt and ERK 1-2 kinase activation suggesting that FKN may induce neuroprotection [55, 58].

Neuronal apoptosis in HAD, which might be caused by either indirect effects of released neurotoxins and neuromodulators from activated astrocytes and microglia or direct effects of HIV proteins such gp120, gp41, Vpr, Tat, Nef, Vpu on neurons or a combination of both. Among shed viral proteins from infected cells, gp120 has been shown in the cerebrospinal fluid and in the brain of patients with HIV encephalitis and dementia [60, 61, 62]. The direct effects of the neurotoxic potential of gp120 has been studied in detail, in the absence of other contaminating cell types, using different types of neurons such as rodent cortical, hippocampal and retinal ganglion neurons [68, 69, 70, 77, 78]. Studies have indicated that HIV envelope protein and other viral proteins shed by infected cells may change intracellular signaling and can induce apoptosis [71, 72, 73, 78]. The exact mechanism by which these proteins cause neuronal damage is unknown. It has been shown that the glutamate-mediated cell death caused by gp120 proceeded through the recruitment of Ca^{2+}-dependent enzymes such as nitric oxide synthase and calpain along with membrane lipid peroxidation [79, 80, 81]. HIV gp120 increases cytoplasmic Ca^{+2} in two ways: facilitating glutamate neurotransmission increasing Ca^{+2} conductance and activating the IP3 pathway, facilitating Ca^{+2} release from the smooth endoplasmic reticulum [82, 83]. Recently, it was shown that injection of gp120 induces neuronal apoptosis which can be prevented by inhibition of TNF-α and CXCR4 signaling [63]. TNF-α may modulate neuronal apoptosis by increasing voltage dependent calcium currents [64, 65, 65]. The effect(s) of gp120 to induce apoptosis is regulated by activation of CXCR4 followed by p38 mitogen activated protein kinase downstream signaling, and gp120 also activates caspase 3 and enhances Bax expression [109, 110]. Other evidence of gp120 induced neuronal apoptosis is that transgenic mice expressing gp120, without productive infection, show microglial activation, astrocytosis and altered expression of immunoproteins and increased blood brain barrier permeability [66, 67].

HIV-1 vpr is a regulatory protein and required for effective infection. Vpr is also detected in CSF of patient with HAD. It was shown that HIV-1 Vpr can induce cell cycle arrest followed by neuronal apoptosis in both human and NTera2 neurons as measured by increasing activaton of caspase 8 [114, 115].

So far, it is generally accepted that HIV infection in the CNS can cause neuropathological changes through indirect effects of infected cells on neurons [74]. Indirect evidence of neuronal apoptosis triggered by gp120 *in vitro* seems to be related to the induction of secretion of neurotoxic factors, such as cytokines, eicosanoids, excitotoxins and free radicals [24]. After infection of brain cells by HIV, secretion of neurotoxins from infected cells may cause multicellular complex interactions between the CNS cells. It has been shown that neurotoxins secreted from HIV infected cells can cause metabolically alteration in the CNS cells [75]. Most of the apoptotic cells in the CNS found are not HIV infected cells but surrounding cells, suggesting that soluble factors may be involved. Proinflammatory cytokines secreted from infected or activated cells may directly induce cell death [76].

5. Possible mechanisms of cellular death and roles of microglia and astrocytes

Reactive astrogliosis and microglia is another major characteristics of ADC. [24, 87, 92]. Astrocytes may be involved in the etiology of HAD, which may serve as reservoir for non productive HIV infection and have preventive roles against neurotoxins secreted by HIV infected and activated microglia. The significantly lowered levels of proinflammatory molecules in co-cultures of activated macrophages and astrocytes compared to cultures of macrophages without astrocytes indicate that astrocytes may have a protective role [84, 85, 86].

Activated microglia and macrophages, whether HIV infected or not, are capable of producing viral proteins such as gp120, Tat, Nef, Vpr [62, 97, 98]. Elevated serum levels of proinflammatory cytokines (TNF, IFN-γ, IL-1β, arachidonic acid), inducible nitric oxide synthase, quinolate, PAF, glutamate and quinolinic acid in cerebrospinal fluid have been shown to have high correlation with HIV- dementia [71, 99-104]. Studies reported that cellular factors secreted by microglia and macrophages as well as viral proteins such gp120, Vpr, Tat promote neuronal toxicity via the NMDA type glutamate receptor [90, 91]. Activation of the NMDA receptor may initiate caspase activation or promote calcium influx. This effect could be blocked with anti-NMDA receptor blockers. PAF released from cultured microglia in response to TNF stimulation can induce neuronal apoptosis via Bcl-2 independent pathways [93, 94]. Elevated PAF also induces Ca influx, arachidonic acid release and chemotaxis [93, 95]. Increased levels of prostaglandin E_2 (PGE_2) in the cerebrospinal fluid of patients with HAD suggests that PGE_2 may play a role in progression of dementia [99].

Activated microglia in patients with HAD contains increased expression of TNF-α and TNFR and IL-1β and IL-1β converting enzyme (Caspase 1) [88, 89]. Oxidative stress has a role in neuronal apoptosis in patients with dementia [105, 106]. Nitric oxide synthase, arachidonic acid and P50 enzymes are sources of reactive oxygen species (ROS) in the brain and increased expression of inducible NOS correlated with expression of gp41 [89, 96]. Post mortem studies from pediatric patients with HIV indicate that caspase 3 expression caused by reactive oxygen intermediates were produced in mitochodria, although this activation was independent from Bcl2/Bax pathways [111, 112]. It has been shown that increased expression of Bcl-2 protects cells from HIV induced apoptosis [90, 113].

Additionally, increased production of mitochondrial reactive oxygen species led to caspase 8 activation in patients with HAD [107, 108]. HIV-1 infected monocytes may induce cell adhesion molecules E-selectin and vascular cell adhesion molecules (VCAM-1) on the brain microvascular endothelial cells. Studies showed that secretion of TNF and IL-1β from HIV infected brains induced expression of adhesion molecules on BMVECs. These cell adhesion molecules are known as mediators for transendothelial migration of monocytes [82, 116].

A number of studies indicate that patients with HAD have many clinical signs in common with dopaminergic disorders [5, 117, 118]. Autopsy studies of patients with HAD indicate that HIV infected cells, including macrophages and multinucleated giant cells, are found infiltrating in dopamine rich basal ganglia [5, 119] It has been shown that biogenic amin metabolite, homovanillic acid (HVA) levels are more diminished in patients with HAD compared to the patients with AIDS [120, 121]. A limited number of studies also indicate that cholinergic systems may be involved in the pathogenesis of HAD [5, 122]. Overall, results indicate that dopaminergic systems may be involved in the pathogenesis of HAD.

6. Therapeutic strategies

Introduction of highly active antiretroviral therapy (HAART) has decreased mortality rates and development of dementia. HAART played a major role in improving the life quality and cognitive functions for individuals with HIV infection [123, 124]. However, extended survival of infected people leaves them more vulnerable to drug resistant neurological impairment and development of dementia [117]. With the increasing resistance of HIV strains to antiretrovirals there has been a resurgence in the frequency of HIV encephalitis and HIV leukoencephalopathy [5]. Other limitations observed with HAART are that most of the drugs used in combinations of HAART have a very low ability to penetrate into the CNS. These drugs became less effective in reducing viral load and eliminating higher replication rates of HIV in the CNS [125, 126, 127]. Minor cognitive motor disorders are now a more common neurological problem since HAART was introduced. The prolonged survival of HIV infected patients is more susceptible exposure to HIV virions and proteins because of the CNS may serve as a reservoir for HIV-1 protected from the impact of HAART. Additionally, costs of HAART are still major obstacles for the treatment of HAD.

Based on an increased knowledge of the pathogenesis of HAD, several potential experimental therapeutics to reduce CNS damage are under trial. L-type voltage dependent Ca^{+2} channel antagonist, nimodipine, is one of the promising therapeutics. This drug binds to calcium channels to inhibit cellular depolarization that occurs when extracellular glutamate concentrations are increased. Unlike other NMDA receptor antagonists tested, Memantine, has been proven for safety and effectiveness. Memantine enters through open NMDA receptors stimulated by excessive glutamate and blocks receptor activation. *In vivo* and *in vitro* studies indicate that memantine prevents gp120 induced neuronal injury [128, 129]. It has been shown that nitroglycerin has protective effects against over stimulation of NMDA receptors [98]. The mechanism of nitroglycerin is similar to memantine as it prevents neurons from the effects of over stimulation of the NMDA receptor [133].
Additionally, some chemokines are important potential therapeutic target in the fight against HIV infection. Antagonists of CXCR4 and CCR5 may inhibit HIV entry [42, 43, 44]. In particular, CXCR4 and its ligand, SDF-1 may play a crucial role in the inhibition of gp120 induced neuroapoptosis. Chemokine receptor, CX3CR1, and its ligand, fractalkine (FKN) have been prevented neurons from gp120 induced apoptosis.

Alternatively, antioxidant therapy may help to prevent the development of neurocognitive symptoms and neuronal apoptosis in the CNS [105, 130]. Finally, p38 MAPK inhibitors have been shown to reduce neuronal apoptosis [131, 132].

7. Summary and future directions

Advances in research on HIV allowed researchers to better understand the molecular mechanisms of HAD. Neuronal apoptosis is essentially an irreversible process, but in fact, it has been shown that HAART improves cognitive functions. This indicates that virus induced neurological changes can be reversed. Knowing when neurological damage becomes irreversible is an important question in this field. Latency of HIV in the CNS cells is another important consideration for researchers. Greater understanding of activation and reactivation of HIV in the CNS will lead to development of more effective therapeutics. Ultimately, studies on HIV and the pathogenesis of HAD will improve the quality of life and life expectancy of patients with HIV and reduce the complications of HIV infection.

Acknowledgement

Author acknowledges critical reading of Julio Martin and University of Pennsylvania Post Doctoral Editing Club's editor Jennifer Kent during preparation of this manuscript. Author dedicates this chapter to Dr. Shahid Jameel, virology group leader in ICGEB, New Delhi India.

References:

[1] Dewhurst S., Gelbard HA., Fine SM. Neuropathogenesis of AIDS.Mol Med Today. 1996 Jan;2(1):16-23.

[2] Holmberg SD., Horsburgh CR., Ward JW., Jaffe HW. Biologic factors in the sexual transmission of human immunodeficiency virus. J Infect Dis. 1989 Jul;160(1):116-25.

[3] Padian NS., Shiboski SC., Glass SO., Vittinghoff E. Heterosexual transmission of human immunodeficiency virus (HIV) in Northern California: results from a ten-year study. Am J Epidemiol. 1997 Aug 15;146(4):350-7

[4] Cashion MF., Banks WA., Bost KL., Kastin AJ. Transmission routes of HIV-1 gp120 from brain to lymphoid tissues. Brain Res. 1999 Mar 20;822(1-2):26-33

[5] Koutsilier E., ttet Meulen V., Riederer P. Neurotransmission in HIV associated dementia: a short review. J Neural Transm. 2001;108(6):767-75.

[6] Reger M, Welsh R, Razani J, Martin DJ, Boone KB. A meta-analysis of the neuropsychological sequelae of HIV infection. J Int Neuropsychol Soc. 2002 Mar;8(3):410-24.

[7] Janssen RS., Nwanyanwu OC., Selik R.M., Stehr-Green JK. Epidemiology of human immunodeficiency virus encephalopathy in the United States. Neurology. 1992 Aug; 42 (8): 1472-6.

[8] Janssen RS .Epidemiology of human immunodeficiency virus infection and the neurologic complications of the infection. Semin Neurol. 1992 Mar;12(1):10-7

[9] McArthur JC., Sacktor N., Selnes O. Human immunodeficiency virus associated dementia.Semin Neurol. 1999;19(2):129-5

[10] Barre-Sinoussi F., Chermann JC., Rey F., Nugeyre MT., Chamaret S., Gruest J., Dauguet C., Axler-Blin C., Vezinet-Brun F., Rouzioux C., Rozenbaoum W., Montagnier L. Isolation of a T-lymphotropic retrovirus from a patient at risk for acquired immune deficiency syndrome (AIDS). Science. 1983 May 20;220(4599):868-71

[11] Gallo RC. Salahuddin SZ., Popovic M., Shearer GM., Kaplan M., Haynes., BF., Palker TJ., Redfield R., Oleske J., Safai B. Frequent detection and isolation of cytopathic retroviruses (HTLV-III) from patients with AIDS and at risk for AIDS.Science. 1984 May 4;224(4648):500-3.

[12] Wain-Hobson S., Sonigo P., Danor O., Cole S., Alizon M., Nucleotide sequence of the AIDS virus, LAV.Cell. 1985 Jan;40(1):9-17

[13] Muesing MA., Smith DH., Cabradilla CD., Benton CV., Lasky LA., Capon DJ.. Nucleic acid structure and expression of the human AIDS/lymphadenopathy retrovirus.Nature. 1985 Feb 7-13;313(6002):450-8

[14] Frankel AD, Young JA HIV-1: fifteen proteins and an RNA. Annu Rev Biochem. 1998;67:1-25

[15] Kedzierska K., Crowee SM. The role of monocytes and macrophages in the pathogenesis of HIV-1 infection.Curr Med Chem. 2002 Nov;9(21): 1893-903.

[16] Gorry PR., Taylor J., Holm GH., Mehle A., Morgan T., Cayabyab M., Farzan M., Wang H., Bell JE., Gabuzda D., Increased CCR5 affinity and reduced CCR5/CD4 dependence of a neurovirulent primary human immunodeficiency virus type 1 isolate.J Virol. 2002 Jun;76(12):6277-92.

[17] Albright A., Shieh JT., Itoh T., Lee B., Pleasure D., O'Connor MJ., Doms RW., Gonzales Scarano F., Microglia express CCR5, CXCR4, and CCR3, but of these, CCR5 is the principal coreceptor for human immunodeficiency virus type 1 dementia isolates.J Virol. 1999 Jan;73(1):205-13.

[18] Liu ZQ., Wood C., Levy JA., Cheng-Mayer C., The viral envelope gene is involved in macrophage tropism of a human immunodeficiency virus type 1 strain isolated from brain tissue. J Virol. 1990 Dec;64(12) :6148-53.

[19] Korber BT., Kunstman KJ., Patterson BK., Furtado M., McEvilly MM., Levy R., Wolinsky SM. Genetic differences between blood- and brain-derived viral sequences from human immunodeficiency virus type 1-infected patients: evidence of conserved elements in the V3 region of the envelope protein of brain-derived sequences. J Virol. 1994 Nov;68(11):7467-81.

[20] Westervelt P., Gendelman HE., Ratner L., Identification of a determinant within the human immunodeficiency virus 1 surface envelope glycoprotein critical for productive infection of primary monocytes. Proc Natl Acad Sci U S A. 1991 Apr 15;88(8):3097-101

[21] Budka H. Neuropathology of human immunodeficiency virus infection. Brain Pathol. 1991 Apr;1(3):163-75

[22] Everall IP., Luthert PJ., Lantos PL., Neuronal loss in the frontal cortex in HIV infection. Lancet. 1991 May 11;337(8750):1119-21.,

[23] Wiley CA., Schrier RD., Morey M., Achim C., Venable JC., Nelson JA., Pathogenesis of HIV encephalitis. Acta Pathol Jpn. 1991 Mar;41(3):192-6.

[24] Kaul M., Garden GA., Lipton SA. Pathways to neuronal injury and apoptosis in HIV-associated dementia.Nature. 2001 Apr 19;410(6831) :988-94.

[25] Chen W., Sulcove J., Frank I., Jaffer S., Ozdener H., Kolson DL. Development of a human neuronal cell model for human immunodeficiency virus (HIV)-infected macrophage-induced neurotoxicity: apoptosis induced by HIV type 1 primary isolates and evidence for involvement of the Bcl-2/Bcl-xL-sensitive intrinsic apoptosis pathway. J Virol. 2002 Sep;76(18):9407-19

[26] Stankoff B Calvez V., Suarez S., Bossi P., Rosenblum O. Plasma and cerebrospinal fluid human immunodeficiency virus type-1 (HIV-1) RNA levels in HIV-related cognitive impairment. Eur J Neurol. 1999 Nov;6(6):669-75.

[27] Foudraine NA., Hoetelmans RM., Lange JM., Wolf F., Portegies P., Cerebrospinal - fluid HIV-1 RNA and drug concentrations after treatment with lamivudine plus zidovudine or stavudine. Lancet. 1998 May 23;351(9115):1547-51
[28] Corasaniti MT., Piccirilli S., Paoletti A., Nistico R., Stirngaro A., Malorni W., Evidence that the HIV-1 coat protein gp120 causes neuronal apoptosis in the neocortex of rat via a mechanism involving CXCR4 chemokine receptor. Neurosci Lett. 2001 Oct 19;312(2):67-70.
[29] Shieh JT., Martin J., Baltuch G., Malim MH., Gonzales Scarano F., Determinants of syncytium formation in microglia by human immunodeficiency virus type 1: role of the V1/V2 domains.J Virol. 2000 Jan;74(2):693-701
[30] Liu HY., Soda Y., Shimizu N., Haraguchi Y., Jinno A., Takeuchi Y., Hoshino H., CD4-Dependent and CD4-independent utilization of coreceptors by human immunodeficiency viruses type 2 and simian immunodeficiency viruses. Virology. 2000 Dec 5;278(1):276-88.,
[31] Peluso R., Haase A., Stowring L., Edwards M., Ventura P. A Trojan Horse mechanism for the spread of visna virus in monocytes. Virology. 1985 Nov;147(1):231-6.
[32] Glass JD., Feddor H., Wesselingh Sl., McArthur JC., Immunocytochemical quantitation of human immunodeficiency virus in the brain: correlations with dementia. Ann Neurol. 1995 Nov;38(5):755-62.
[33] Dewhurst S., Gelbard HA., Fine SM. Neuropathogenesis of AIDS. Mol Med Today. 1996 Jan;2(1):16-23
[34] Galey D., Becker K., Haughey N., Kalehua A., Taub D., Woodward J., Mattson MP., Nath A., Differential transcriptional regulation by human immunodeficiency virus type 1 and gp120 in human astrocytes. J Neurovirol. 2003 Jun;9(3):358-71
[35] Kim TA., Avraham HK., Koh YH., Jiang S., Park IW., Avraham S., HIV-1 Tat-mediated apoptosis in human brain microvascular endothelial cells. J Immunol. 2003 Mar1;170(5):2629-7.
[36] Kanmogne GD., Kennedy RC., Grammas P. HIV-1 gp120 proteins and gp160 peptides are toxic to brain endothelial cells and neurons: possible pathway for HIV entry into the brain and HIV-associated dementia. J Neuropathol Exp Neurol. 2002 Nov;61(11):992-1000
[37] Su ZZ., Kang DC., Chen Y., Pekarskaya O., Chao W., Volsky DJ., Fisher PB., Identification of gene products suppressed by human immunodeficiency virus type 1 infection or gp120 exposure of primary human astrocytes by rapid subtraction hybridization. J Neurovirol. 2003 Jun;9(3):372-89.
[38] Tornatore C., Meyers K., Atwood W. Conant K., Major E., Temporal patterns of human immunodeficiency virus type 1 transcripts in human fetal astrocytes. J Virol. 1994 Jan;68(1):93-102.
[39] Harouse JM., Wroblewska Z., Laughlin MA., Hickey WF., Gonzales-Scarano F. Human choroid plexus cells can be latently infected with human immunodeficiency virus. Ann Neurol. 1989 Apr;25(4):406-11.
[40] Lackner AA., Dandekar S., Gardner MB., Neurobiology of simian and feline immunodeficiency virus infections. Brain Pathol. 1991 Apr;1(3):201-12
[41] Bragg DC., Childers TA., Tompkins MB., Tomkins WA., Meekerr RB. Infection of the choroid plexus by feline immunodeficiency virus. J Neurovirol. 2002 Jun;8(3):211-24.
[42] Bleul CC, Farzan M., Choe H., Parolin C., Clark-Lewis I., Sodrisku J., Springer TA. The lymphocyte chemoattractant SDF-1 is a ligand for ESTR/fusin and blocks HIV-1 entry. Nature. 1996 Aug 29;382(6594):829-33
[43] Cocchi F., DeVico AL., Garzino-Demo A., Arya SK., Gallo RC., Lusso P. Identification of RANTES, MIP-1 alpha, and MIP-1 beta as the major HIV-suppressive factors produced by CD8+ T cells. Science. 1995 Dec 15;270(5243):1811-5.
[44] Oberlin E., Amara A., BachelerieF., Bessia C., Virelizier JL., Moser B., The CXC chemokine SDF-1 is the ligand for LESTR/fusin and prevents infection by T-cell-line-adapted HIV-1. Nature. 1996 Aug 29;382(6594):833-5
[45] Giovanneli A., Limatola C., Ragozzino D., Mileo AM., Ruggieri A., Eusebi F., CXC chemokines interleukin-8 (IL-8) and growth-related gene product alpha (GROalpha) modulate Purkinje neuron activity in mouse cerebellum. J Neuroimmunol. 1998 Dec 1;92(1-2):122-32.
[46] Bezzi P.Domercq M., Brambilla L., Galli R., Schols D., Volterra A. CXCR4-activated astrocyte glutamate release via TNF alpha: amplification by microglia triggers neurotoxicity. Nature Neuroscience. 2001 Jul;4(7):702-10.
[47] Allen NJ., Attwell DA chemokine-glutamate connection Nature Neuroscience 2001 4, 676 - 678
[48] Ohagen A., Ghosh S., He J., Huang K., Chen Y., Shaw G., Gabuzda D., Apoptosis induced by infection of primary brain cultures with diverse human immunodeficiency virus type 1 isolates: evidence for a role of the envelope. J Virol. 1999 Feb;73(2):897-906.
[49] Miller RJ., Meucci O., AIDS and the brain: is there a chemokine connection? Trends Neurosci. 1999 Oct;22(10):471-9

[50] Zheng J. Thylin MR., Ghorpade A., Xiong H., Persidsky Y., Cotter R., Gendelman HE. Intracellular CXCR4 signaling, neuronal apoptosis and neuropathogenic mechanisms of HIV-1-associated dementia. J Neuroimmunol. 1999 Aug 3;98(2):185-200
[51] Klein RS., Willianms KC., Alvarez-Hernandez X., Westmoreland S., Force T., Lackner AA., Luster AD. Chemokine receptor expression and signaling in macaque and human fetal neurons and astrocytes: implications for the neuropathogenesis of AIDS. J Immunol. 1999 Aug 1;163(3):1636-46.
[52] Corasaniti MT., Piccirilli S., Paoletti A. Nistico R., Stirngaro A., Malorni W., Finazzi-Agro A., Bagetta G. Evidence that the HIV-1 coat protein gp120 causes neuronal apoptosis in the neocortex of rat via a mechanism involving CXCR4 chemokine receptor. Neurosci Lett. 2001 Oct 19;312(2):67-70.
[53] Bezzi P., Domercq M., Brambilla L., Galli R., Schols D., De Clercq E. Volterra A. CXCR4-activated astrocyte glutamate release via TNFalpha: amplification by microglia triggers neurotoxicity. Nat Neurosci. 2001 Jul;4(7):702-10.
[54] Biard-Piechaczyk M., Robert-Hebrmann V., Richard V., Roland J., Hipskinf RA., Devaux C., Caspase-dependent apoptosis of cells expressing the chemokine receptor CXCR4 is induced by cell membrane-associated human immunodeficiency virus type 1 envelope glycoprotein (gp120). Virology. 2000 Mar 15;268(2):329-44.
[55] Meucci O., Fatatis A., Simen AA., Miller RJ. Expression of CX3CR1 chemokine receptors on neurons and their role in neuronal survival. Proc Natl Acad Sci U S A. 2000 Jul 5;97(14):8075-80.
[56] Maciejewski-Lenoir D., Chen S., Feng L., Maki R., Bacon KB. Characterization of fractalkine in rat brain cells: migratory and activation signals for CX3CR-1-expressing microglia.J Immunol. 1999 Aug 1;163(3):1628-35.
[57] Tong N., Perry SW., Zhang O., James HJ., Guo H., Brooks A., Bal H., Gelbard HA., Neuronal fractalkine expression in HIV-1 encephalitis: roles for macrophage recruitment and neuroprotection in the central nervous system. J Immunol. 2000 Feb 1;164(3):1333-9.
[58] Meucci O., Fataris A., Simen AA., Bushell TJ., Gray PW., Miller RJ. Chemokines regulate hippocampal neuronal signaling and gp120 neurotoxicity. Proc Natl Acad Sci U S A. 1998 Nov 24;95(24):14500-5.
[59] Shi B. De Girolami U. He J. Wang S. Lorenzo A., Busciglio J. Gabuzda D. Apoptosis induced by HIV-1 infection of the central nervous system.J Clin Invest. 1996 Nov 1;98(9):1979-90.
[60] Buzy J., Brenneman DE., pert CB., Martin A., Slazar A., Ruff MR. Potent gp120-like neurotoxic activity in the cerebrospinal fluid of HIV-infected individuals is blocked by peptide T. Brain Res. 1992 Dec 11;598(1-2):10-8
[61] Jones MV., Bell JE., Nath A. Immunolocalization of HIV envelope gp120 in HIV encephalitis with dementia. AIDS. 2000 Dec 1;14(17):2709-13.
[62] Van de Bovenkamp M. Notter HS., Pereira CF., Interactions of human immunodeficiency virus-1 proteins with neurons: possible role in the development of human immunodeficiency virus-1-associated dementia. Eur J Clin Invest. 2002 Aug;32(8):619-27
[63] Kaul M., Lipton SA. Chemokines and activated macrophages in HIV gp120-induced neuronal apoptosis. Proc Natl Acad Sci U S A. 1999 Jul 6;96(14):8212-6.
[64] Soliven B., Albert J. Tumor necrosis factor modulates Ca2+ currents in cultured sympathetic neurons. J Neurosci. 1992 Jul;12(7):2665-71.
[65] Yu C., Takeda M., Soliven B. Regulation of cell cycle proteins by TNF-alpha and TGF-beta in cells of oligodendroglial lineage.J Neuroimmunol. 2000 Aug 1;108(1-2):2-10.
[66] Banks WA., Kastin AJ., Akerstrom V., HIV-1 protein gp120 crosses the blood-brain barrier: role of adsorptive endocytosis. Life Sci. 1997;61(9):PL119-25.
[67] Cioni C., Annunziata P., Circulating gp120 alters the blood-brain barrier permeability in HIV-1 gp120 transgenic mice. Neurosci Lett. 2002 Sep 27;330(3):299-301.
[68] Dawson VL., Dawson TM., Uhl GR., Synder SH. Human immunodeficiency virus type 1 coat protein neurotoxicity mediated by nitric oxide in primary cortical cultures. Proc Natl Acad Sci U S A. 1993 Apr 15;90(8):3256-
[69] Dreyer EB., Kaiserr PK., Offermann JT., Lipton SA. HIV-1 coat protein neurotoxicity prevented by calcium channel antagonists. Science. 1990 Apr 20;248(4953):364-7.
[70] Lipton SA., Sucher NJ., Kaiser PK., Dreyer EB. Synergistic effects of HIV coat protein and NMDA receptor-mediated neurotoxicity. Neuron. 1991 Jul;7(1):111-8
[71] Yeung MC. Pulliam L., Lau AS. The HIV envelope protein gp120 is toxic to human brain-cell cultures through the induction of interleukin-6 and tumor necrosis factor-alpha. AIDS. 1995 Feb;9(2):137-43.

[72] Bonavia R., Bajetto A., Barbero S., Albini A., Noonan DM., Schettini G., HIV-1 Tat causes apoptotic death and calcium homeostasis alterations in rat neurons. Biochem Biophys Res Commun. 2001 Oct 26;288(2):301-8
[73] Scorziello A., Florio T., Bajeto A., Thallung S., Schettini G., TGF-beta1 prevents gp120-induced impairment of Ca2+ homeostasis and rescues cortical neurons from apoptotic death. J Neurosci Res. 1997 Sep 1;49(5):600-7.
[74] Glass JD., Johnson RT. Human immunodeficiency virus and the brain. Annu Rev Neurosci. 1996;19:1-26
[75] Giulian D., Wendt E., Vaca K., Noonan CA.The envelope glycoprotein of human immunodeficiency virus type 1 stimulates release of neurotoxins from monocytes. Proc Natl Acad Sci U S A. 1993 Apr 1;90(7):2769-73
[76] Pulliam L., Clarke JA., McGuire D., McGrath MS. Investigation of HIV-infected macrophage neurotoxin production from patients with AIDS dementia. Adv Neuroimmunol. 1994;4(3):195-8
[77] Corasaniti MT., Navarra M. Nistico S., Rotiroti D., Maccarrone M., Melino G., Finazzi Agro A. Requirement for membrane lipid peroxidation in HIV-1 gp120-induced neuroblastoma cell death. Biochem Biophys Res Commun. 1998 May 29;246(3):686-9
[78] Catani MV., Corasaniti MT., Navarra M., Nistico G. Finazzi-Agro A. Melino G. gp120 induces cell death in human neuroblastoma cells through the CXCR4 and CCR5 chemokine receptors
[79] Corasaniti MT., Melino G., Navarra M., Garaci E., Finazzi- Agro A., Nistico G., Death of cultured human neuroblastoma cells induced by HIV-1 gp120 is prevented by NMDA receptor antagonists and inhibitors of nitric oxide and cyclooxygenase. Neurodegeneration. 1995 Sep;4(3):315-21.
[80] Corasaniti MT., Navarra M., Catani MV., Melino G., Nistico G., Finazzi-Agro A. NMDA and HIV-1 coat protein, GP120, produce necrotic but not apoptotic cell death in human CHP100 neuroblastoma cultures via a mechanism involving calpain. Biochem Biophys Res Commun. 1996 Dec 4;229(1):299-304.
[81] Nagano S., Takeda M. Ma L., Soliven B. Cytokine-induced cell death in immortalized Schwann cells: roles of nitric oxide and cyclic AMP. J Neurochem. 2001 Jun;77(6):1486-95.
[82] Scorziello A., Floriao T., Bajetto A. , Schettini G. Intracellular signalling mediating HIV-1 gp120 neurotoxicity. Cell Signal. 1998 Feb;10(2):75-84.
[83] Galicia O., Sanchez-Alavez M., Mendez Diaz M.,Nav arro L., Prospero-Garcia O. [HIV glycoprotein 120: possible etiological agent of AIDS-associated dementia Rev Invest Clin. 2002 Sep-Oct;54(5):437-52.
[84] Nottet HS., Jett M., Flanagan CR., Zhai OH., Persidsky Y., Schwartz J., Aregulatory role for astrocytes in HIV-1 encephalitis. An overexpression of eicosanoids, platelet-activating factor, and tumor necrosis factor-alpha by activated HIV-1-infected monocytes is attenuated by primary human astrocytes. J Immunol. 1995 Apr 1;154(7):3567-81
[85] Tornatore C., Chandra R., Berger JR., Major EO. HIV-1 infection of subcortical astrocytes in the pediatric central nervous system. Neurology. 1994 Mar;44(3 Pt 1):481-7.
[86] Hori K., Burd PR., Furuke K., Kutza J., Weih KA, Clousse KA. Human immunodeficiency virus-1-infected macrophages induce inducible nitric oxide synthase and nitric oxide (NO) production in astrocytes: astrocytic NO as a possible mediator of neural damage in acquired immunodeficiency syndrome. Blood. 1999 Mar 15;93(6):1843-50.
[87] Garden GA Microglia in human immunodeficiency virus-associated neurodegeneration. Glia. 2002 Nov;40(2):240-5
[88] Sippy BD., Hofman FM., Wallach D., Hinton DR., Increased expression of tumor necrosis factor-alpha receptors in the brains of patients with AIDS. J Acquir Immune Defic Syndr Hum Retrovirol. 1995 Dec 15;10(5):511-21
[89] Zhao ML., Kim MO., Morgelli S., Lee SC. Expression of inducible nitric oxide synthase, interleukin-1 and caspase-1 in HIV-1 encephalitis.J Neuroimmunol. 2001 Apr 2;115(1-2):182-9
[90] Doble A. The role of excitotoxicity in neurodegenerative disease: implications for therapy. Pharmacol Ther. 1999 Mar;81(3):163-22
[91] Nishida K. Markey SP., Kustova Y., Morse HC., Sei Y. Increased brain levels of platelet-activating factor in a murine acquired immune deficiency syndrome are NMDA receptor-mediated. J Neurochem. 1996 Jan;66(1):433-5et al 1996
[92] Ghorpade A, Holter S, Borgmann K, Persidsky R, Wu L. HIV-1 and IL-1beta regulate Fas ligand expression in human astrocytes through the NF-kappaB pathway. J Neuroimmunol. 2003 Aug;141(1-2):141-9
[93] Westmoreland SV., Kolson D., Gonzales-Scarano F. Toxicity of TNF alpha and platelet activating factor for human NT2N neurons: a tissue culture model for human immunodeficiency virus dementia.J Neurovirol. 1996 Apr;2(2):118-26.

[94] Perry SW. Hamilton JA., Tjoelker LW., Dbaibo G. Glebard HA. Platelet-activating factor receptor activation. An initiator step in HIV-1 neuropathogenesis. J Biol Chem. 1998 Jul 10;273(28):17660-4.

[95] Del Sorbo L., DeMartino A. Biancone L., Bussolati B., Conaldi PG. Camussi G. The synthesis of platelet-activating factor modulates chemotaxis of monocytes induced by HIV-1 Tat.Eur J Immunol. 1999 May;29(5):1513-21

[96] Adamson DC., McArthur JC., Dawson TM., Dawson VL. Rate and severity of HIV-associated dementia (HAD): correlations with Gp41 and iNOS. Mol Med. 1999 Feb;5(2):98-109.

[97] Eugenin EA., D'Avers TG., Lopez L., Calceron TM., Berman JW. MCP-1 (CCL2) protects human neurons and astrocytes from NMDA or HIV-tat-induced apoptosis. J Neurochem. 2003 Jun;85(5):1299-311.

[98] Lipton SA., Similarity of neuronal cell injury and death in AIDS dementia and focal cerebral ischemia: potential treatment with NMDA open-channel blockers and nitric oxide-related species. Brain Pathol. 1996 Oct;6(4):507-17.

[99] Griffin DE., Wesselingh SL., McArthur JC. Elevated central nervous system prostaglandins in human immunodeficiency virus-associated dementia. Ann Neurol. 1994 May;35(5):592-7

[100] Smith DG, Guillemin GJ, Pemberton L, Kerr S, Nath A, Smythe GA, Brew BJ. Quinolinic acid is produced by macrophages stimulated by platelet activating factor, Nef and Tat. J Neurovirol. 2001 Feb;7(1):56-60

[101] Jiang ZG., Pigge C., Heyes MP., Murphy C., Markey SP. Glutamate is a mediator of neurotoxicity in secretions of activated HIV-1-infected macrophages. J Neuroimmunol. 2001 Jul 2;117(1-2):97-107.

[102] Gendelman HE., Zheng J., Coulter CL., Ghorpade A., Che M., Sindells S. Suppression of inflammatory neurotoxins by highly active antiretroviral therapy in human immunodeficiency virus-associated dementia. J Infect Dis. 1998 Oct;178(4):1000-7.

[103] Vecchiet J., Dalessandro M., Travasi F., Falasca K., Pizzigallo E. Interleukin-4 and interferon-gamma production during HIV-1 infection and changes induced by antiretroviral therapy. Int J Immunopathol Pharmacol. 2003 May-Aug;16(2):157-66

[104] Schulz TF. Kaposi's sarcoma-associated herpesvirus (human herpesvirus 8): epidemiology and pathogenesis. J Antimicrob Chemother. 2000 Apr;45 Suppl T3:15-27.

[105] Turchan J., Pocernish Cb., Gairola C., Chauhan A., Nath A., Oxidative stress in HIV demented patients and protection ex vivo with novel antioxidants. Neurology. 2003 Jan 28;60(2):307-14.

[106] Toborek M., Lee YW., Pu H., Malecki A., Flora G., Nath A. HIV-Tat protein induces oxidative and inflammatory pathways in brain endothelium.J Neurochem. 2003 Jan;84(1):169-79.

[107] Banki K, Hutter E, Gonchoroff NJ, Perl A. Molecular ordering in HIV-induced apoptosis. Oxidative stress, activation of caspases, and cell survival are regulated by transaldolase. J Biol Chem. 1998 May 8;273(19):11944-53

[108] Accomero P. Raddizzani M., Care A. Mattia G. Chiodoni C. Colomo MP. HIV/gp120 and PMA/ionomycin induced apoptosis but not activation induced cell death require PKC for Fas-L upregulation. FEBS Lett. 1998 Oct 9;436(3):461-5.

[109] Ullrich CK., Groopman JE., Ganju RK. HIV-1 gp120- and gp160-induced apoptosis in cultured endothelial cells is mediated by caspases. Blood. 2000 Aug 15;96(4):1438-42.

[110] Biard-Piechaczyk M., Robert-Hebmann V., Richard V., Roland J., Hipskind RA., Devaux C., Caspase-dependent apoptosis of cells expressing the chemokine receptor CXCR4 is induced by cell membrane-associated human immunodeficiency virus type 1 envelope glycoprotein (gp120). Virology. 2000 Mar 15;268(2):329-44.

[111] James HJ., Sharer LR., Zhang Q., Wang HG., Epstein LG., Reed JC., Gelbard HA. Expression of caspase-3 in brains from paediatric patients with HIV-1 encephalitis. Neuropathol Appl Neurobiol. 1999 Oct;25(5):380-6.

[112] Banki K. Hutter E., Gonchoroff NJ., Perl A. Molecular ordering in HIV-induced apoptosis. Oxidative stress, activation of caspases, and cell survival are regulated by transaldolase. J Biol Chem. 1998 May 8;273(19):11944-53.

[113] Strack PR., Frey MW., Rizzo CJ., Cordova B., Korant BD. Apoptosis mediated by HIV protease is preceded by cleavage of Bcl-2. Proc Natl Acad Sci U S A. 1996 Sep 3;93(18):9571-6

[114] Patel CA., Mukhtar M., Pomerantz RJ. Human immunodeficiency virus type 1 Vpr induces apoptosis in human neuronal cells. J Virol. 2000 Oct;74(20):9717-26.

[115] Stewart SA, Poon B, Song JY, Chen IS.Human immunodeficiency virus type 1 vpr induces apoptosis through caspase activation. J Virol. 2000 Apr;74(7):3105-11

[116] Nottet HS., Persidsky Y., Sasse Sasseville VG, Nukuna AN, Bock P, Zhai QH, Sharer LR, McComb RD, Swindells S, Soderland C, Gendelman HE Mechanisms for the transendothelial migration of HIV-1-infected monocytes into brain. J Immunol. 1996 Feb 1;156(3):1284-95

[117] Czub S, Koutsilieri E, Sopper S, Czub M, Stahl-Hennig C, Muller JG, Pedersen V, Gsell W, Heeney JL, Gerlach M, Gosztonyi G, Riederer P, ter Meulen V. Enhancement of central nervous system pathology in early simian immunodeficiency virus infection by dopaminergic drugs. Acta Neuropathol (Berl). 2001 Feb;101(2):85-91.

[118] Nath A. Pathobiology of human immunodeficiency virus dementia. Semin Neurol. 1999;19(2):113-27.

[119] Navia BA., Cho ES., Peito CK., Price RW., The AIDS dementia complex: II. Neuropathology. Ann Neurol. 1986 Jun;19(6):525-35.

[120] Kramer EL., Sanger JJ. Brain imaging in acquired immunodeficiency syndrome dementia complex. Semin Nucl Med. 1990 Oct;20(4):353-63

[121] Berger JR., Kumar M., Kumar A., Fernandez JB., Levin B. Cerebrospinal fluid dopamine in HIV-1 infection. AIDS. 1994 Jan;8(1):67-71.

[122] Koutsilieri E., Czub S., Scheller C., Sopper S. Tatschner T., Riederer P. Brain choline acetyltransferase reduction in SIV infection. An index of early dementia? Neuroreport. 2000 Aug 3;11(11):2391-3.

[123] Suarez S., Baril L., Stankoff B., Khellaf M., Dubois B., Lubetzki C. Hauw JJ. Outcome of patients with HIV-1-related cognitive impairment on highly active antiretroviral therapy. AIDS. 2001 Jan 26;15(2):195-200

[124] Sacktor N. The epidemiology of human immunodeficiency virus-associated neurological disease in the era of highly active antiretroviral therapy. J Neurovirol. 2002 Dec;8 Suppl 2:115-21

[125] Farinpour R., Miller EN., Satz P., Selnes OA., Cohen BA., Visscher BR. Psychosocial risk factors of HIV morbidity and mortality: findings from the Multicenter AIDS Cohort Study (MACS).J Clin Exp Neuropsychol. 2003 Aug;25(5):654-70.

[126] Enting RH., Hoetelmans RM., Lange JM., Burger DM., Portegies P. Antiretroviral drugs and the central nervous system. AIDS. 1998 Oct 22;12(15):1941-55

[127] Cunningham PH., Smith DG., Satchell C., Cooper DA., Brew B. Evidence for independent development of resistance to HIV-1 reverse transcriptase inhibitors in the cerebrospinal fluid. AIDS. 2000 Sep 8;14(13):1949-54.

[128] Nath A., Anderson C., Jones M., Maragos W., Booze R., Mattson M. Neurotoxicity and dysfunction of dopaminergic systems associated with AIDS dementia. J Psychopharmacol. 2000;14(3):222-7.

[129] Holden CP., Haughey NJ., Nath A., Geiger JD. Role of Na+/H+ exchangers, excitatory amino acid receptors and voltage-operated Ca2+ channels in human immunodeficiency virus type 1 gp120-mediated increases in intracellular Ca2+ in human neurons and astrocytes. Neuroscience. 1999;91(4):1369-78.

[130] Shor-Posner G., Lecusay R., Morales G., Campa A., Miguez Burbano MJ. Neuroprotection in HIV-positive drug users: implications for antioxidant therapy. J Acquir Immune Defic Syndr. 2002 Oct 1;31 Suppl 2:S84-8.

[131] Ghatan S. Larner S., Kinoshita Y., Hetman M., Patel L. Morrison RS. p38 MAP kinase mediates bax translocation in nitric oxide-induced apoptosis in neurons. J Cell Biol. 2000 Jul 24;150(2):335-47

[132] Bhat NR., Zhang P., Lee JC., Hogan EL. Extracellular signal-regulated kinase and p38 subgroups of mitogen-activated protein kinases regulate inducible nitric oxide synthase and tumor necrosis factor-alpha gene expression in endotoxin-stimulated primary glial cultures. J Neurosci. 1998 Mar 1;18(5):1633-41.

[133] Jain KK. Evaluation of memantine for neuroprotection in dementia. Expert Opin Investig Drugs. 2000 Jun;9(6):1397-406.

Frontiers in Neurodegenerative Disorders and Aging: Fundamental Aspects, Clinical Perspectives and New Insights
T. Özben and M. Chevion (Eds.)
IOS Press, 2004

Olfactory Dysfunction in Neurodegenerative Diseases

M. Hakan Özdener* and Nancy E. Rawson*
Monell Chemical Senses Center, University Science Center
3500 Market Street Philadelphia, Pennsylvania, USA

Abstract: Interest in olfactory dysfunction has increased tremendously in the past decade, in part due to observations that chemosensory impairment is an early symptom of many neurodegenerative diseases. Several features of the olfactory system make it particularly relevant to understanding neurodegeneration/regeneration. First, while being vulnerable to environmental and infectious exposure, the olfactory system has the unique property of ongoing replacement of the olfactory sensory neurons under physiological conditions and following injury. Second, the receptor neurons residing in the periphery are developmentally related to those of the central nervous system, yet are accessible relatively noninvasively via biopsy from living subjects. Third, olfactory performance can easily be tested in a variety of ways that provide insight into the function of brain areas involved in detection, identification and memory. In addition to providing insights into the etiology or diagnosis of disease, a better understanding of olfactory neurobiology is needed to develop ways to treat olfactory dysfunction, which affects both quality of life and personal safety. At least 3,000,000 Americans suffer from chemosensory disorders, and that is likely to increase as the aging segment of the population grows. Olfactory impairment represents a danger to the individuals resulting from inability to detect hazards, such as natural gas and spoiled food, and threatens quality of life through the loss of enjoyment of foods and fragrances. The neurological systems responsible for olfactory function represent perhaps the most diverse, complex and adaptable components of the nervous system. The loss in olfaction result from changes at both the anatomical and molecular level. The loss can be caused by aging, toxins, infectious agents, environmental factors and a variety of diseases. Understanding the neurobiology of this sensory system may help us to develop new diagnostic measures and treatments for neurodegenerative disease as well as to improve the quality of life for millions of people who are handicapped by their inability to detect the flavors and fragrances around them.

1. Introduction

Olfactory impairment is a common occurrence in aging and may be an early signal of neurodegenerative diseases. Olfactory loss caused by aging and diseases affects both quality of life and personal safety. Aging, as well as viral infections, neurodegenerative diseases, head injuries, chronic sinusitis infections and nasal obstructions are the most common causes of olfactory disorders [73]. In addition, at least one third of older people report dissatisfaction

*Address for reprint and other correspondence: M. Hakan Özdener and Nancy E. Rawson. Monell Chemical Senses Center, University Science Center. 3500 Market Street Philadelphia, Pennsylvania USA 19104 USA
e-mail: hozdener@monell.org and rawson@monell.org

with their sense of taste or smell [1, 70]. The impact of sensory loss on elders is not only physiological but also emotional. The sense of smell and its capacity is critical for most mammals in terms of identification and evaluation of food, mates and territories, and in general for the maintenance of a good quality of life. The susceptibility of elderly people to aging and diseases, particularly neurodegenerative diseases, is varied. Therefore, complaints about sensory functions should be considered seriously as possible indicators of neurodegenerative diseases or other underlying conditions. The population of elderly is increasing as a result of improved health care throughout the world, and the attention of the medical and scientific community has focused on prevention and treatment of age-related diseases and dysfunctions. Olfactory dysfunction can lead to changes of dietary habits that may in turn exacerbate disease states or contribute to nutritional deficiencies [72, 73]. Although diagnosis of taste and smell disorders has improved considerably over the last two decades, treatment of these disorders is still limited to conditions with discernible and reversible causes [71, 72].

Taste and smell are fundamental sensory systems responsible for the perception of aroma and flavor. Olfactory function is commonly measured based on either detection sensitivity (threshold), identification or discrimination of odors. These tests can be performed fairly easily and may be useful tools to improve diagnosis of conditions in which olfactory loss is an early symptom, such as Alzheimer's dementia, Parkinson's disease and other neurodegenerative disorders.

Unlike the central nervous system (CNS) neurons and other sensory neurons, olfactory neurons are unique in their ability to be replaced after injury. These primary receptor neurons are developmentally related to those of the CNS, yet are accessible for study from living patients. Studies of the cellular processes underlying the regenerative capacity of the peripheral and central components of the olfactory system are leading to new therapeutic approaches in the treatment of spinal cord injury (90, 91), stroke (92, 93) and may also contribute to the treatment or prevention of neurodegenerative diseases. In this chapter, we will review recent progress made in understanding olfactory function and olfactory dysfunction in neurodegenerative diseases and aging.

2. Anatomy and cellular features of the olfactory system

This sensory system is able to detect and discriminate an enormous variety of volatile molecules with great sensitivity and specificity. Tens of thousands of chemicals can be detected, many at concentrations as low as a few parts per trillion [94, 95]. This feat is accomplished through anatomical, cellular and molecular features that are designed to amplify, encode and integrate a vast array of incoming olfactory information.

The olfactory epithelium is localized to the interior surface of the nasal cavity and consists primarily of three basic cell types: olfactory receptor neurons (ORNs), supporting cells, and basal cells [2]. Post mortem biopsies, anatomical studies and explant cultures of olfactory neurons from different parts of the nasal cavity show that sensory epithelium extends from the olfactory cleft down to varying degrees onto the superior aspect of the medial turbinate [3, 4, 5]. The turbinate structures are cartilaginous ridges covered with respiratory epithelium, a non-sensory ciliated columnar epithelial tissue also populated with mucus secreting goblet cells. This structure increases the surface area available for both warming and humidifying incoming air, as well as funneling volatile chemicals up into the sensory epithelium. Human olfactory receptor neurons have a generally similar morphology to those of other vertebrates, although there is variation among species [6]. The receptor cell is comprised of a cell body with an apical dendrite terminating in a knob containing multiple nonmotile cilia. The cilia project into the mucus overlying the nasal epithelium where they have direct contact with volatile chemicals in the air. Basally, an axon projects through the cribriform plate to synapse with the dendrites of mitral cells in the olfactory bulb. The mitral cells project via the olfactory nerve (cranial nerve I) to the entorhinal cortex, as well as regions involved in emotion and memory, such as the amygdala and hippocampus. Several types of interneurons modulate mitral cell activity, including periglomerular cells, tufted cells and granule cells. Granule cells are dopaminergic/GABAergic interneurons that are involved in signal processing and modulation [105, 106].

3. Transduction Mechanisms

During the past decade, tremendous advances in our understanding of the initial events in olfactory transduction have been made. The discovery of a large family of genes encoding G-protein-coupled receptors with seven transmembrane domains that apparently represent odorant receptors is a cornerstone in this progress. Each olfactory receptor is responsive to a range of stimuli. Odorant binding leads to a depolarizing current within the cilia of the bipolar receptor cells that ultimately triggers the action potentials that collectively provide the neural code that is deciphered by higher brain centers (83). Most of the olfactory receptor proteins are linked to the stimulatory guanine nucleotide-binding protein [G_{olf}]. When stimulated, it activates the enzyme adenylate cyclase to produce the second messenger adenosine monophosphate (cAMP) [96]. cAMP diffuses through the cell and activates cellular depolarization via the opening of cyclic-nucleotide-gated ionic channels [83]. Another possible mechanism is that some odorants also activate cyclic guanosine monophosphate (cGMP), which is believed to play a role in the modulation of the sensitivity of olfactory receptor neurons, such as during adaptation [83]. In addition, recent evidence indicates that some odorants may activate phospholipase C to produce the second messenger inositol trisphosphate [IP_3], which may also modulate the activity of the cAMP pathway via the activity of phosphoinositol-3 kinase [85]. Medications, diseases or disorders that interfere with or alter the ability of these transduction pathways to operate can influence olfactory performance. Also, as this tissue is available via biopsy from live subjects, functional studies may suggest specific genetic or pathologic alterations related to early symptoms or causes of neurodegenerative disease [21].

4. Neuroregeneration in the olfactory system

The exposure of ORNs to the external environment makes these primary sensory neurons vulnerable to injury from environmental insults such toxins, infectious agents and trauma. However, unlike the central nervous system (CNS) neurons and other sensory neurons, ORNs can be replaced after injury. The average lifecycle of an ORN is approximately 30-120 days [8]. This replacement process begins with a population of multi-potent basal neuroepithelial precursor cells which undergo successive stages of differentiation to a fully mature ORN. It is also thought that these cells may differentiate along a non-neuronal pathway, although there may be separate populations of precursor cells as well [107, 108, 109, 110]. Following olfactory nerve injury or toxic exposure, reconstitution of neuroepithelial cells and establishment of connections within the olfactory bulb can be enhanced by growth factors including retinoic acid, IGF-1, TGF-α, TGF-β and FGF2 [9, 10, 11 12, 49]. Apoptotic cell death has been observed in cells representing all stages of neurogenesis (e.g. in proliferating neuronal precursors, immature olfactory receptor neurons, and mature olfactory receptor neurons) implying that apoptotic regulation of neuronal numbers may occur at multiple stages of the neuronal lineage [83, 84]. Remarkably, central components of the olfactory system may also be replaced. A population of proliferating stem cells arising in the subventricular zone migrates into the olfactory bulb where they differentiate into granule cells [50, 51]. This process appears to continue throughout life, although the impact on olfaction and the mechanisms controlling proliferation and differentiation of these cells are unknown.

5. Age associated olfactory loss

Detailed information about the prevalence of chemosensory disorders has been limited. An initial report by the National Institutes of Health (NIH) from the late 1970s indicated that more than 2 million adults in the United States had a disorder of smell or taste. Another survey conducted by the National Geographic Society in 1987 showed that 1% of their 1.2 million respondents could not smell 3 or more of 6 odorants using a 'scratch and sniff' test. This study indicated that age was an important factor with a decline beginning in the second decade of life [20]. A recent study conducted by the NIH collaborating with the National Center for Health Statistics (NCHS) in 1993 to acquire information on the prevalence of smell/taste problems, showed a prevalence of 2.7 million (1.4%) U.S. adults with olfactory problems. The prevalence rates increased exponentially with age. Almost 40% of respondents with a chemosensory problem (1.5 million) were 65 years of age or greater [71, 74]. The ability to detect, discriminate and identify odors is most sensitive to age and disease related dysfunction [19, 20]. In spite of the widespread age-related prevalence of olfactory loss, remarkably little is known about the specific mechanisms responsible and no treatments are currently available.

Several features of olfactory system are particularly susceptible to age and disease associated changes that may lead to functional deficits. Changes at both the anatomical and molecular level may contribute to this loss. Local injury from physical or chemical causes, damage to neural projections, disturbance of the cycle of neurogenesis resulting from general malnutrition, infectious diseases, metabolic disturbances, drugs, or radiation, or alteration of the composition of the mucus due to medication are possible major causative reasons to be determined in the pathogenesis of olfactory dysfunction [73]. The composition of mucus is critical to proper ORN function and may change with hydration, which is often reduced in the elderly, as well as from age-related diseases or associated medications. Reduction and/or alteration in olfactory function may also be due to changes at the level of the receptor cell. For instance, an age-related loss of selectivity was observed in a study of odorant response characteristics of ORNs dissociated from biopsies [114]. It was found that age-related changes in ion channel distribution [111, 112] or other components of the intracellular signaling cascades [113] could result in receptor cell dysfunction. Although the extent of olfactory epithelium is reduced with aging [21, 98], it remains unclear whether this accounts for age-related olfactory loss, as studies indicate that olfactory function is not affected even with substantial reduction of the olfactory epithelial area [21, 22]. Other anatomical changes, such as altered vascular and mucosal composition and peptidergic innervation, could lead to reduced sensitivity through indirect mechanisms or changes in the transport and clearance of odorants [97]. Sensory dysfunction may be a consequence of chronic health conditions such as diabetes, cancer, radiation, surgery and dentures. However, in most cases, the cause of olfactory loss is unknown and the development of treatments will require a better understanding of the mechanisms underlying this sensory impairment.

6. Olfactory impairment and neurodegenerative diseases

Scientists and physicians have paid increasing attention to the olfactory system and its function during the last decade, largely because of: (a) advances in our understanding of the histocompatibility basis for the receptor mechanisms, (b) evidence that the receptor cells undergo neurogenesis and both programmed and induced cell death, (c) important technical and practical developments in psychophysical measurement, and (d) the accessibility of these cells relatively noninvasively from living subjects [14, 15, 16, 17, 18]. These developments have led to the development of standardized olfactory testing that can assess detection sensitivity (threshold) and the ability to identify odors. These tests can be easy to perform and may be useful in improving diagnosis [80]. Since the first observation of olfactory function impairment in Parkinson disease [23] and senile dementia [24], olfactory function testing has revealed compromised olfactory function in a number of neurodegenerative diseases such Alzheimer's disease [25, 26 27, 28], Parkinson's disease [29, 30], Huntington's disease [31], HIV associated dementia [32, 33] and amyotrophic lateral sclerosis [57].

7. Alzheimer's Disease and Down Syndrome

Olfactory impairment and neuroanatomical changes in the central portions of the olfactory system occur early in the development of Alzheimer's disease (AD), and olfactory testing has been explored as a diagnostic aide [79, 81, 98]. Patients with AD perform more poorly on tests of odor identification [99, 100] and exhibit altered olfactory evoked response potentials compared to age-matched controls [101]. Olfactory tests alone, however, are insufficient to discriminate AD from Parkinson's disease and careful consideration of cognitive function is required to insure reliable results [102].

It is generally accepted that the classic AD neuropathology occurs in the entorhinal cortex very early in the development of the disease [103]. This observation led some to speculate that a causative agent might enter the brain via the nasal epithelium leading to the idea that histological studies of biopsies of the olfactory neuroepithelium might be useful as an early diagnostic tool. However, more comprehensive studies indicate that the density of plaques and tangles in the olfactory bulb is less severe, and studies of the peripheral olfactory epithelium have been inconsistent. In general, phosphorylated tau and neurofilament proteins are not observed in the perikarya of the olfactory neurons but are evident within the axons and dendrites of these cells [13, 104]. Several studies have reported AD-specific neuropathology within the olfactory epithelium [7, 34, 81] but others, using different markers, have noted similar features in non-AD and healthy olfactory tissue from elderly controls. In addition, studies that have included tissue from patients with other types of dementia or neurological disease have failed to identify any marker present in the olfactory epithelium that would serve to reliably distinguish AD from other conditions such as Parkinson's disease or vascular dementia [35, 36]. Consistent with these findings, while we have observed some functional differences in preliminary studies of ORNs obtained via biopsy from patients with early stage AD, these neurons appeared normal morphologically and were able to respond to odorants [21, 82]. Further studies of olfactory neuronal cell function may prove more useful than histology alone in understanding the alteration in cellular metabolism or signaling that herald the onset of this type of disease.

Patients with Down syndrome display neuropathological features similar in some respects to those seen in AD. For example, individuals with Down syndrome had significant deficits in olfactory functioning compared to the control groups [78]. The Alcohol Sniff Test (AST), a rapid screen for olfactory function, revealed olfactory deficits in children with Down syndrome [43]. Another study also indicated that olfactory deficits may provide a sensitive and early indicator of the deterioration and progression of the brain in older patients with Down syndrome [44].

8. Parkinson's Disease

Impairment in olfactory function is a well-documented abnormality in patients with Parkinson's disease (PD) [64]. The cellular and molecular mechanisms for this deficit are unknown but likely relate to impairment at several levels of the olfactory system. Olfactory impairment in PD was not related to the degree of motor dysfunction, or the disease duration, but was related to disease severity [30, 58, 59, 60, 65]. Interestingly, Hawkes et al. proposed that idiopathic PD may start in the olfactory system prior to damage in the basal ganglia [61]. Another study indicated that olfactory testing may be useful for differential diagnosis between PD and progressive supranuclear palsy (PSP) [63]. Both PD and PSP have similar motor symptoms and PSP is commonly misdiagnosed as PD, although they are distinct neuropathological entities [21, 63]. In one study, olfactory dysfunction was seen in patients with an abnormal reduction in striatal dopamine transporter binding who subsequently developed clinical parkinsonism. None of 23 normosmic relatives of these patients developed signs or symptoms of parkinsonism [86]. These observations indicate that olfactory deficits may precede clinical motor signs in PD and support a practical clinical application in the early diagnosis/prognosis of the disease.

PD-related olfactory dysfunction may relate to the function of dopamine receptors in both central [105, 115, 116, 117] and peripheral components of the system [37, 38, 39, 40]. Centrally, dopamine modulates synaptic activity in the olfactory bulb and entorhinal cortex, influences the activity of several ion channels and enzymes involved in olfactory transduction, and has been reported to induce apoptosis and modulate differentiation of olfactory neurons *in vitro* [86, 87, 88]. These effects are mediated via D2 receptors in the periphery [88], and D1 and D2 receptors on mitral/tufted and juxta-glomerular cells in the olfactory bulb [66]. The dopaminergic granule cells in the olfactory bulb derive from stem cells that migrate throughout life from the subventricular zone. These stem cells are being studied as a potential source for dopaminergic replacement cells via transplant [62].

9. Human Immunodeficiency Virus (HIV) infection and AIDS

HIV-associated dementia is a leading cause of neurodegenerative disorders among individuals under 30 years [89]. HIV-1 infects the central nervous system (CNS) and 7-25% of patients with CNS infection develop dementia and at least 50% of them develop mild neurocognitive impairment. Several studies have shown that patients with neurocognitive impairment caused by HIV infection had diminished odor sensitivity [52, 53, 54]. Impaired olfactory function may serve as an early marker of HIV associated neurological impairment [55] and could be helpful to evaluate the impact of therapeutic agents. Schiffman also reported that HIV positive patients had significantly impaired menthol detection compared to controls. It is likely that the chemosensory losses found in HIV patients reflect both central and peripheral deficits [56]. It was reported that out of 207 HIV-infected patients, 70% of them (n=144) reported that chemosensory complaints were associated with a poor quality of life [75]. Wasting with reduced caloric intake is an increasingly common clinical manifestation of AIDS. The perceptions of taste and smell play an important role in stimulating caloric intake and flavor enhancement of food can have a significant positive impact on nutritional status in hospitalized patients [56]. Significant taste and smell losses in HIV infected subjects may be of clinical significance in the development or progression of HIV associated wasting and are thus worthy of clinical consideration and treatment [76].

10. Creutzfeldt-Jacob disease

Taste and smell loss was reported as an early sign of Creutzfeldt-Jacob disease [67]. The pathologic prion protein (PrPSc) was found in the neuroepithelium of the olfactory mucosa in patients with sporadic Creutzfeldt-Jacob disease [68]. This result indicates that olfactory biopsy may provide diagnostic information, and further studies are warranted.

11. Huntington's disease and Multiple Sclerosis

Patients with Huntington's disease exhibit significant deficits in odor identification, but odor recognition memory was not found to be affected [69, 79]. In an animal model of the disease, the olfactory system exhibited early and significant accumulation of huntingtin-containing aggregates, which may account for the early olfactory impairment [77].

Olfactory dysfunction may also be an early indicator of disease progression in multiple sclerosis. The Cross Cultural Smell Identification test utilized in patients with multiple sclerosis indicated that these patients scored significantly worse than control groups. They also found a significant correlation between smell alteration and symptoms of anxiety and depression and the severity of neurological impairments [47].

In several studies, the neuropathology as based on plaque numbers was directly related to olfactory function [41, 42]. As plaque numbers declined or increased in the inferior frontal and temporal lobes, olfactory function declined or improved in correlation [45, 46, 48]. While these reports are suggestive of olfactory involvement and potential utility in diagnostic approaches for these diseases, no studies have been done to directly investigate the neuropathology or cell/molecular basis for the olfactory impairment.

12. Summary and future directions

The olfactory system is a fundamental sensory system responsible for the perception of flavor and fragrance. Olfaction is critical for most mammals for the maintenance of a good quality of life. Although diagnosis of smell disorders caused by aging and neurodegenerative diseases has improved considerably over the last two decades, treatment of these disorders is still limited to conditions with discernible and reversible causes. The medical community often overlooks sensory complaints. Understanding the biological basis for olfactory system disorders can help us to develop new approaches to improve the quality of flavor experience for those with impaired ability. In addition, studies of olfaction and ORN function may lend new insight into the etiology of neurodegenerative disease. Future research is needed for a better understanding of chemosensory mechanisms, establishing improved diagnostic procedures, and disseminating knowledge about chemosensory disorders among practitioners and the general public [71, 72].

Acknowledgement

Authors acknowledge critical reading by the University of Pennsylvania Postdoctoral Editing Club's editor Jennifer Kent during preparation of this manuscript.

References

[1] Pelchat ML You can teach an old dog new tricks: olfaction and responses to novel foods by the elderly. Appetite. 2000 Oct;35(2):153-60.2003
[2] Graziadei PP Cell dynamics in the olfactory mucosa. Tissue Cell. 1973;5(1):113-31
[3] Rawson NE, Gomez G, Cowart B, Brand JG, Lowry LD, Pribitkin EA, Restrepo D Selectivity and response characteristics of human olfactory neurons. J Neurophysiol. 1997 Mar;77(3):1606-13.
[4] Nibu K, Li G, Zhang X, Rawson NE, Restrepo D, Kaga K, Lowry LD, Keane WM, Rothstein JL. Olfactory neuron-specific expression of NeuroD in mouse and human nasal mucosa.Cell Tissue Res. 1999 Dec;298(3):405-14.
[5] Gomez G, Rawson NE, Hahn CG, Michaels R, Restrepo D Characteristics of odorant elicited calcium changes in cultured human olfactory neurons.J Neurosci Res. 2000 Dec 1;62(5):737-49.
[6] Schild D., Restrepo D., Transduction mechanisms in vertebrate olfactory receptor cells. Physiol Rev. 1998 Apr;78(2):429-66.
[7] Yamagishi M, Ishizuka Y, Seki K. Pathology of olfactory mucosa in patients with Alzheimer's disease. Ann Otol Rhinol Laryngol. 1994 Jun;103(6):421-7
[8] Astic L, Saucier D. Neuronal plasticity and regeneration in the olfactory system of mammals: morphological and functional recovery following olfactory bulb deafferentation. Cell Mol Life Sci. 2001 Apr;58(4):538-45
[9] Costanzo RM Regeneration of olfactory receptor cells. Ciba Found Symp. 1991;160:233-42
[10] Schwob JE, Neural regeneration and the peripheral olfactory system. Anat Rec. 2002 Feb 15;269(1):33-49
[11] Federico G, Maremmani C, Cinquanta L, Baroncelli GI, Fattori B, Saggese G.. Mucus of the human olfactory epithelium contains the insulin-like growth factor-I system which is altered in some neurodegenerative diseases. Brain Res. 1999 Jul 24;835(2):306-14.
[12] Amoore JE. Specific anosmia: a clue to the olfactory code. Nature. 1967 Jun 10;214(93):1095-8.
[13] Talamo BR, Rudel R, Kosik KS, Lee VM, Neff S, Adelman L, Kauer JS. Pathological changes in olfactory neurons in patients with Alzheimer's disease. Nature. 1989 Feb 23;337(6209):736-9.
[14] Rawson NE, Gomez G Cell and molecular biology of human olfaction. Microsc Res Tech. 2002 Aug 1;58(3):142-51.

[15] Amoore JE. Evidence for the chemical olfactory code in man.Ann N Y Acad Sci. 1974 Sep 27;237(0):137-43
[16] Menashe I, Man O, Lancet D, Gilad Y Different noses for different people. Nat Genet. 2003 Jun;34(2):143-4.
[17] Wysocki CJ, Dorries KM, Beauchamp GK Ability to perceive androstenone can be acquired by ostensibly anosmic people. Proc Natl Acad Sci U S A. 1989 Oct;86(20):7976-8.
[18] Beauchamp GK, Yamazaki K. Chemical signalling in mice. Biochem Soc Trans. 2003 Feb;31(Pt 1):147-51.
[19] Deems DA., and Doty RL. Age-related changes in the phenyl ethyl alcohol odor detection threshold. Trans Pa Acad Ophthalmol Otolaryngol. 1987;39(1):646-50
[20] Wysocki CJ., and Gilbert AN., National Geographic Smell Survey. Effects of age are heterogenous. Ann N Y Acad Sci. 1989;561:12-28
[21] Rawson NE, Gomez G, Cowart B, Restrepo D.The use of olfactory receptor neurons (ORNs) from biopsies to study changes in aging and neurodegenerative diseases.Ann N Y Acad Sci. 1998 Nov 30;855:701-7.
[22] Loo AT, Youngentob SL, Kent PF, Schwob JE.The aging olfactory epithelium: neurogenesis, response to damage, and odorant-induced activity. Int J Dev Neurosci. 1996 Nov;14(7-8):881-900.
[23] Ansari KA, Johnson A Olfactory function in patients with Parkinson's disease. J Chronic Dis. 1975 Oct;28(9):493-7.
[24] Waldton S Clinical observations of impaired cranial nerve function in senile dementia. Acta Psychiatr Scand. 1974;50(5):539-47.
[25] Koss E, Weiffenbach JM, Haxby JV, Friedland RP, Olfactory detection and identification performance are dissociated in early Alzheimer's disease. Neurology. 1988 Aug;38(8):1228-32
[26] Morgan CD, Nordin S, Murphy C., Odor identification as an early marker for Alzheimer's disease: impact of lexical functioning and detection sensitivity. J Clin Exp Neuropsychol. 1995 Oct;17(5):793-803.
[27] Murphy C, Gilmore MM, Seery CS, Salmon DP, Lasker BR. Olfactory thresholds are associated with degree of dementia in Alzheimer's disease. Neurobiol Aging. 1990 Jul-Aug;11(4):465-9
[28] Rezek DL. Olfactory deficits as a neurologic sign in dementia of the Alzheimer type. Arch Neurol. 1987 Oct;44(10):1030-2.
[29] Korten JJ, Meulstee J. Olfactory disturbances in Parkinsonism. Clin Neurol Neurosurg. 1980;82(2):113-8.
[30] Doty RL, Deems DA, Stellar S. Olfactory dysfunction in parkinsonism: a general deficit unrelated to neurologic signs, disease stage, or disease duration. Neurology. 1988 Aug;38(8):1237-44
[31] Moberg PJ, Pearlson GD, Speedie LJ, Lipsey JR, Strauss ME, Folstein SE. Olfactory recognition: differential impairments in early and late Huntington's and Alzheimer's diseases. J Clin Exp Neuropsychol. 1987 Dec;9(6):650-64.
[32] Razani J, Murphy C, Davidson TM, Grant I, McCutchan A. Odor sensitivity is impaired in HIV-positive cognitively impaired patients. Physiol Behav. 1996 Apr-May;59(4-5):877-81.
[33] Hornung DE, Kurtz DB, Bradshaw CB, Seipel DM, Kent PF, Blair DC, Emko P. The olfactory loss that accompanies an HIV infection. Physiol Behav. 1998 Jun 15;64(4):549-56.
[34] Lee JH, Goedert M, Hill WD, Lee VM, Trojanowski JQ. Tau proteins are abnormally expressed in olfactory epithelium of Alzheimer patients and developmentally regulated in human fetal spinal cord. Exp Neurol. 1993 May;121(1):93-105.
[35] Crino PB, Martin JA, Hill WD, Greenberg B, Lee VM, Trojanowski JQ. Beta-Amyloid peptide and amyloid precursor proteins in olfactory mucosa of patients with Alzheimer's disease, Parkinson's disease, and Down syndrome. Ann Otol Rhinol Laryngol. 1995 Aug;104(8):655-61.
[36] Yamagishi M, Ishizuka Y, Seki K.Definitive diagnosis of Alzheimer's disease using olfactory mucosal biopsyNippon Jibiinkoka Gakkai Kaiho. 1994 Jan;97(1):51-60.
[37] Herve D, Levi-Strauss M, Marey-Semper I, Verney C, Tassin JP, Glowinski J, Girault JA G(olf) and Gs in rat basal ganglia: possible involvement of G(olf) in the coupling of dopamine D1 receptor with adenylyl cyclase. J Neurosci. 1993 May;13(5):2237-48.
[38] Berkowicz DA, Trombley PQ. Dopaminergic modulation at the olfactory nerve synapse. Brain Res. 2000 Feb 7;855(1):90-9.
[39] Trombley PQ, Shepherd GM Synaptic transmission and modulation in the olfactory bulb. Curr Opin Neurobiol. 1993 Aug;3(4):540-7.
[40] Vargas G, Lucero MT Dopamine modulates inwardly rectifying hyperpolarization-activated current (Ih) in cultured rat olfactory receptor neurons. J Neurophysiol. 1999 Jan;81(1):149-58.

[41] Zivadinov R, Zorzon M, Monti Bragadin L, Pagliaro G, Cazzato G. Olfactory loss in multiple sclerosis. J Neurol Sci. 1999 Oct 15;168(2):127-30.

[42] Zorzon M, Ukmar M, Bragadin LM, Zanier F, Antonello RM, Cazzato G, Zivadinov R. Olfactory dysfunction and extent of white matter abnormalities in multiple sclerosis: a clinical and MR study. Mult Scler. 2000 Dec;6(6):386-90.

[43] Davidson TM, Freed C, Healy MP, Murphy C Rapid clinical evaluation of anosmia in children: the Alcohol Sniff Test.Ann N Y Acad Sci. 1998 Nov 30;855:787-92.

[44] Murphy C and Jinich S Olfactory dysfunction in Down's Syndrome. Neurobiol Aging.1996 Jul-Aug;17(4):631-7

[45] Doty RL, Li C, Mannon LJ, Yousem DM Olfactory dysfunction in multiple sclerosis.N Engl J Med. 1997 Jun 26;336(26):1918-9

[46] Doty RL, Li C, Mannon LJ, Yousem DM., Olfactory dysfunction in multiple sclerosis: relation to longitudinal changes in plaque numbers in central olfactory structures. Neurology. 1999 Sep 11;53(4):880-2.

[47] Zivadinov R, Zorzon M, Monti Bragadin L, Pagliaro G, Cazzato G. Olfactory loss in multiple sclerosis. J Neurol Sci. 1999 Oct 15;168(2):127-30

[48] Doty RL, Li C, Mannon LJ, Yousem DM Olfactory dysfunction in multiple sclerosis. Relation to plaque load in inferior frontal and temporal lobes. Ann N Y Acad Sci. 1998 Nov 30;855:781-6.

[49] Yee KK, Rawson NE. Retinoic acid enhances the rate of olfactory recovery after olfactory nerve transsection. Brain Res Dev Brain Res. 2000; 124:129-132

[50] Englund U, Bjorklund A, Wictorin K.Migration patterns and phenotypic differentiation of long-term expanded human neural progenitor cells after transplantation into the adult rat brain. Brain Res Dev Brain Res. 2002 Mar 31;134(1-2):123-41.

[51] Fricker RA, Carpenter MK, Winkler C, Greco C, Gates MA, Bjorklund A. Site-specific migration and neuronal differentiation of human neural progenitor cells after transplantation in the adult rat brain. J Neurosci. 1999 Jul 15;19(14):5990-6005.

[52] Brody D, Adler LA, Kim T, Angrist B, Rotrosen J.Effects of buspirone in seven schizophrenic subjects. J Clin Psychopharmacol. 1990 Feb;10(1):68-9.

[53] Hornung DE, Kurtz DB, Bradshaw CB, Seipel DM, Kent PF, Blair DC, Emko P.The olfactory loss that accompanies an HIV infection. Physiol Behav. 1998 Jun 15;64(4):549-56.

[54] Razani J, Murphy C, Davidson TM, Grant I, McCutchan A. Odor sensitivity is impaired in HIV-positive cognitively impaired patients. Physiol Behav. 1996 Apr-May;59(4-5):877-81

[55] Serby MJ, Larson PM, Kalkstein D. Olfaction and neuropsychiatry In: Serby, MJ. Chobor KL eds. Science of Olfaction. New York: Springer-Verlag; 1992:559-584

[56] Heald AE, Schiffman SS. Taste and smell. Neglected senses that contribute to the malnutrition of AIDS. N C Med J. 1997 Mar-Apr;58(2):100-4

[57] Ahlskog JE, Waring SC, Petersen RC, Esteban-Santillan C, Craig UK, O'Brien PC, Plevak MF, Kurland LT. Olfactory dysfunction in Guamanian ALS, parkinsonism, and dementia. Neurology. 1998 Dec;51(6):1672-7.

[58] Adler CH, Gwinn KA, Newman S. Olfactory function in restless legs syndrome. Mov Disord. 1998 May;13(3):563-5.

[59] Doty RL, Bromley SM, Stern MB. Olfactory testing as an aid in the diagnosis of Parkinson's disease: development of optimal discrimination criteria. Neurodegeneration. 1995 Mar;4(1):93-7.

[60] Wszolek ZK, Markopoulou K., Olfactory dysfunction in Parkinson's disease. Clin Neurosci. 1998;5(2):94-101.

[61] Hawkes CH, Shephard BC, Daniel SE. Is Parkinson's disease a primary olfactory disorder? QJM. 1999 Aug;92(8):473-80.

[62] Parati EA, Bez A, Ponti D, Sala S, Pozzi S, Pagano SF. Neural stem cells. Biological features and therapeutic potential in Parkinson's disease. J Neurosurg Sci. 2003 Mar;47(1):8-17.

[63] Doty RL, Golbe LI, McKeown DA, Stern MB, Lehrach CM, Crawford D. Olfactory testing differentiates between progressive supranuclear palsy and idiopathic Parkinson's disease. Neurology. 1993 May;43(5):962-5.

[64] Sobel N, Thomason ME, Stappen I, Tanner CM, Tetrud JW, Bower JM, Sullivan EV, Gabrieli JDAn impairment in sniffing contributes to the olfactory impairment in Parkinson's disease. Proc Natl Acad Sci U S A. 2001 Mar 27;98(7):4154-9.

[65] Tissingh G, Berendse HW, Bergmans P, DeWaard R, Drukarch B, Stoof JC, Wolters EC. Loss of olfaction in de novo and treated Parkinson's disease: possible implications for early diagnosis. Mov Disord. 2001 Jan;16(1):41-6.
[66] Wilson DA, Sullivan RM. The D2 antagonist spiperone mimics the effects of olfactory deprivation on mitral/tufted cell odor response patterns. J Neurosci. 1995; 15:5574-5581.
[67] Reuber M, Al-Din AS, Baborie A, Chakrabarty A. New variant Creutzfeldt-Jakob disease presenting with loss of taste and smell. J Neurol Neurosurg Psychiatry. 2001 Sep;71(3):412-3.
[68] Zanusso G, Ferrari S, Cardone F, Zampieri P, Gelati M, Fiorini M, Farinazzo A, Gardiman M, Cavallaro T, Bentivoglio M, Righetti PG, Pocchiari M, Rizzuto N, Monaco S. Detection of pathologic prion protein in the olfactory epithelium in sporadic Creutzfeldt-Jakob disease .N Engl J Med. 2003 Feb 20;348(8):711-9.
[69] Nordin S, Paulsen JS, Murphy C. Sensory- and memory-mediated olfactory dysfunction in Huntington's disease.J Int Neuropsychol Soc. 1995 May;1(3):281-90.
[70] Winkler S, Garg AK, Mekayarajjananonth T, Bakaeen LG, Khan E. Depressed taste and smell in geriatric patients. J Am Dent Assoc. 1999 Dec;130(12):1759-65.
[71] Spielman AI. Chemosensory function and dysfunction Crit Rev Oral Biol Med. 1998;9(3):267-91.
[72] Bromley SM. Smell and taste disorders: a primary care approach. Am Fam Physician. 2000 Jan 15;61(2):427-36, 438.
[73] Schiffman SS. Taste and smell in disease (second of two parts). N Engl J Med. 1983 Jun 2;308(22):1337-43.
[74] Hoffman HJ, Ishii EK, MacTurk RH Age-related changes in the prevalence of smell/taste problems among the United States adult population. Results of the 1994 disability supplement to the National Health Interview Survey (NHIS). Ann N Y Acad Sci. 1998 Nov 30;855:716-22.
[75] Heald AE, Pieper CF, Schiffman SS Taste and smell complaints in HIV-infected patients. 1998 Sep 10;12(13):1667-74.
[76] Graham CS, Graham BG, Bartlett JA, Heald AE, Schiffman SS. Taste and smell losses in HIV infected patients. Physiol Behav. 1995 Aug;58(2):287-93.
[77] Menalled LB, Sison JD, Dragatsis I, Zeitlin S, Chesselet MF Time course of early motor and neuropathological anomalies in a knock-in mouse model of Huntington's disease with 140 CAG repeats. J Comp Neurol. 2003 Oct 6;465(1):11-26.
[78] Nijjar RK, Murphy C. Olfactory impairment increases as a function of age in persons with Down syndrome Neurobiol Aging. 2002 Jan-Feb;23(1):65-73.
[79] Bacon Moore AS, Paulsen JS, Murphy C., A test of odor fluency in patients with Alzheimer's and Huntington's disease. J Clin Exp Neuropsychol. 1999 Jun;21(3):341-51.
[80] Murphy C Loss of olfactory function in dementing disease. Physiol Behav. 1999 Apr;66(2):177-82.
[81] Arnold SE, Smutzer GS, Trojanowski JQ, Moberg PJ Cellular and molecular neuropathology of the olfactory epithelium and central olfactory pathways in Alzheimer's disease and schizophrenia. Ann N Y Acad Sci. 1998 Nov 0;855:762-75.
[82] Rawson NE., and et al unpublished data
[83] Doty RL Olfaction. Annual Review of Psychology 2001 Feb Vol. 52: 423-452.
[84] Holcomb JD, Mumm JS, Calof AL Apoptosis in the neuronal lineage of the mouse olfactory epithelium: regulation in vivo and in vitro. Dev Biol. 1995 Nov;172(1):307-23.
[85] Zhainazarov AB, Doolin R, Herlihy JD, Ache BW. Odor-stimulated phosphatidylinositol 3-kinase in lobster olfactory receptor cells. J Neurophysiol. 2001 Jun;85(6):2537-44.
[86] Berendse HW, Booij J, Francot CM, Bergmans PL, Hijman R, Stoof JC, Wolters EC Subclinical dopaminergic dysfunction in asymptomatic Parkinson's disease patients' relatives with a decreased sense of smell. Ann Neurol. 2001 Jul;50(1):34-41.
[87] Coronas V, Feron F, Hen R, Sicard G, Jourdan F, Moyse E- In vitro induction of apoptosis or differentiation by dopamine in an immortalized olfactory neuronal cell line. J Neurochem. 1997 Nov;69(5):1870-81.
[88] Koster NL, Norman AB, Richtand NM, Nickell WT, Puche AC, Pixley SK, Shipley MT Olfactory receptor neurons express D2 dopamine receptors. J Comp Neurol. 1999 Sep 6;411(4):666-73.
[89] Wilkie FL, Goodkin K, Khamis I, Van Zuilen MH, Lee D, Lecusay R, Concha M, Symes S, Suarez P, Eisdorfer C. Cognitive Functioning in Younger and Older HIV-1-Infected Adults. J Acquir Immune Defic Syndr. 2003 Jun 1;33(2):S93-S105.

[90] Huang H, Chen L, Wang H, Xiu B, Li B, Wang R, Zhang J, Zhang F, Gu Z, Li Y, Song Y, Hao W, Pang S, Sun J.Influence of patients' age on functional recovery after transplantation of olfactory ensheathing cells into injured spinal cord injury. Chin Med J (Engl). 2003 Oct;116(10):1488-91.
[91] Resnick DK, Cechvala CF, Yan Y, Witwer BP, Sun D, Zhang S.Adult olfactory ensheathing cell transplantation for acute spinal cord injury. J Neurotrauma. 2003 Mar;20(3):279-85.
[92] Parent JM. Injury-induced neurogenesis in the adult mammalian brain. Neuroscientist. 2003 Aug;9(4):261-72.
[93] Arlotta P, Magavi SS, Macklis JD. Induction of adult neurogenesis: molecular manipulation of neural precursors in situ. Ann N Y Acad Sci. 2003 Jun;991:229-36.
[94] Walker JC, Hall SB, Walker DB, Kendal-Reed MS, Hood AF, Niu XF.Human odor detectability: new methodology used to determine threshold and variation. Chem Senses. 2003 Nov;28(9):817-26.
[95] Angioy AM, Desogus A, Barbarossa IT, Anderson P, Hansson BS. Extreme sensitivity in an olfactory system. Chem Senses. 2003 May;28(4):279-84.
[96] Lowe G, Nakamura T, Gold GH. Adenylate cyclase mediates olfactory transduction for a wide variety of odorants. Proc Natl Acad Sci U S A. 1989 Jul;86(14):5641-5.
[97] Ohta Y, Ichimura K Changes in epidermal growth factor receptors in olfactory epithelium associated with aging. Ann Otol Rhinol Laryngol. 2000 Jan;109(1):95-8.
[98] Loo AT, Youngentob SL, Kent PF, Schwob JE. The aging olfactory epithelium: neurogenesis, response to damage, and odorant-induced activity.Int J Dev Neurosci. 1996 Nov;14(7-8):881-900.
[99] McCaffrey RJ, Duff K, Solomon GS. Olfactory dysfunction discriminates probable Alzheimer's dementia from major depression: a cross-validation and extension. J Neuropsychiatry Clin Neurosci. 2000 Winter;12(1):29-33.
[100] Rezek DL.Olfactory deficits as a neurologic sign in dementia of the Alzheimer type. Arch Neurol. 1987 Oct;44(10):1030-2.
[101] Warner MD, Peabody CA, Flattery JJ, Tinklenberg JR.Olfactory deficits and Alzheimer's disease. Biol Psychiatry. 1986 Jan;21(1):116-8.
[102] Thesen T, Murphy C.Age-related changes in olfactory processing detected with olfactory event-related brain potentials using velopharyngeal closure and natural breathing. Int J Psychophysiol. 2001 Mar;40(2):119-27.
[103] Mesholam RI, Moberg PJ, Mahr RN, Doty RL.Olfaction in neurodegenerative disease: a meta-analysis of olfactory functioning in Alzheimer's and Parkinson's diseases.Arch Neurol. 1998 Jan;55(1):84-90.
[104] Reyes PF, Deems DA, Suarez MG. Olfactory-related changes in Alzheimer's disease: a quantitative neuropathologic study.Brain Res Bull. 1993;32(1):1-5.
[105] Trombley PQ, Shepherd GM. Synaptic transmission and modulation in the olfactory bulb. Curr Opin Neurobiol. 1993; 3:540-547.
[106] Brunig I, Sommer M, Hatt H et al. Dopamine receptor subtypes modulate olfactory bulb gamma-aminobutyric acid type A receptors. Proc Natl Acad Sci U S A. 1999; 96:2456-2460.
[107] DeHamer MK, Guevara JL, Hannon K et al. Genesis of olfactory receptor neurons in vitro: regulation of progenitor cell divisions by fibroblast growth factors. Neuron. 1994; 13:1083-1097.
[108] Calof AL, Mumm JS, Rim PC et al. The neuronal stem cell of the olfactory epithelium. J Neurobiol. 1998; 36:190-205.
[109] Calof AL, Bonnin A, Crocker C et al. Progenitor cells of the olfactory receptor neuron lineage. Microsc Res Tech. 2002; 58:176-188.
[110] Huard JM, Youngentob SL, Goldstein BJ et al. Adult olfactory epithelium contains multipotent progenitors that give rise to neurons and non-neural cells. J Comp Neurol. 1998; 400:469-486.
[111] Thibault O, Hadley R, Landfield PW Elevated postsynaptic [Ca2+]i and L-type calcium channel activity in aged hippocampal neurons: relationship to impaired synaptic plasticity. J Neurosci. 2001 Dec 15;21(24):9744-56.
[112] Tanaka Y, Ando S. Age-related changes in the subtypes of voltage-dependent calcium channels in rat brain cortical synapses. Neurosci Res. 2001 Feb;39(2):213-20.
[113] Palego L, Giromella A, Mazzoni MR, Marazziti D, Naccarato AG, Giannaccini G, Cassano GB, Lucacchini A. Gender and age-related variation in adenylyl cyclase activity in the human prefrontal cortex, hippocampus and dorsal raphe nuclei. Neurosci Lett. 2000 Jan 21;279(1):53-6.
[114] Rawson NE, Gomez G, Cowart B et al. The use of olfactory receptor neurons (ORNs) from biopsies to study changes in aging and neurodegenerative diseases. Ann N Y Acad Sci. 1998; 855:701-7.:701-707.

[115] Church AC, Bunney BS, Krieger NR. Neuronal localization of dopamine-sensitive adenylate cyclase within the rat olfactory tubercle. Brain Res. 1982; 234:369-376
[116] Baker H, Farbman AI. Olfactory afferent regulation of the dopamine phenotype in the fetal rat olfactory system. Neuroscience. 1993; 52:115-134
[117] Mijnster MJ, Isovich E, Flugge G et al. Localization of dopamine receptors in the tree shrew brain using [3H]-SCH23390 and [125I]-epidepride. Brain Res. 1999; 841:101-113

Frontiers in Neurodegenerative Disorders and Aging: Fundamental Aspects, Clinical Perspectives and New Insights
T. Özben and M. Chevion (Eds.)
IOS Press, 2004

Aspects of the Cell Biology of Prions

Albert Taraboulos
Department of Molecular Biology, the Hebrew University-Hadassah Medical School, P.O.Box 12272, Jerusalem 91120, Israel. Email: taraboul@cc.huji.ac.il

Abstract: Prions are unusual pathogens that cause the invariably fatal transmissible spongiform encephalopaties (TSE). The central event of prion propagation is the refolding of the normal cell surface protein PrP^C into the "prion" conformer, PrP^{Sc}, which in turn serves as a template for further conversion. The mechanistic and cell biological details of this event are still poorly understood. Here, we review the concept of prions and the properties of the prion proteins, and address two aspects of their cellular metabolism. (i) The early steps of PrP^C biosynthesis and folding in the secretory pathway have recently come into focus. The formation of PrP "aggresomes" under certain conditions, and their relevance to the spontaneous prion diseases, is discussed. (ii) A second topic relates to prions and "rafts". Rafts are microdomains of the membrane that are enriched in cholesterol and in sphingolipids (SLs), and that are involved in a wide variety of cellular processes. Evidence that rafts control the formation of prions, and the possible mechanisms involved, are also addressed.

1. Introduction

1.1 TSE and prions

The transmissible spongiform encephalopaties (TSE), such as scrapie of sheep, and Creutzfeldt-Jakob disease (CJD) and kuru of humans, have long been known for their peculiar characteristics, two of which stand out (reviewed in [2, 3]): First, their etiology is multiple. Thus, they can be infectious (kuru, scrapie, CJD, and bovine spongiform encephalopathy, or BSE), demonstrating the presence of an infectious agent. However, they can also be inherited in a mendelean fashion (such as familial CJD, and also Gerstman-Sträussler-Scheinker disease, or GSS), suggesting their linkage to a host gene. Indeed, the known familial prion diseases are all linked to mutations in the PrP gene of the host. Finally, the TSEs can also appear sporadically in the population at large (most CJD cases). Most intriguingly, the brains of the sporadic and genetic patients (who were never infected from exogenous sources) contained infectious material that can often transmit the disease to experimental animals (*spontaneous* prions). A second unusual character of TSEs is the resistance of the infectious agent to treatments that modify nucleic acids, but leave proteins intact (such as low doses of uv or ionizing irradiation, etc). These peculiarities of TSE are elegantly explained by current versions of the prion model for TSEs [5] [6]. The *protein-only* model of prions stipulates that

(i) prions are composed primarily of PrP^{Sc}, an abnormal conformer of the *host encoded* glycoprotein PrP^{C}; in this view, prions thus lack genes of nucleic acids , and (ii) that prions propagate by the template-assisted refolding of PrP^{C} (the substrate) into PrP^{Sc} (both template and product). To explain the inherited prion diseases, one has to make additional suppositions as to the properties of mutant PrP. For instance, some mutations might destabilize PrP^{C} and cause its occasional misfolding into a PrP^{Sc} conformation that might initiate a prion disease.

The TSEs are not the only disorders that are characterized by insoluble protein deposits. However, they occupy a unique place among these 'conformational diseases' [7] owing to their transmissibility and mechanism of propagation (for a review, see [2].

Exactly how PrP^{C} is transformed into PrP^{Sc} is not yet known. Based on the observed formation of fibrils by amyloidogenic peptides *in vitro*, a seeding-polymerization model for the propagation of prions was proposed [8]. In this model, the active "catalytic" prion (i.e. the particle that imposes its tertiary structure on PrP^{C}) is a large amyloidic PrP^{Sc} fibril, that works by accreting more PrP^{C} monomers. However, data on UV inactivation of prion infectivity, as well as ultrafiltration data, suggest that the infectious agent may be as small as a PrP dimer, indicating that large amyloidic fibrils may not be needed as a catalytic prion. Rather, the conversion reaction might involve heterodimers of interacting PrP^{C} and PrP^{Sc} [6]. Attempts to form PrP^{Sc} *de novo* in the test tube have been partially successful [9]. When PrP^{C} is mixed with excess PrP^{Sc} or PrP synthetic peptides in suitable conditions, PrP^{C} acquires prionlike properties such as a partial resistance to proteolysis. However, whether *bona fide* prions are produced in such *in vitro* reactions remains to be determined.

The information that prions bequeath their "progeny" is thus encrypted in the folding pattern of PrP^{Sc}. Prions can therefore be viewed as a *self-propagating switch* between two protein conformations: a "normal" conformation that comes out of the cellular folding machinery (PrP^{C}), and an abnormal "prion" conformation that is acquired post-translationally (PrP^{Sc}). While this phenomenon was first discovered in a pathogen of mammals, it is now clear that the prion way of "propagation" is used by Nature elsewhere. Non-PrP based prionlike phenomena have been found in yeast and fungi, where they may in some cases perform a physiological role (see for instance [10]). Most fascinatingly, a prionlike "switch" may also function in the establishment and maintenance of long term memory in aplysia [11]. However, these most interesting discoveries are beyond the scope of this review.

1.2 The prion proteins

Mammalian prions propagate by refolding the normal prion protein of the host, PrP^{C}, into a β-sheet rich abnormal conformation (PrP^{Sc}). PrP^{Sc} is in turn the only known component of prions and serves as a template for further conversion [6, 9]. The two PrP "isoforms" share the same covalent structure (including a glycophosphatidyl inositol (GPI) anchor, a disulfide bridge, and two N-linked sugars (Fig. 1)), but possess contrasting biochemical properties [12], which help identify and separate them in experimental settings. PrP^{Sc} possesses a protease-resistant core, called PrP27-30 (Fig. 1), is insoluble in detergents, and tends to form amyloidic fibrillary structures, or "prion rods", when extracted from membranes [13]. Native PrP^{Sc} also differs from PrP^{C} in that it reacts poorly with all [14, 15] but three [16] [17] [18] existing PrP antibodies. These biochemical properties are used as "surrogate" characteristics to differentiate between PrP^{C} and PrP^{Sc} instead of animal bioassays. Recent advances indicate that these biochemical criteria have to be broadened to include partially aggregated, protease-sensitive PrP^{Sc} species [15] [19]. Structural motifs that bind copper, heparin [20], and sphingolipids

(SLs) [21] have been mapped within PrP (Fig. 1). The functions of PrP^C have not yet been established, but it may store or shuttle Cu^{++} or Zn^{++}, function as a weak superoxide dismutase (reviewed in [22]), or transduce signals when engaged by an unidentified extracellular ligand [23] [24]. PrP^C is expressed by a variety of cell types. In contrast, the formation, metabolism, and pathogenesis of PrP^{Sc} can only be studied in a few cell types susceptible to prions, such as N2a mouse neuroblastoma [25] and GT1 mouse hypothalamic [26] [27] cell lines [28]. Infection of N2a cells with mouse prions (RML strain) has resulted in the establishment of a persistently infected cell line, ScN2a, many subclones and variants of which now exist in several laboratories. These cells produce both PrP^{Sc} and prion infectivity.

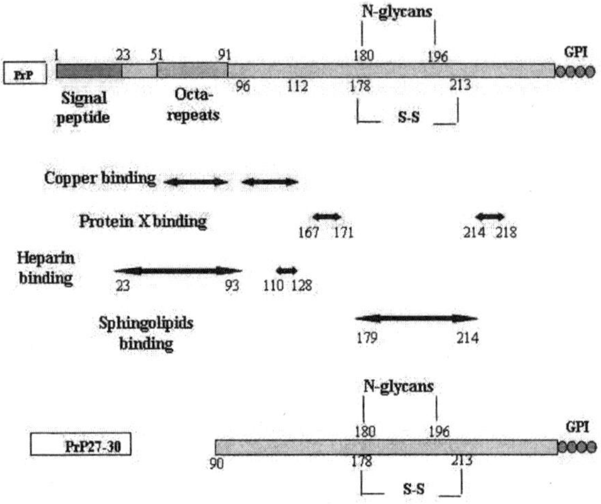

Figure 1. Representation of PrP, PrP27-30, and various binding sites.

1.3 Cell Biology of Prions

Experimental setup: Experiments usually involve N2a and ScN2a cells or other pairs of infected and uninfected cells. To study each of these isoforms separately in ScN2a cells, one must first separate them from each other by taking advantage of their disparate properties. For instance, proteinase K is routinely used to digest away PrP^C and protease-sensitive PrP^{Sc} from cell lysates, while converting protease-resistant PrP^{Sc} to PrP27-30 (the protease-resistant core). As mentioned above, the resulting PrP27-30 must then be denatured (usually with boiling SDS or with chaotropic salts) before it can be recognized by most PrP antibodies.

PrP metabolism: The cell biology of PrP has been delineated (Fig. 2, reviewed by [29]). Most PrP^C is translocated into the ER lumen where the signal peptide is cleaved and the C-terminal hydrophobic region is replaced by the GPI anchor. The interaction of PrP with the folding and the quality control (QC) mechanisms in the ER have attracted much recent attention (see 3. below). Most mature PrP^C molecules are exported to the cell surface to which they are attached by their GPI anchor. They are subsequently internalized and recycled to the cell surface [30] via pathways that may include both clathrin- and non-clathrin coated pits.

Like many GPI-anchored protein (GPI-APs), the PrP isoforms reside in lipid rafts (see 2. below) [31] [4] [32] [1], which play a decisive role in their metabolism [33]. PrP^C degradation, which occurs on rafts, starts with the removal of a N-terminal region by non-acidic endoproteases [4] of the disintegrin family [34]. This first step of PrP^C degradation is very interesting in that it appears to remove aa sequences that are absolutely essential for the ability of PrP^C to form PrP^{Sc}. By doing so, it thus exerts a protective antiprion effect, and in this sense it behaves like the α-secretase of Alzheimer's disease, which severs the amyloid precursor protein (APP) in the middle of the amyloidogenic sequences and thereby prevents the formation of the β-amyloid.

The formation of PrP^{Sc} takes place after PrP^C has left the ER, possibly on the cell surface or in endocytic compartments [35] [36]. N-linked glycosylation is not needed for the efficient conversion of PrP^C into PrP^{Sc}. Importantly, in scrapie-infected ScN2a cells only a small a minority (ca 5%) of GPI-anchored PrP^C molecules is transformed into protease-resistant PrP^{Sc} ($t1/2$ = ca 7h) [37]. Within 1 h of its formation, PrP^{Sc} is N-terminally trimmed by acid proteases to yield PrP27-30 [38] [39] and accumulate primarily in lysosomes [40].

PrP carrying some of the pathogenic mutations (that cause prion diseases in humans) have intrinsic prionlike properties even in the absence of exogenous infection [41], but they do not form *bona fide* PrP^{Sc} in cultured cells (in contrast to their ability to initiate prion diseases in transgenic mice).

PrP-associated molecules: There is an intense interest in identifying cellular molecules that interact with the PrP isoforms, especially those that assist the formation of PrP^{Sc}. Chief among them are cholesterol and sphingolipids (SLs), which crucially influence the metabolism of prions (either through rafts or by direct interactions with PrP, see 2. below). Other PrP-interacting species include: (i) the laminin receptor (LR/LRP) [42], stress-induced protein 1 [43], and cellular heparan sulfates (HS) proteoglycans [44]. Transgenetic studies have also indicated the existence of a host PrP^{Sc} cofactor, "Protein X" [45] (Fig. 1).

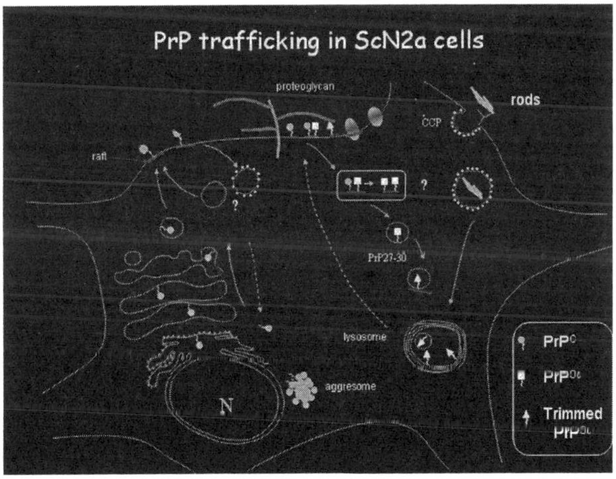

Figure 2: Cellular trafficking of the PrP isoforms. Uninfected cells contain only PrP^C, whereas both PrP^C and PrP^{Sc} are found in cells infected with prions.

1.4 This review

Here we review two very different aspects of PrP metabolism: (i) the formation of PrP "aggresomes" in cells treated with the immunosuppressant drug, cyclosporin A (CsA), and the possible significance of this finding for GSS, and (ii) the interaction of PrP with rafts, which seem to control the formation of PrP^{Sc}.

2. Prion Propagation Requires Cholesterol/Sphingolipid Rafts

2.1 What are rafts?

Lipid rafts are dynamic membrane microdomains that are thought to assemble through the packing of sphingolipids (SLs), which are the preponderantly saturated, and cholesterol [46]. Although most biophysical properties of rafts, such as their sizes and stability, remain controversial, their discovery is probably one of the most important recent developments in Cell Biology. Rafts are implicated in cell signaling (e.g., in the immunological synapse), in protein sorting and trafficking (e.g. folate potocytosis), and also in pathologies such as Alzheimer's disease (AD) [47] and prion diseases (see below) (reviewed in [48]. Rafts and their components are studied through a variety of methods including: (i) their association with buoyant membrane complexes ("DRMs") that are insoluble in certain non-ionic detergents such as Triton X-100 (TX-100) [49], (ii) their segregation from non-raft membrane proteins in co-patching experiments [50], and (iii) by other methods, including chemical crosslinking [51] and fluorescent resonance energy transfer (FRET). Caveolae, small (50 nm) saccules that hang beneath the plasma membrane of some cell types, may be a subset of rafts which are caveolin-coated. They occur only in cells that express one of three known caveolin isoforms. Caveolae are not essential for the formation of PrP^{Sc} [1].

2.2 Rafts control PrP^{Sc} metabolism

To characterize the role of rafts in the metabolism of PrP in N2a and ScN2a cells, we asked the following questions: (i) Are both PrP isoforms found in rafts? (ii) Are they found in the *same* rafts? (iii) Is PrP^{Sc} still formed if PrP is removed from rafts by manipulating the C-terminal GPI anchoring signal? (iv) What happens to the metabolism of PrP if the lipid composition of rafts is altered by pharmacological agents? Our findings are summarized below.

(i) PrP^{C} is attached to rafts: GPI-APs tend to accumulate within rafts [49] primarily (but not only) because the glycolipid has a high affinity for these domains. To determine if the PrP isoforms associate with rafts, we used floatation density gradients. We found that both the PrP isoforms associate with TX-100-DRMs. The association of PrP with rafts was also demonstrated by using a detergent-free method originally developed for the isolation of caveolae [32]. PrP^{C} appears to differ from archetypical GPI-APs in that it is often only a 'part-time' raft resident, as evidenced by its reduced partitioning in detergent-insoluble complexes [52] [53] in some cell types. Raft association of GPI-APs may vary during their trafficking, as judged by detergent insolubility [54]. Importantly, we observed that the flotation of PrP^{C} differs widely among cell types, and also among subclones of N2a cells. In particular, flotation of PrP^{C} was vastly more robust in cured ScN2a cell (Fig. 3). Whether this improved flotation is causally related to the vast susceptibility of these cells to re-infection remains to be seen.

Variability among N2a subclones is a recurrent observation in this field, and includes their widely disparate susceptibility to prion infection [55], and their caveolin content.

That PrP^{C} is found in rafts was not unexpected since most if not all GPI-APs are bound to these domains. In contrast, there were no *a priori* reasons to assume that PrP^{Sc} would be found in these domains as well. Although PrP^{Sc} possesses a GPI tail, it has not yet been determined that it is anchored to membranes through this moiety has not been determined. Unlike PrP^{Sc} and most other GPI proteins, PrP^{Sc} cannot be detached from the cellular membranes with the GPI-specific phospholipase PIPLC. Our results thus suggest that PrP^{Sc} is indeed attached to membranes through its GPI anchor. The finding that all the PrP players of the prion reaction are found in rafts strongly suggests that the formation of prions takes place in these membrane microdomains.

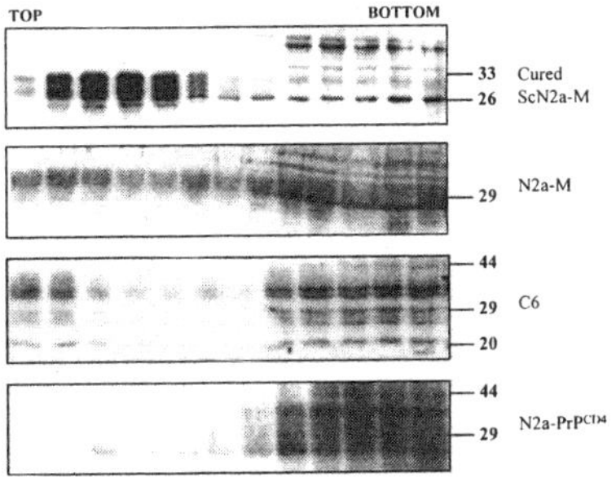

Figure 3. Vastly increased flotation of PrP^{C} in cured ScN2a cells. The indicated cells were lysed in 1% TX-100, subjected to a flotation assay in Nycodenz [1], and PrP in the fractions was detected by western immunoblotting. PrP^{CD4} was included as a non-raft marker [4]. All PrP^{C} completely floated in cured ScN2a cells, as opposed to the other lines. (ScN2a were cured with pentosan sulfate)

(ii) PrP^{C} and PrP^{Sc} mostly reside on disparate rafts. Since PrP^{C} is primarily a cell-surface molecule, while PrP^{Sc} is found mainly in lysosomes, it was reasonable to assume that the rafts in which proteins reside might possess different properties. We thus looked for experimental conditions that would separate these putatively disparate rafts. We indeed found that when the TX-100 cell lysates were incubated at 37°C (rather than 4°C) prior to the flotation gradient [1], or when CHAPS [56] served as a detergent, PrP^{C} migrates to lower density fractions, whereas PrP^{C} was found primarily in heavier regions of the gradient (Fig. 4). However, some PrP^{Sc} was still found in light rafts, and further studies will be needed to determine if catalytic fractions of PrP^{Sc} are found in overlapping light rafts.

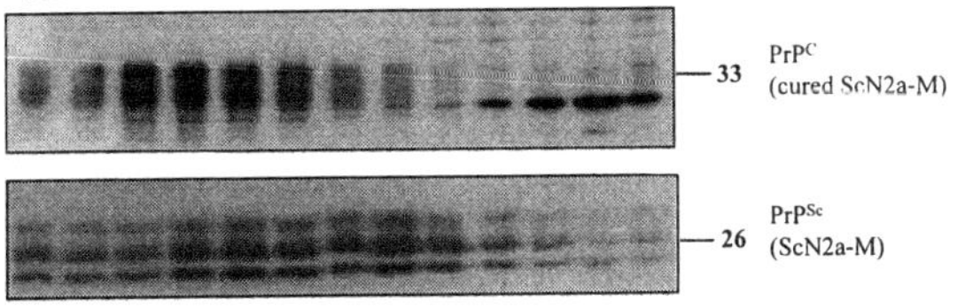

Figure 4. PrP^{C} and PrP^{Sc} float to different fractions in CHAPS-Nycodenz equilibrium gradients. The PrP^{Sc} samples were proteolyzed prior to western analysis

(iii) Removing PrP from Rafts Prevents PrP^{Sc} formation. To disconnect PrP from rafts, we swapped the GPI anchoring signal at the carboxyterminus of the PrP gene with the transmembrane and cytosolic regions of mouse CD4. The resulting chimeric gene (which was epitopically tagged) was then transfected into ScN2a cells, which provided endogenous prions. We determined that the transgene was expressed in these cells and formed chimeric PrP^{C}-CD4 and that PrP^{C}-CD4 was absent from TX-100-insoluble, buoyant fractions of the gradient, and thus was not in rafts. Most interestingly, chimeric PrP^{C}-CD4 did not acquire protease-resistance in these cells, i.e., was unable to form PrP^{Sc} [4]. This finding again suggests that being in rafts is essential for PrP^{C} molecules to form PrP^{Sc}. An obvious caveat of this approach is that adding a rigid TM tail to PrP might prevent the subsequent conformational changes that are required for the formation of PrP^{Sc}. Additional constructs with other TM sequences, all originating from non-raft proteins, subsequently failed to form PrP^{Sc} in ScN2a cells [57]. However, there are several TM-anchored (non-GPI) proteins that reside in rafts, and it will be interesting to see if PrP fused to such rafts TM sequences is able to form PrP^{Sc}.

(iv) Modifying Cellular Choelsterol and Spingolipids Modulates PrP^{Sc} synthesis. We reasoned that if PrP^{Sc} forms on rafts, then the lipid composition of these domains might modulate the formation of PrP^{Sc}. Indeed, several function that have been assigned to rafts have been shown to depend on normal levels of cholesterol and sphingolipids, the two major lipid constituents of rafts. For instance, folate potocytosis was vastly reduced both when compactin was used to deplete cellular cholesterol, and when fumonisin B1 was used to reduce the level of cellular SLs. We used a similar pharmacological approach to study the role of rafts in the formation of PrP^{Sc}. When cells were depleted of cholesterol by use of either lovastatin or β-cyclodextrin, PrP^{Sc} synthesis was vastly reduced [4]. With SLs, the situation was more complex and more interesting. Depending on the type of the SL targeted in the experiment, PrP^{Sc} levels could be either decreased or increased [33]. Thus, cholesterol and sphingolipids play distinguishable roles in the metabolism of PrP^{Sc}.

In addition, filipin [58] and amphotericin B [59], which are both cholesterol-binding agents, reduce PrP^{Sc} in cultured cells. Indirect evidence includes the inactivation of neuronal nitric acid synthase (nNOS), a cytosolic, facultative raft resident, during prion infection [60].

2.3 How do rafts control PrP^{Sc} formation?

How do rafts encourage the formation of prions? An attractive possibility is that rafts help laterally crowd 'seed' PrP^{Sc} and 'substrate' PrP^{C}, thereby fostering their interaction and facilitating PrP^{Sc} formation. Crowding could be exacerbated by endocytosis, such as in the case of BACE1 and APP [47]. Putative prion accessory molecules might also be made more available by such lateral clustering. Direct measurements will be needed to verify whether the PrP isoforms are indeed found in high lateral density within the cell membrane.

Rafts could also control PrP^{C} through entirely different mechanisms. For instance, there is growing evidence that rafts and caveolae are associated with specific internalization pathways. Thus, being in rafts, the PrP could gain access to propitious PrP^{Sc} biosynthetic compartments.

Finally, there could also be a direct interaction of raft cholesterol and SL with PrP, that can lead to PrP destabilization and refolding [61] [62] (disputed by [63]). The finding of sphingolipids [64] in highly purified prion rods suggests that these lipids may be a structural component of prions particles.

2.4 *Does lipid disequilibrium contribute to prion pathogenesis?*

The association of PrP^{Sc} with rafts may also have pathological implications. Prion diseases are characterized by a profound pathogenesis that includes neuronal vacuolation and death, leading to *status spongiosus*. In spite of many studies performed with synthetic amyloidogenic PrP peptides [65] [66] [67], the mechanisms leading to the pathogenesis of *bona* fide prions remain unknown. Seminal transplantation experiments [68] have shown that PrP^{Sc} leaking from transplanted brain tissue has little toxicity in $PrP^{0/0}$ tissues, whereas it is strongly pathogenic for tissue that expresses PrP^{C}, which are able to produce PrP^{Sc}. Based on this observation, we have previously suggested that *endogenously* made PrP^{Sc}, a large part of which is attached to membranes, may be much more cytotoxic than *exogenous* prions.

It is possible that toxic effects of membranal PrP^{Sc} could be mediated through abnormal rafts. When exogenous prion rods are administered to cultured cells, these cells take them up very efficient [69]. However, very little, if any, of this material becomes attached to membranes (unpublished results). In contrast, endogenous PrP^{Sc} is attached to a special variety of rafts [1] (Fig. 4). We propose that PrP^{Sc} could form lateral aggregates on the membrane (the aggregation status of PrP^{Sc} on membranes is unknown). By mobilizing raft lipids to these aggregates, PrP^{Sc} would (i) promote the formation of large, constitutively patched rafts, perhaps thereby causing a constant and abnormal signal transduction (like in the case of Ab-induced PrP patching [23] [24], and (ii) disrupt the homeostasis of raft lipids, and especially of SL and cholesterol. Whether abnormal accumulation of lipids in such pathological rafts could play a role in the pathogenicity of prions remains however to be determined.

3. Does Cytosolic PrP Contribute to the Etiology of Spontaneous Prion Diseases?

3.1 *There is PrP in the cytosol.*

Because misfolded PrP is potentially so toxic, it is very important to understand its early biosynthetic steps, including its translocation into the ER lumen, and the folding pathways and QC mechanisms involved in its maturation. Most PrP^{C} molecules are entirely luminal, implying that they have translocated into the ER lumen. However, the existence of a minority of cytosolic PrP molecules has been recognized a long ago, implying the possibility of incomplete ER translocation or, alternatively, of mechanisms that export PrP^{C} molecules back from the ER into the cytosol. The existence of PrP in the cytosol of a subset of neurons has also been demonstrated by immunocytochemical methods [70]. Here we review some aspects of cytosolic PrP.

The ER-associated degradation (ERAD)–proteasome pathway is involved in the degradation of incorrectly folded secreted or membrane proteins, which are forbidden to exit the ER through vesicular traffic (reviewed in [71]). Damaged proteins are dislocated through the ER membrane back to the cytosol through a modified sec61p translocon. The translocated molecule is then deglycosylated by a cytosolic *N*-glycanase, usually ubiquitylated, and presented to the 26S proteasome for degradation. Covalent attachment of ubiquitin or polyubiquitin chains to lysine residues of proteins often results in the formation of a series of species that are separated by M_r increments of 8.6 kDa, thus forming a "M_r ladder".

3.2 Pathways leading to cytosolic PrP.

To see if ERAD plays a role in the export of PrP molecules to the cytosol, we used proteasome inhibitors [72]. Cells incubated with ALLN or lactacystin accumulated both detergent-soluble and insoluble PrP species. The insoluble fraction, which comprises misfolded and aggregated PrP^C, included a major unglycosylated 26 kDa PrP species as well as minor additional species with (i) a 19 kDa protease-resistant core akin to that of *bona fide* PrP^{Sc}, and (ii) a M_r 'ladder' that contained ubiquitylated PrP, demonstrating its cytosolic location. This suggested that wild-type PrP^C molecules are indeed subjected to ERAD, which can provide a source for cytosolic PrP. This result, as well as similar findings by other investigators [73], were later challenged in an elegant study by the Harris group [74]. Using an antiserum prepared against the N-terminal region of PrP, these investigators showed that the major 26kDa species that accumulates in the cytosol of ALLN-treated cells possesses an uncleaved signal peptide. This suggested that the 26kDa species had never accessed the ER. These findings thus suggest one pathway for cytosolic PrP^C. Whether ERAD is involved in the biogenesis the other insoluble PrP species remains to be seen.

There are several reasons that cytosolic PrP might be cytotoxic. (i) PrP contains a NH_2-proximal nuclear localization signal (NLS) [75]. PrP has been reported in the nucleoli of prion-infected cells [76]. The pathogenic mutant Y145stop has also been detected in the nucleus following proteasome inhibition [77]. Possible consequences of PrP in the nucleus remain to be determined. PrP could also exert deleterious effects in the cytosol. PrP binds to glial fibrillary acidic protein (GFAP) [78]. Cytosolic PrP could bind to GFAP and initiate deleterious interactions. It is pertinent to note that one of the hallmarks of prion diseases is the activation of glia and the increased synthesis of GFAP (see {Kretzschmar, 1993 #93} for a review).

3.3 PrP aggresomes in cells treated with cyclosporin A.

Little is known of the chaperones and foldases that assist the folding of PrP^C or that escort it through QC. Since two proline substitutions (P102L and P105L) are linked with familial GSS [79], we wondered whether *cis–trans* isomerization of peptidylprolyl bonds might participate either in the folding of PrP^C or in its disposal. During the folding of many proteins, the isomerization of X-Pro bonds is accelerated by ubiquitous peptidylprolyl isomerases (PPIases), including the cyclophilins [80]. Cyclosporin A (CsA), a fungal peptide used as an immunosuppressant, specifically inhibits the cyclophilin family. We thus used CsA to study the importance of cyclophilins in the metabolism of PrP. When N2a-M cells (that overexpress an epitopically labeled mouse PrP) were treated with 25μg/ml CsA for 24h, protease-resistant PrP deposited in a single juxtanuclear focus. This distribution was strikingly different from the diffuse PrP deposits seen with proteasome inhibitors, and contained no detectable ubiquitylation. This juxtanuclear dot was reminiscent of "proteolysis centers" [81], or "aggresomes", that were described several years ago as microtubule-dependent inclusion bodies located at the centrosome [82, 83]. To determine how similar the CsA-induced PrP dots are to previously described aggresomes, we used criteria defined by these investigators. By immunofluorescent microscopy, the PrP dots were confined within vimentin cages, and they co-localized with γ-tubulin, a marker for centrosomes. Furthermore, their formation was prevented by the microtubule depolymerizing agent, nocodazole. Finally, immuno-electron microscopy (EM) identified these deposits as aggresomes [84]. To the best of our knowledge, this is the first instance of a wild-type cellular protein accumulating in stable aggresomes.

Western blots showed the induction, in CsA-treated cells, of a novel 25kDa PrP species which was (i) detergent insoluble, (ii) partially protease-resistant, but were not detectably ubiquitylated.

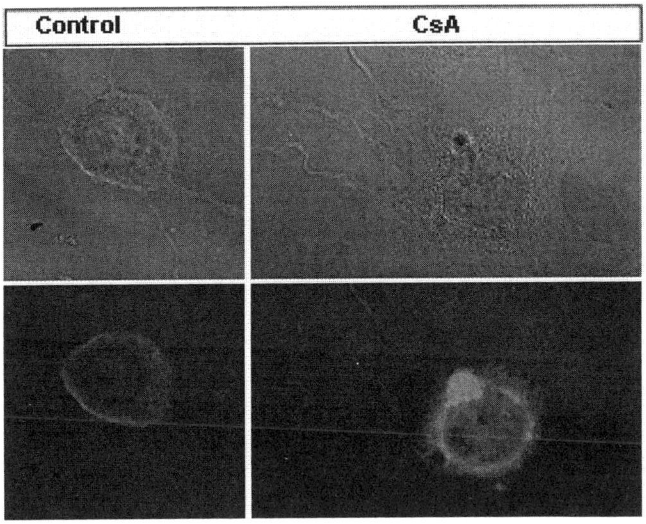

Figure 5. PrP aggresomes in CsA-treated N2a cells. N2a-M cells were treated for 24h with 25μg/ml CsA,. They were then permeabilized, and PrP was detected by immunofluorescence microscopy. In about 10% of the CsA-treated cells, PrP formed a single juxtanuclear dot that was identified as an aggresomes

These results suggested that cyclophilins may play a role in the early metabolism of PrP. To see which prolines interact with cyclophilins, we constructed three mutants on the mouse PrP platform: P101L and P104L (the homologues of the disease-linked mutations in humans), and the double mutant P101L,P104L. These mutants are expected to be refractive to cyclophilin action at the mutated prolines, in which case they would display "local" CsA-like effects. In untreated cells, immunofluorescence microscopy revealed no difference in the distribution of these mutants as compared to wt PrP. Surprisingly, however, when the cells were treated with ALLN, both P101L and P104L formed diffuse perinuclear structures, and the double mutant even produced some *bona fide*, vimentin-caged aggresomes [84]. One way to explain these findings is that a minority of mutant PrP molecules (especially the double mutant) are constantly exported to the cytosol, perhaps through QC mechanisms, where they have the potential to form aggresomes. At steady state these molecules are, however, digested by the proteasome-ubiquitin system. However, in the presence of ALLN, these molecules accumulate and form aggresomes.

These observations rise the possibility that weakening of PPIase or of proteasome activity during aging may contribute to the development of sporadic prion diseases by inducing potentially toxic PrP deposits in neurons. Similarly, familial GSS might, in some cases, be initiated by proteasomal malfunction that enables the aggregation of proline-substituted mutant PrP to form 'prion seeds' within aggresomes.

4. Conclusions

TSEs have revealed a novel biological principle, that of proteinaceous conformational switches or prions. In the cell this principle acquires a fascinating complexity. The two aspects of PrP metabolism that we have addressed here relate to two different manifestations of TSEs.

- The interaction of PrP with rafts appears to be essential for the *de novo* formation of PrP^{Sc}. It is thus particularly relevant to the *infectious* phase of prions, where a PrP^{Sc} seed already exists in luminal compartments.
- In contrast, the study of PrP^{C} folding and of cytosolic PrP relates to the etiology of the *spontaneous* (familial and sporadic) phases of TSEs, and may help explain why these diseases appear preferentially in older individuals.

References

[1] Naslavsky, N., et al., *Characterization of detergent-insoluble complexes containing the cellular prion protein and its scrapie isoform.* J Biol Chem, 1997. **272**(10): p. 6324-31.

[2] Prusiner, S.B., *Prions.* Proc Natl Acad Sci U S A, 1998. **95**(23): p. 13363-83.

[3] McKintosh, E., S.J. Tabrizi, and J. Collinge, *Prion diseases.* J Neurovirol, 2003. **9**(2): p. 183-93.

[4] Taraboulos, A., et al., *Cholesterol depletion and modification of COOH-terminal targeting sequence of the prion protein inhibit formation of the scrapie isoform.* J Cell Biol, 1995. **129**(1): p. 121-32.

[5] Prusiner, S.B., *Novel proteinaceous infectious particles cause scrapie.* Science, 1982. **216**(4542): p. 136-44.

[6] Prusiner, S.B., et al., *Transgenetic studies implicate interactions between homologous PrP isoforms in scrapie prion replication.* Cell, 1990. **63**(4): p. 673-86.

[7] Carrell, R.W. and D.A. Lomas, *Conformational disease.* Lancet, 1997. **350**(9071): p. 134-8.

[8] Come, J.H., P.E. Fraser, and P.T. Lansbury, Jr., *A kinetic model for amyloid formation in the prion diseases: importance of seeding.* Proc Natl Acad Sci U S A, 1993. **90**(13): p. 5959-63.

[9] Kocisko, D.A., et al., *Cell-free formation of protease-resistant prion protein.* Nature, 1994. **370**(6489): p. 471-4.

[10] Uptain, S.M. and S. Lindquist, *Prions as protein-based genetic elements.* Annu Rev Microbiol, 2002. **56**: p. 703-41.

[11] Si, K., S. Lindquist, and E.R. Kandel, *A neuronal isoform of the aplysia CPEB has prion-like properties.* Cell, 2003. **115**(7): p. 879-91.

[12] Meyer, R.K., et al., *Separation and properties of cellular and scrapie prion proteins.* Proc Natl Acad Sci U S A, 1986. **83**(8): p. 2310-4.

[13] McKinley, M.P., et al., *Scrapie prion rod formation in vitro requires both detergent extraction and limited proteolysis.* J Virol, 1991. **65**(3): p. 1340-51.

[14] Serban, D., et al., *Rapid detection of Creutzfeldt-Jakob disease and scrapie prion proteins.* Neurology, 1990. **40**(1): p. 110-7.

[15] Safar, J., et al., *Eight prion strains have PrP(Sc) molecules with different conformations.* Nat Med, 1998. **4**(10): p. 1157-65.

[16] Korth, C., P. Streit, and B. Oesch, *Monoclonal antibodies specific for the native, disease-associated isoform of the prion protein.* Methods Enzymol, 1999. **309**: p. 106-22.

[17] Paramithiotis, E., et al., *A prion protein epitope selective for the pathologically misfolded conformation.* Nat Med, 2003. **9**(7): p. 893-9.

[18] Serbec, V.C., et al., *Monoclonal Antibody against a Peptide of Human Prion Protein Discriminates between Creutzfeldt-Jacob's Disease-affected and Normal Brain Tissue.* J Biol Chem, 2004. **279**(5): p. 3694-8.

[19] Tzaban, S., et al., *Protease-sensitive scrapie prion protein in aggregates of heterogeneous sizes.* Biochemistry, 2002. **41**(42): p. 12868-75.

[20] Warner, R.G., et al., *Identification of the heparan sulfate binding sites in the cellular prion protein.* J Biol Chem, 2002. **277**(21): p. 18421-30.

[21] Mahfoud, R., et al., *Identification of a common sphingolipid-binding domain in Alzheimer, prion, and HIV-1 proteins.* J Biol Chem, 2002. **277**(13): p. 11292-6.

[22] Brown, D.R. and J. Sassoon, *Copper-dependent functions for the prion protein.* Mol Biotechnol, 2002. **22**(2): p. 165-78.

[23] Cashman, N.R., et al., *Cellular isoform of the scrapie agent protein participates in lymphocyte activation.* Cell, 1990. **61**(1): p. 185-92.

[24] Mouillet-Richard, S., et al., *Signal transduction through prion protein.* Science, 2000. **289**(5486): p. 1925-8.

[25] Butler, D.A., et al., *Scrapie-infected murine neuroblastoma cells produce protease-resistant prion proteins.* J Virol, 1988. **62**(5): p. 1558-64.

[26] Mellon, P.L., et al., *Immortalized hypothalamic gonadotropin-releasing hormone neurons.* Ciba Found Symp, 1992. **168**: p. 104-17; discussion 117-26.

[27] Schatzl, H.M., et al., *A hypothalamic neuronal cell line persistently infected with scrapie prions exhibits apoptosis.* J Virol, 1997. **71**(11): p. 8821-31.

[28] Solassol, J., C. Crozet, and S. Lehmann, *Prion propagation in cultured cells.* Br Med Bull, 2003. **66**: p. 87-97.

[29] Harris, D.A., *Trafficking, turnover and membrane topology of PrP.* Br Med Bull, 2003. **66**: p. 71-85.

[30] Shyng, S.L., M.T. Huber, and D.A. Harris, *A prion protein cycles between the cell surface and an endocytic compartment in cultured neuroblastoma cells.* J Biol Chem, 1993. **268**(21): p. 15922-8.

[31] Gorodinsky, A. and D.A. Harris, *Glycolipid-anchored proteins in neuroblastoma cells form detergent-resistant complexes without caveolin.* J Cell Biol, 1995. **129**(3): p. 619-27.

[32] Vey, M., et al., *Subcellular colocalization of the cellular and scrapie prion proteins in caveolae-like membranous domains.* Proc Natl Acad Sci U S A, 1996. **93**(25): p. 14945-9.

[33] Naslavsky, N., et al., *Sphingolipid depletion increases formation of the scrapie prion protein in neuroblastoma cells infected with prions.* J Biol Chem, 1999. **274**(30): p. 20763-71.

[34] Vincent, B., et al., *The disintegrins ADAM10 and TACE contribute to the constitutive and phorbol ester-regulated normal cleavage of the cellular prion protein.* J Biol Chem, 2001. **276**(41): p. 37743-6.

[35] Caughey, B. and G.J. Raymond, *The scrapie-associated form of PrP is made from a cell surface precursor that is both protease- and phospholipase-sensitive.* J Biol Chem, 1991. **266**(27): p. 18217-23.

[36] Borchelt, D.R., A. Taraboulos, and S.B. Prusiner, *Evidence for synthesis of scrapie prion proteins in the endocytic pathway.* J Biol Chem, 1992. **267**(23): p. 16188-99.

[37] Borchelt, D.R., et al., *Scrapie and cellular prion proteins differ in their kinetics of synthesis and topology in cultured cells.* J Cell Biol, 1990. **110**(3): p. 743-52.

[38] Caughey, B., et al., *N-terminal truncation of the scrapie-associated form of PrP by lysosomal protease(s): implications regarding the site of conversion of PrP to the protease-resistant state.* J Virol, 1991. **65**(12): p. 6597-603.

[39] Taraboulos, A., et al., *Synthesis and trafficking of prion proteins in cultured cells.* Mol Biol Cell, 1992. **3**(8): p. 851-63.

[40] McKinley, M.P., et al., *Ultrastructural localization of scrapie prion proteins in cytoplasmic vesicles of infected cultured cells.* Lab Invest, 1991. **65**(6): p. 622-30.

[41] Lehmann, S. and D.A. Harris, *Mutant and infectious prion proteins display common biochemical properties in cultured cells.* J Biol Chem, 1996. **271**(3): p. 1633-7.

[42] Rieger, R., et al., *The human 37-kDa laminin receptor precursor interacts with the prion protein in eukaryotic cells.* Nat Med, 1997. **3**(12): p. 1383-8.

[43] Zanata, S.M., et al., *Stress-inducible protein 1 is a cell surface ligand for cellular prion that triggers neuroprotection.* Embo J, 2002. **21**(13): p. 3307-16.

[44] Ben-Zaken, O., et al., *Cellular heparan sulfate participates in the metabolism of prions.* J Biol Chem, 2003. **278**(41): p. 40041-9.

[45] Telling, G.C., et al., *Prion propagation in mice expressing human and chimeric PrP transgenes implicates the interaction of cellular PrP with another protein.* Cell, 1995. **83**(1): p. 79-90.

[46] Simons, K. and E. Ikonen, *Functional rafts in cell membranes.* Nature, 1997. **387**(6633): p. 569-72.

[47] Ehehalt, R., et al., *Amyloidogenic processing of the Alzheimer beta-amyloid precursor protein depends on lipid rafts.* J Cell Biol, 2003. **160**(1): p. 113-23.

[48] Simons, K. and R. Ehehalt, *Cholesterol, lipid rafts, and disease.* J Clin Invest, 2002. **110**(5): p. 597-603.

[49] Brown, D.A. and J.K. Rose, *Sorting of GPI-anchored proteins to glycolipid-enriched membrane subdomains during transport to the apical cell surface.* Cell, 1992. **68**(3): p. 533-44.

[50] Harder, T., et al., *Lipid domain structure of the plasma membrane revealed by patching of membrane components.* J Cell Biol, 1998. **141**(4): p. 929-42.

[51] Friedrichson, T. and T.V. Kurzchalia, *Microdomains of GPI-anchored proteins in living cells revealed by crosslinking.* Nature, 1998. **394**(6695): p. 802-5.

[52] Madore, N., et al., *Functionally different GPI proteins are organized in different domains on the neuronal surface.* Embo J, 1999. **18**(24): p. 6917-26.

[53] Sunyach, C., et al., *The mechanism of internalization of glycosylphosphatidylinositol-anchored prion protein.* Embo J, 2003. **22**(14): p. 3591-601.

[54] Fivaz, M., et al., *Differential sorting and fate of endocytosed GPI-anchored proteins.* Embo J, 2002. **21**(15): p. 3989-4000.

[55] Bosque, P.J. and S.B. Prusiner, *Cultured cell sublines highly susceptible to prion infection.* J Virol, 2000. **74**(9): p. 4377-86.

[56] Rouvinski, A., et al., *Both raft- and non-raft proteins associate with CHAPS-insoluble complexes: some APP in large complexes.* Biochem Biophys Res Commun, 2003. **308**(4): p. 750-8.

[57] Kaneko, K., et al., *COOH-terminal sequence of the cellular prion protein directs subcellular trafficking and controls conversion into the scrapie isoform.* Proc Natl Acad Sci U S A, 1997. **94**(6): p. 2333-8.

[58] Marella, M., et al., *Filipin prevents pathological prion protein accumulation by reducing endocytosis and inducing cellular PrP release.* J Biol Chem, 2002. **277**(28): p. 25457-64.

[59] Mange, A., et al., *Amphotericin B inhibits the generation of the scrapie isoform of the prion protein in infected cultures.* J Virol, 2000. **74**(7): p. 3135-40.

[60] Ovadia, H., et al., *Effect of scrapie infection on the activity of neuronal nitric-oxide synthase in brain and neuroblastoma cells.* J Biol Chem, 1996. **271**(28): p. 16856-61.

[61] Kazlauskaite, J., et al., *Structural changes of the prion protein in lipid membranes leading to aggregation and fibrillization.* Biochemistry, 2003. **42**(11): p. 3295-304.

[62] Sanghera, N. and T.J. Pinheiro, *Binding of prion protein to lipid membranes and implications for prion conversion.* J Mol Biol, 2002. **315**(5): p. 1241-56.

[63] Fantini, J., *How sphingolipids bind and shape proteins: molecular basis of lipid-protein interactions in lipid shells, rafts and related biomembrane domains.* Cell Mol Life Sci, 2003. **60**(6): p. 1027-32.

[64] Klein, T.R., et al., *Prion rods contain small amounts of two host sphingolipids as revealed by thin-layer chromatography and mass spectrometry.* Biol Chem, 1998. **379**(6): p. 655-66.

[65] Florio, T., et al., *Prion protein fragment 106-126 induces apoptotic cell death and impairment of L-type voltage-sensitive calcium channel activity in the GH3 cell line.* J Neurosci Res, 1998. **54**(3): p. 341-52.

[66] Bonetto, V., et al., *Synthetic miniprion PrP106.* J Biol Chem, 2002. **277**(35): p. 31327-34.

[67] Hanan, E., S.A. Priola, and B. Solomon, *Antiaggregating antibody raised against human PrP 106-126 recognizes pathological and normal isoforms of the whole prion protein.* Cell Mol Neurobiol, 2001. **21**(6): p. 693-703.

[68] Brandner, S., et al., *Normal host prion protein (PrPC) is required for scrapie spread within the central nervous system.* Proc Natl Acad Sci U S A, 1996. **93**(23): p. 13148-51.

[69] Schonberger, O., et al., *Novel heparan mimetics potently inhibit the scrapie prion protein and its endocytosis.* Biochem Biophys Res Commun, 2003. **312**(2): p. 473-9.

[70] Mironov, A., Jr., et al., *Cytosolic prion protein in neurons.* J Neurosci, 2003. **23**(18): p. 7183-93.

[71] McCracken, A.A. and J.L. Brodsky, *Evolving questions and paradigm shifts in endoplasmic-reticulum-associated degradation (ERAD).* Bioessays, 2003. **25**(9): p. 868-77.

[72] Yedidia, Y., et al., *Proteasomes and ubiquitin are involved in the turnover of the wild-type prion protein.* Embo J, 2001. **20**(19): p. 5383-91.

[73] Ma, J. and S. Lindquist, *Wild-type PrP and a mutant associated with prion disease are subject to retrograde transport and proteasome degradation.* Proc Natl Acad Sci U S A, 2001. **98**(26): p. 14955-60.

[74] Drisaldi, B., et al., *Mutant PrP is delayed in its exit from the endoplasmic reticulum, but neither wild-type nor mutant PrP undergoes retrotranslocation prior to proteasomal degradation.* J Biol Chem, 2003. **278**(24): p. 21732-43.

[75] Basler, K., et al., *Scrapie and cellular PrP isoforms are encoded by the same chromosomal gene.* Cell, 1986. **46**(3): p. 417-28.

[76] Pfeifer, K., et al., *Kinetics of expression of prion protein in uninfected and scrapie-infected N2a mouse neuroblastoma cells.* Cell Biochem Funct, 1993. **11**(1): p. 1-11.

[77] Zanusso, G., et al., *Proteasomal degradation and N-terminal protease resistance of the codon 145 mutant prion protein.* J Biol Chem, 1999. **274**(33): p. 23396-404.
[78] Oesch, B., et al., *Identification of cellular proteins binding to the scrapie prion protein.* Biochemistry, 1990. **29**(24): p. 5848-55.
[79] Hsiao, K., et al., *Linkage of a prion protein missense variant to Gerstmann-Straussler syndrome.* Nature, 1989. **338**(6213): p. 342-5.
[80] Hamilton, G.S. and J.P. Steiner, *Immunophilins: beyond immunosuppression.* J Med Chem, 1998. **41**(26): p. 5119-43.
[81] Wojcik, C., et al., *Ubiquitin-mediated proteolysis centers in HeLa cells: indication from studies of an inhibitor of the chymotrypsin-like activity of the proteasome.* Eur J Cell Biol, 1996. **71**(3): p. 311-8.
[82] Johnston, J.A., C.L. Ward, and R.R. Kopito, *Aggresomes: a cellular response to misfolded proteins.* J Cell Biol, 1998. **143**(7): p. 1883-98.
[83] Wigley, W.C., et al., *Dynamic association of proteasomal machinery with the centrosome.* J Cell Biol, 1999. **145**(3): p. 481-90.
[84] Cohen, E. and A. Taraboulos, *Scrapie-like prion protein accumulates in aggresomes of cyclosporin A-treated cells.* Embo J, 2003. **22**(3): p. 404-17.

Author Index